Principles of Finance for Health Information and Informatics Professionals

Susan White, PhD, CHDA

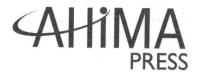

ISBN: 978-1-58426-297-8
AHIMA Product No.: AB204011

AHIMA Staff:
Jessica Block, MA, Assistant Editor
Claire Blondeau, MBA, Managing Editor
Adrienne Cook, JD, Developmental Editor
Katie Greenock, MS, Editorial and Production Coordinator
Jason O. Malley, Director, Creative Content Development

For more information about AHIMA Press publications, including updates, visit http://www.ahima.org/publications/updates.aspx.

American Health Information Management Association
233 North Michigan Avenue, 21st Floor
Chicago, Illinois 60601-5809
ahima.org

Brief Contents

BRIEF CONTENTS

Contents

CHAPTER ONE   Introduction to Healthcare Finance   1

CHAPTER TWO   Understanding Financial Statements   27

CHAPTER THREE   Financial Performance Measurement   49

CHAPTER FOUR   Budgets   103

CHAPTER FIVE   Variance Analysis   145

CHAPTER SIX   Third-Party Contract Analysis   167

About the Downloadable Ancillaries

For Students

The downloadable ancillary materials that accompany this book include selected chapter tables and case study data in Excel file format. The formulas presented in the book are built into these files so that users can manipulate the data. Go to http://ahimapress.org/White2978, click the Downloadable Ancillaries link, and enter case-sensitive password **S204011ab** to download the files.

For Instructors

AHIMA provides supplementary materials for educators who use this book in their classes. Materials include the student materials listed above, as well as an instructor manual with lesson plans and test banks for each chapter, Power-Point notes for lectures, and complete answer keys. Visit http://www.ahima.org/publications/educators.aspx for further instruction. If you have any questions regarding the instructor materials, please contact AHIMA Customer Relations at (800) 335-5535 or submit a customer support request at https://secure.ahima.org/contact/contact.aspx.

About the Author

Susan White, PhD, CHDA, is a clinical associate professor in the HIM department at the Ohio State University. She teaches classes in statistics, data analytics, healthcare finance, and computer applications. Prior to joining OSU, Dr. White was vice president of research and development for Cleverley + Associates and vice president of data operations for CHIPS/Ingenix. Dr. White has written numerous books and articles regarding the benchmarking of healthcare facilities and the appropriate use of claims data. She has published articles in the areas of outcomes assessment and risk adjustment using healthcare financial and clinical data analysis, hospital benchmarking, and claims data mining. Dr. White earned her PhD in statistics from the Ohio State University in 1991.

Acknowledgments

I would like to thank my family and coworkers for their patience during the writing of this text. Special thanks to Melanie Brodnik, PhD, RHIA, who allowed me to take the time to develop the text and served as a valuable mentor through the publishing process. I would also like to thank the OSU HIMS class of 2012 for their indulgence in test-driving the draft version of this text during their finance class. Editors Claire Blondeau, MBA, and Adrienne Cook, JD, should be commended for their unending patience in answering my questions and keeping this project on track.

Finally, thank you to Nadinia Davis, the technical editor for this text. She provided valuable feedback and suggestions for revisions to the content and structure of the text. Her keen eye and healthcare finance experience in both the classroom and the field strengthened the quality of this manuscript.

Foreword

As the healthcare ecosystem in the United States continues to evolve, the one constant that does not show any signs of abating is its complexity. In fact, the issues and financial prophecies surrounding healthcare are so complex, they are often misunderstood by the general public as well as policy makers. This book takes the complex web of healthcare finance and carefully deconstructs each major element, giving the reader a superb foundation for understanding how healthcare finance works today as well as the pressures that are baked into the status quo.

As the pricing and discounting orthodoxies for healthcare providers are highly variant to each payer in their payer mix, gaining a real understanding of a provider's revenue situations and trends is particularly challenging. The author does an excellent job of familiarizing the reader with financial performance metrics that are relevant for healthcare providers. Further, key analytic approaches such as common-size analysis are explained and allow for a comparative understanding of performance among provider organizations. The book does an excellent job of illustrating how governmental and private insurance payers contract and pay for services. All the current methods as well as the evolving payment methods are explained in straightforward language. The complexities of contracting and the pitfalls that lead to poor performing contracts are clearly delineated.

This work is comprehensive in providing overall economic context for US healthcare as well as a substantive understanding of revenue management, cost management, variance management, and contracting. This is a fulsome overview of healthcare finance and its challenges. I wholeheartedly recommend this book for anyone seeking to understand our healthcare system or for any executive responsible for leadership in a provider organization.

Mary A. Tolan, MBA
President, Chief Executive Officer & Director
at Accretive Health, Inc.;
Trustee, University of Chicago

Introduction to Healthcare Finance

Learning Objectives

➥ Understand the US healthcare environment
➥ Understand the importance of payer mix in healthcare
➥ Study trends in insurance types
➥ Understand community benefit

Key Terms

Advance beneficiary notice (ABN)
Affordable Care Act (ACA)
Bad debt
Balance bill
Catholic Health Association (CHA)
Centers for Medicare and Medicaid
   Services (CMS)
Charity care
Commercial payer
Community benefit
Consumers
Cost shifting
Federal Poverty Guidelines (FPG)
For-profit
Government payer
Gross domestic product (GDP)
Gross revenue
High-deductible health plan

Margin
Medicaid
Medicare
Not-for-profit
Payer
Payer mix
Premium
Private payer
Product
Profit
Self-pay
State Children's Health Insurance
   Program (SCHIP)
Third-party payer
TRICARE
Underinsured
US Census Bureau

The US Healthcare Environment

Before studying healthcare finance, it is important to understand the US healthcare environment, including the role of healthcare in the US economy.

1

Providers operating in the US healthcare system have a unique set of financial pressures. The variety of payment methodologies and payers involved in the US system makes it one of the most complex healthcare delivery systems in the world. The term **payer** in the healthcare industry refers to the entity that reimburses the provider for care.

The Importance of Healthcare in the US Economy

Healthcare expenditures make up a significant portion of the US economy. According to **Medicare** actuaries, national healthcare expenditures represented 16.2 percent of the **gross domestic product** (GDP) in 2007 (Sisko et al. 2009, w347). The GDP is a statistic that economists use to measure the value of all products a country produces. Analyzing healthcare dollars expended relative to the GDP allows year-to-year comparisons.

To help put this in perspective, in 2007 approximately $1,870 per capita was spent on healthcare in the United States. The amount of our GDP and per capita rates have grown dramatically from 13.7 percent in 1993 and are projected to continue to grow to 20.3 percent in 2018 (Sisko et al. 2009). Figure 1.1 shows the trend and future projections for both figures. These estimates do not reflect the impact of the health reform legislation that was enacted in 2010. The per capita expenditures are projected to increase at a higher rate than the percentage of GDP resulting from a projected slower growth in the economy caused by the recent recession.

Figure 1.1   US national health expenditures per capita and as percentage of GDP

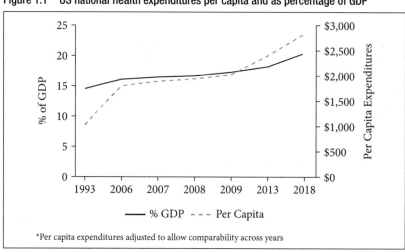

*Per capita expenditures adjusted to allow comparability across years

Source: Sisko et al. 2009, w347.

The Organisation for Economic Co-operation and Development (OECD) collects data for a variety of countries on a number of economic issues. According to its 2008 statistics, the most recent available, the percentage of the GDP represented by healthcare expenditures in the United States is significantly higher than that observed in other countries. Figure 1.2 shows that the US percentage of GDP spent on healthcare in 2008 far exceeds that of the other countries shown. France, Canada, Germany, Austria, and New Zealand all hover around 10 percent. Healthcare in the United States is a significant part of our economy. It is important to acknowledge that fact in studying healthcare finance and measurement of the financial position of healthcare providers.

Before studying the financial management of healthcare, it is also important to understand the basic business model. Like most industries, the healthcare system in the United States includes suppliers (providers) and **consumers** (patients) of a **product** (healthcare). There is one critical difference in the US healthcare system: The consumer rarely directly pays for the product at the

Figure 1.2   Healthcare expenditures by country as percentage of GDP

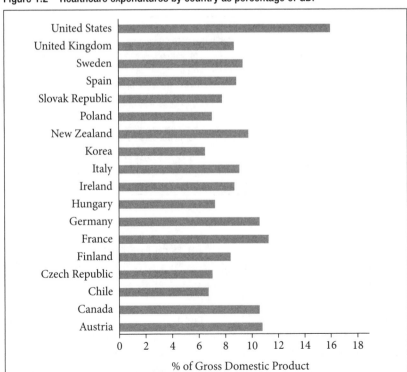

Source: OECD n.d.

Table 1.1   Health insurance terms

Term	Definition
Coinsurance	Cost sharing in which the policyholder or certificate holder pays a preestablished percentage of eligible expenses after the deductible has been met; the percentage may vary by type or site of service.
Copayment	Cost sharing in which the policyholder or certificate holder pays a fixed dollar amount (flat fee) per service, supply, or procedure that is owed to the healthcare facility by the patient. The fixed amount that the policyholder pays may vary by type of service, such as $15 per prescription or $20 per physician visit.
Deductible	The amount of cost, usually annual, the policyholder must incur (and pay) before the insurance plan will assume liability for the remaining covered expenses.
Enrollee	The primary insured individual on an insurance policy.
Health maintenance organization (HMO)	A healthcare system that assumes both the financial risks associated with providing comprehensive medical services (insurance and service risk) and the responsibility for healthcare delivery in a particular geographic area to HMO members, usually in return for a fixed, prepaid fee. Financial risk may be shared with the providers participating in the HMO.
Indemnity plan	A type of medical plan that reimburses the patient and/or provider as expenses are incurred.
Preferred provider organization (PPO) plan	An indemnity plan where coverage is provided to participants through a network of selected healthcare providers (such as hospitals and physicians). The enrollees may go outside the network, but this would incur larger costs in the form of higher deductibles, higher coinsurance rates, or nondiscounted charges from the providers.
Premium	The amount of money that a policyholder or certificate holder must periodically pay an insurer in return for healthcare coverage.
Reimbursement	Compensation or payment for healthcare services.
Third-party administrator (TPA)	An individual or firm hired by an employer to handle claims processing, pay providers, and manage other functions related to the operation of health insurance. The TPA is not the policyholder or the insurer.

Source: AHIMA 2010.

time of service delivery. There are as many as four participants in the delivery of healthcare services in the United States. Table 1.1 lists a number of health insurance terms that are helpful in understanding these relationships.

Figure 1.3 depicts the relationships among the patient, the employer, the **third-party payer,** and the provider. There are transactions and communication among all four parties. Relationship (1) represents transactions between the consumer or patient and the provider. Healthcare services are provided to the patient. The patient contacts the provider to arrange services and is responsible for payment if the patient does not have insurance coverage for the service.

Figure 1.3   US healthcare business model

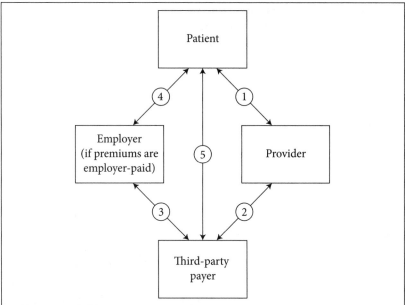

If the patient does have coverage, then the patient pays any copayments that may be required under the third-party payer coverage parameters. Relationship (2) represents transactions between the provider and the third-party payer. The provider submits an invoice to the third-party payer for services the patient received. The third-party payer submits payment on behalf of the patient based on any contractual relationship it may have with the provider.

Relationship (3) represents the transactions between the third-party payer and the patient's employer. If the patient's healthcare coverage is a benefit of employment, then the employer may pay all or a portion of the **premium** to the third-party payer on behalf of the patient. If the patient pays the third party directly, then the transactions are directly between the patient and the third-party payer; relationship (5) is a better representation of those transactions. Relationship (5) also represents the payment of any precertifications that may be required by the patient's health plan prior to service. Relationship (4) represents the transactions between the patient and the patient's employer. If the patient is responsible for a portion of the premium paid to the third-party payer, then that sum is collected via payroll processing. Another healthcare-related transaction between the patient and the patient's employer may be the selection of a plan. Many larger employers provide a menu of health plans with varying benefits and premium levels that employees may choose from.

Figure 1.3 helps in the presentation of the complexities inherent in the US healthcare system. Understanding the various relationships and parties that are involved in the delivery of healthcare in the United States provides a valuable context for the study of healthcare finance issues.

Payer Mix

Payers are typically segmented into three categories: Private, government, and self-pay. **Private payers** include employer-sponsored plans where the employer may be self-insured or may contract with a health insurance company to provide coverage for their employees. Individuals may also purchase plans through **commercial** insurance companies. The collection of payers that remit payments to a provider is called the **payer mix.** The payer mix that is active at a particular healthcare provider is an important driver of financial decision making and performance.

Government payers include Medicare, **Medicaid, TRICARE, State Children's Health Insurance Program** (SCHIP), and other healthcare programs administrated by federal, state, or local government agencies (see table 1.2). Medicare is a federal program that provides coverage for the elderly and disabled populations. Medicaid is a state-funded program that provides health insurance coverage to low-income individuals who meet state and federal criteria. TRICARE is the program that provides health insurance to active and retired military personnel and their families. SCHIP provides health insurance coverage for children without another source of coverage but whose families do not qualify for Medicaid.

Self-pay patients pay the provider directly for their care. The self-pay population typically includes people who do not qualify or have not applied for government healthcare coverage and those who choose to self-insure due to the availability of sufficient resources to pay for healthcare out of their own

Table 1.2   Government health insurance programs

Program	Sponsor	Who Is Eligible?
Medicare	Federal government	Individuals over 65 or those with permanent disabilities
Medicaid	Federal/state cost sharing	Low income—eligibility varies by state
TRICARE	Federal government	Retired military and their families
SCHIP	Federal/state cost sharing	Uninsured children in families not eligible for Medicaid

Source: Casto and Layman 2011.

pockets. Many low-income self-pay patients are eligible for some sort of government-funded coverage. Many providers have internal programs dedicated to assisting patients in accessing that coverage. Insured patients may be financially responsible or considered self-pay for services that are not covered under their particular insurance plan. For instance, cosmetic procedures are typically not considered a covered service and are therefore paid out-of-pocket by the patient. Insurance companies may also **balance bill** patients for services that are not completely covered or not considered medically necessary. Providers that participate in the Medicare program may not balance bill Medicare patients for noncovered services without first notifying them and requiring them to sign an **advance beneficiary notice** (ABN) that ensures that the patients understand they are financially liable for the noncovered service.

A provider with a high percentage of private-pay patients will generally have a greater potential for financial success than one with a higher percentage of government payers or self-pay patients. This is because government payers offer a lower level of reimbursement and most self-pay patients are unable to make full payment. The level of reimbursement received from government payers is lower than that received from commercial payers for providing the same care to their beneficiaries (Fox and Pickering 2008, 1). Providers must make up the losses on the government-paid portion of their services by negotiating higher rates with private insurance companies. This practice is referred to as **cost shifting** because the cost of caring for government insurance beneficiaries is shifted to the private insurance market. According to a 2008 report provided to the American Hospital Association (AHA) by Milliman (Fox and Pickering 2008, 2), an estimated $88.8 billion in healthcare costs shifted from Medicare and Medicaid to commercial payers in the hospital and physician setting.

The **US Census Bureau** compiled healthcare coverage figures based on the 2010 Current Population Survey Annual Social and Economic Supplement (DeNavas-Walt et al. 2010). In that survey, participants are asked a series of questions regarding health insurance coverage. According to this survey, an estimated 16.7 percent of the US population had no health insurance coverage in 2008. This figure increased from 13.7 percent in 2000. Of those with insurance coverage, approximately two-thirds have some form of private insurance that is purchased through their employer or directly from an insurance company.

Figure 1.4 depicts the percentage of healthcare expenditures by source of funds from 1960 to 2008. These data come from the Centers for Medicare and Medicaid Services (CMS) office of the actuary and are used for policy analysis and development (CMS 2010). In 1960, nearly 75 percent of all healthcare

Figure 1.4   Trend in source of funds for healthcare expenditures: 1960–2008

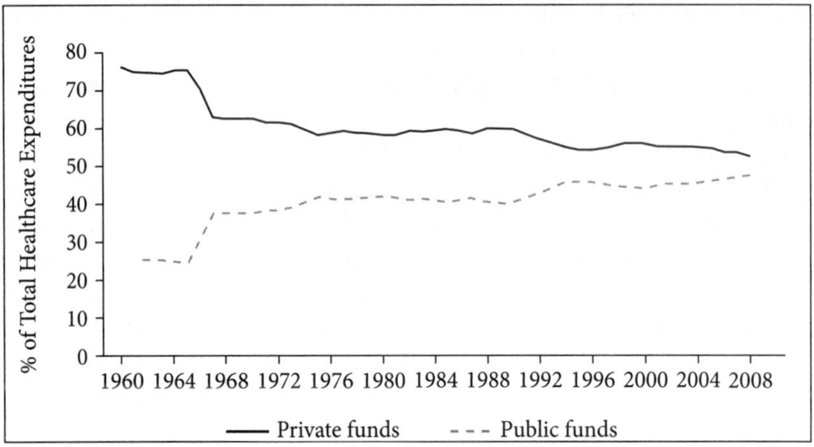

Source: CMS 2010, national health expenditure data.

expenditures were funded by private dollars. Note that there was a dramatic shift in 1966 due to the creation of the Medicare program. In 2008, 53 percent of healthcare expenditures were from private funds; the percentage due to public funds grew to 47 percent. The Census Bureau estimates that in 2008 approximately 29 percent of the population was covered under a government health plan, but government health plans represented 47 percent of all healthcare expenditures in the United States during 2008 (DeNavas-Walt et al. 2010).

Both government and private health insurance payers are motivated to provide a comprehensive set of benefits to subscribers at a reasonable cost. Private payers must compete with each other to attract subscribers and employers by offering robust benefits for a low premium cost. Government payers have less market pressure but are monitored closely by Congress to ensure that constituents are not dissatisfied with the level of coverage they receive for their investment. Payers in turn must work to keep their cost of care under control. Both types of payers have components of their payment systems that work very well at controlling costs and providing appropriate care to patients. The relationship between the payer and the provider of services is also different for these two categories of payer.

Providers do not have the ability to negotiate payment terms and rates with government payers. The payment methodology for Medicare is determined via the federal rule-making process. Adjustments to the Medicare payment system are announced on an annual basis. Providers may make comments on the changes before they become final, but the comment process is not a negotiation, and the **Centers for Medicare and Medicaid Services** (CMS), the government agency that administers Medicare, is not obligated to act on provider comments. The provider does have some control over the payment level in that it participates in quality measurement and other value-based purchasing programs that are now part of the Medicare program.

Providers do negotiate with commercial third-party payers. The payment terms, including methodology, included/excluded services, and the timing of payments, are all up for negotiation. Providers must substantiate that the rates they desire are defensible and that they are providing good-quality care at a fair price. Provider contracts with third-party payers may include incentives for cost containment, utilization, quality measurement, or any combination of these.

Financial Impact of the Uninsured

The proportion of the population that is not covered under either government or private health insurance is growing. The uninsured population is primarily made up of three pools:

1. Individuals who work for firms that do not offer their employees health insurance
2. Individuals who are employed less than full time and are therefore not eligible for employer-sponsored benefits
3. Individuals who are unemployed but do not qualify for government healthcare coverage

The Centers for Disease Control and Prevention (CDC) estimates, based on the January–June 2010 National Health Interview Survey, that 43.9 percent of the near poor from ages 18 to 65 are uninsured (Martinez and Cohen 2010). This is more than the 34.9 percent of that population that is covered by private health insurance. Due to state and federal programs such as SCHIP, this survey found that only 8.2 percent of the children with parents in the near poor category were uninsured.

This growth in the uninsured population causes a financial strain on the entire US healthcare system. Hospitals have greater difficulty collecting payment for services provided, which can compromise their financial position. Individuals who are **underinsured** also cause a financial strain on both themselves and their providers. Underinsured individuals may have plans with lifetime limits or low coverage limits that reimburse the provider for only a portion of the care provided to the patient. The patient is left with the remaining balance.

In addition to growth in the uninsured population, there has been a significant increase in the number of individuals with **high-deductible health plans** (Martinez and Cohen 2010). High-deductible health plans are a less costly type of coverage for employers to provide. Deductibles as high as $5,000 or more leave the patient self-insured or essentially uninsured for a significant portion of the care provided. These plans can cause financial hardship for both the patient and the provider, which will have more difficulty collecting the patient's portion of the reimbursement. Education is needed so that patients covered under high-deductible plans understand the coverage parameters and strategies to plan for the potential payment of the deductible. Subscribers to high-deductible health plans are often considered part of the underinsured population, since a portion of their healthcare costs are left unpaid when they cannot pay the deductible amount.

Health reform efforts represent an attempt to reduce the proportion of the population that is uninsured and underinsured. On March 23, 2010, the **Affordable Care Act** (ACA) was signed into law. This legislation included a number of initiatives intended to extend coverage and eliminate many of the practices of health insurers that compromised the level of coverage offered to individuals.

This legislation had an immediate effect on the number of uninsured by allowing adult children to stay on their parents' health plan until age 26. The law also eliminated the exclusion of children from health plans due to pre-existing conditions. This provision will be extended to adults in 2014 with the creation of health exchanges. The ACA also banned lifetime limits on insurance plans, which should reduce the number of underinsured individuals (Martinez and Cohen 2010). The ACA does not solve all of the issues of healthcare delivery and payment in the US healthcare system but does address some of the larger issues that impact the consumer.

Hospitals: For-Profit versus Not-for-Profit

Hospital providers fall into two broad categories: **not-for-profit** and **for-profit.** For-profit hospitals are typically owned by large corporate systems or smaller investor-owned corporations. Not-for-profit hospitals may be further segmented into those that are publicly funded and those that are privately funded. Publicly funded hospitals are funded by a government entity (federal, state, county, etc.) and provide a substantial level of service to individuals in poverty. Not-for-profit hospitals are sometimes referred to as voluntary hospitals. Privately funded not-for-profit hospitals also often have a mission to provide healthcare to the poor, but they are funded by private entities. Many privately funded not-for-profit hospitals are sponsored by religious groups. Many of the largest hospitals in the country are actually not-for-profit. Table 1.3 lists the top 10 hospitals in the United States based on number of beds, according to the CMS Hospital Cost Report Information System (HCRIS). Only Methodist Hospital in San Antonio is listed as a for-profit hospital. The remaining nine are not-for-profit organizations.

Definitions

Profit is the amount of revenue or income that is collected minus the cost to produce the item or service. If the revenue received for a product is more than the cost to produce, then the profit is a positive number. In the business world, profitability is a key indicator of the success of a firm. Profitability may also be measured as a profit margin (often referred to as simply "margin"). **Margin** is the profit a firm earns divided by the revenue. It may be interpreted as the percentage of the revenue that does not go to cover expenses. Since margin is standardized for the size of the firm by dividing it by the revenue, it is a measure that allows for comparison among firms of various sizes. The formula for calculating margin is presented in figure 1.5.

The term "not-for-profit" does not necessarily mean that a facility does not or cannot make a profit in providing services to patients. Not-for-profit status means that the facility is exempt from federal, state, and local taxes. In exchange for the tax-exempt status, organizations must operate under a stricter set of rules than their for-profit counterparts. Not-for-profit hospitals, like all charitable organizations, are defined based on section 501(c)(3) of the US tax code. The

Table 1.3   Top 10 largest US hospitals by number of beds

Hospital Name	Location	Ownership/Control	Number of Beds
Florida Hospital	Orlando, FL	Voluntary not-for-profit, other	1,869
New York-Presbyterian Hospital	New York, NY	Voluntary not-for-profit, other	1,800
Jackson Memorial	Miami, FL	Governmental not-for-profit	1,564
Clarian Health Partners, Inc.	Indianapolis, IN	Governmental not-for-profit	1,395
Montefiore Medical Center	Bronx, NY	Voluntary not-for-profit, other	1,383
Baptist Health System	San Antonio, TX	Voluntary not-for-profit, church	1,378
Methodist Hospital	San Antonio, TX	For-profit, corporation	1,369
UPMC—Presbyterian	Pittsburgh, PA	Voluntary not-for-profit, other	1,263
Methodist H/C Memphis Hospital	Memphis, TN	Voluntary not-for-profit, other	1,219
Orlando Regional	Orlando, FL	Voluntary not-for-profit, other	1,218

Source: CMS HCRIS Data File 2010.

Figure 1.5   Profit formulas

$$\text{Profit} = \text{Revenue} - \text{Expense}$$

$$\text{Profit margin} = \frac{\text{Revenue} - \text{Expense}}{\text{Revenue}}$$

tax code enumerates the circumstances under which a hospital may be exempt from federal tax. The Internal Revenue Service (IRS) website (IRS 2010a) provides the following list of requirements for a tax-exempt organization:

Exemption Requirements—Section 501(c)(3) Organizations

To be tax-exempt under section 501(c)(3) of the Internal Revenue Code, an organization must be organized and operated exclusively for exempt purposes set forth in section 501(c)(3), and none of its earnings may inure to any private shareholder or individual. In addition, it may not be an action organization, *i.e.,* it may not attempt to influence legislation as a substantial part of its activities and it may not participate in any campaign activity for or against political candidates.

Organizations described in section 501(c)(3) are commonly referred to as *charitable organizations*. Organizations described in section 501(c)(3), other than testing for public safety organizations, are eligible to receive tax-deductible contributions in accordance with Code section 170.

The organization must not be organized or operated for the benefit of private interests, and no part of a section 501(c)(3) organization's net earnings may inure to the benefit of any private shareholder or individual. If the organization engages in an excess benefit transaction with a person having substantial influence over the organization, an excise tax may be imposed on the person and any organization managers agreeing to the transaction.

Section 501(c)(3) organizations are restricted in how much political and legislative (*lobbying*) activities they may conduct. For a detailed discussion, see Political and Lobbying Activities. For more information about lobbying activities by charities, see the article Lobbying Issues; for more information about political activities of charities, see the FY-2002 CPE topic Election Year Issues.

Most state and local governments adopt the same definitions to determine whether a hospital is exempt from taxes in their jurisdictions. According to 2008 Medicare Cost Report data filed by acute care facilities, 52 percent of hospitals were not-for-profit. Another 18 percent were classified as owned by federal, state, or city governments. Only 30 percent of all hospitals were classified as for-profit or proprietary (see figure 1.6).

Figure 1.6   Distribution of hospital type

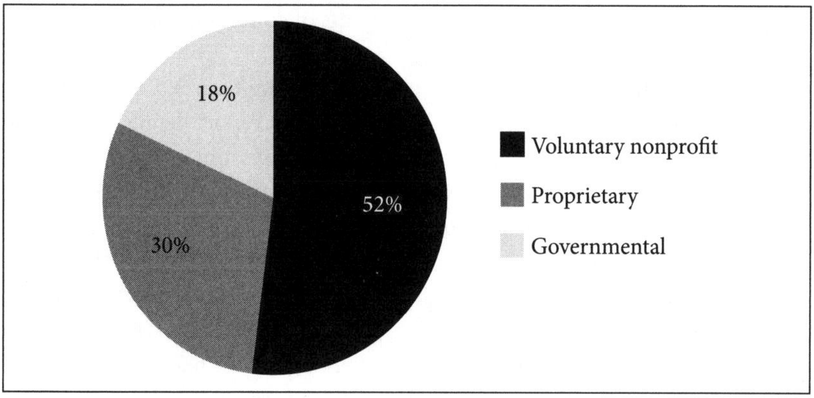

Source: 2008 Medicare Cost Reports.

The distinction between for-profit and not-for-profit hospitals is primarily based on how any excess income (profit) from providing patient care is distributed. In for-profit entities, the profits are distributed to shareholders. In not-for-profit entities, the profits are not redistributed but are used for reinvesting in the facility, paying salaries, and funding the cost of care. According to the IRS definition (IRS 2010a), excessive compensation for employees may call the not-for-profit status of a hospital into question or cause an excise tax to be levied on the organization. This may be an issue for facilities that employ physicians in executive positions. In return for providing healthcare services to the community, the not-for-profit hospital is exempt from income, property, and sales tax. The mission of a not-for-profit hospital is to provide healthcare to the community.

Recently, many not-for-profit hospitals and healthcare systems have been under increased scrutiny to determine if they are indeed providing a service to the community. Quantifying the benefits provided to the community is a difficult task but a necessary one if not-for-profit hospitals are going to continue to enjoy the benefits associated with their status.

Measuring Community Benefit

Community benefit or value is a term used to describe the positive impact that a not-for-profit hospital has on the community it serves. The basic premise is that a hospital should be providing a real and valuable service to the community in order to earn or justify the tax exemptions it is awarded. Many components of community value are not quantifiable and therefore are very difficult to measure. The IRS (IRS 2010c) recently revised the primary tax form that all not-for-profit entities must file in order to provide a method for hospitals to report the measurable components of community benefit.

All not-for-profit entities with gross revenue of more than $25,000 in a fiscal year must file IRS Form 990 on an annual basis to report details about their operations (IRS 2010b). **Gross revenue** is the total amount of money an organization takes in. Because the IRS requires electronic filing of the 990 form, initially hospitals were not able to supply additional documentation to support the assertion that they were providing significant services to their community. The description of community benefit is often included in a hospital's annual report. Beginning in 2009 (for tax year 2008), the IRS (IRS 2010b; IRS 2010c) redesigned Form 990 and added Schedule H, which allows hospitals to report the value of their community benefit activities. Before the creation of Schedule H, there were no formal guidelines for reporting community benefits. Schedule H includes the following parts:

Part I—Charity Care and Certain Other Community Benefits at Cost
Part II—Community Building Activities
Part III—Bad Debt, Medicare, and Collection Practices
Part IV—Management Companies and Joint Ventures
Part V—Facility Information
Part VI—Supplemental Information

Part I requests information about the hospital's **charity care** policy. This portion of the form is based on community reporting guidelines developed by the **Catholic Health Association** (CHA) and Voluntary Hospital Association (VHA). Questions include the criteria for free or reduced-cost care. The **Federal Poverty Guidelines** (FPG) are used to determine if a patient is eligible for discounted services. The hospital reports the percentage of FPG for eligibility (100 percent, 150 percent, 200 percent, and so on) for both free and discounted care. If the hospital does not use the FPG to determine eligibility, then it must describe its criteria in Part VI.

Part I of the form also requests detailed information about the cost of charity care provided by the hospital. The data reported are displayed in figure 1.7. Preparing the data for this portion of the form is a major project for providers that did not report community value data prior to this 2009 IRS requirement (Williams 2008). An accurate reporting of the cost of charity care and other community programs will aid hospitals in building a compelling case to justify their tax-exempt status.

Part III of Schedule H allows hospitals to report **bad debt** and payment short-falls from Medicare. The IRS did not include this in the first drafts of the form. Comments from representatives of the AHA noted that an accounting of uncollectable funds was important in evaluating the full value of services provided to the community (Reid Hatton 2008). This section of the form also requests information about the hospital's debt-collection policy.

The data reported on Form 990 provide an unprecedented amount of information to the public for assessing the community value of not-for-profit hospitals. Feedback from hospitals states that the form takes a significant amount of time and effort to complete and may not include information regarding all programs and services provided to the community. Hospitals continue to report program information in their annual reports and on their websites to ensure that the public understands their level of commitment and the service they provide to the surrounding community. The full IRS Form 990 Schedule H is presented in Appendix 1.1.

Other Providers

The healthcare system includes a wide variety of providers beyond hospitals. Other types of facilities include skilled nursing facilities (SNFs), ambulatory surgery centers (ASCs), intermediate care facilities (ICFs), and home health

Figure 1.7   Form 990 Schedule H Part I

7 Financial Assistance and Certain Other Community Benefits at Cost						
Financial Assistance and Means-Tested Government Programs	(a) Number of activities or programs (optional)	(b) Persons served (optional)	(c) Total community benefit expense	(d) Direct offsetting revenue	(e) Net community benefit expense	(f) Percent of total expense
a Financial Assistance at cost (from Worksheets 1 and 2)						
b Unreimbursed Medicaid (from Worksheet 3, column a)						
c Unreimbursed costs—other means-tested government programs (from Worksheet 3, column b)						
d **Total** Financial Assistance and Means-Tested Government Programs						
Other Benefits						
e Community health improvement services and community benefit operations (from Worksheet 4)						
f Health professions education (from Worksheet 5)						
g Subsidized health services (from Worksheet 6)						
h Research (from Worksheet 7)						
i Cash and in-kind contributions to community groups (from Worksheet 8)						
j **Total.** Other Benefits						
k **Total.** Add lines 7d and 7j						

Source: IRS 2010b.

agencies (HHAs). Physician practices and multispecialty clinics are also major components of the healthcare provider spectrum. The management of financial performance at these providers requires attention to the same key indicators as at hospitals. Many of the financial concepts discussed in the text are immediately transferable to these other settings.

Summary

Healthcare makes up a major portion of the US economy. To understand the importance of measuring the financial performance of healthcare entities, we need to study the topic of healthcare finance in the context of the healthcare delivery system. Significant external forces such as payer mix, uninsured patients, and the economy can impact a healthcare entity's financial position. Many hospitals and other healthcare providers operate as not-for-profit entities. They must balance the requirements of maintaining their not-for-profit status with the need to support operations financially.

CHECK YOUR UNDERSTANDING

1. In 2008, the majority of hospitals were for-profit organizations. (True/False)
2. Not-for-profit hospitals should bring in only enough revenue to cover their costs. (True/False)
3. Healthcare providers with a higher proportion of private-pay patients tend to perform better financially. (True/False)
4. The percentage of the GDP made up by healthcare expenditures is higher in Canada than in the United States. (True/False)
5. The growth in the number of uninsured adults in the United States does not have an impact on the financial performance of a healthcare organization. (True/False)
6. Underinsured patients are those who:
   a. Are self-insured
   b. Pay a large portion of their own health insurance premiums
   c. Have high deductibles and lifetime limits on benefits
   d. Work for firms that do not provide healthcare coverage
7. Since 1960, the proportion of US healthcare expenditures paid by government health insurance coverage has:
   a. Increased
   b. Decreased
   c. Not changed

8. Since 1993, per capita US healthcare expenditures have:
   a. Increased
   b. Decreased
   c. Not changed
9. Which of the following is not a community benefit that is reported on Schedule H of the IRS 990 form?
   a. Interest expense
   b. Unreimbursed Medicaid expenses
   c. Charity care
   d. Research
10. The criteria for providing charity care for a patient is often based on:
   a. Comparing the patient's income to the Federal Poverty Guidelines
   b. Type of procedure performed
   c. Patient's age
   d. None of these

References

111th Congress. 2010. HR 3590: Patient Protection and Affordable Care Act. http://www.govtrack.us/congress/bill.xpd?bill=h111-3590.

AHIMA. 2010. *2010 Pocket Glossary of Health Information Management and Technology,* 2nd ed. Chicago: AHIMA.

Casto, A., and E. Layman. 2011. *Principles of Healthcare Reimbursement*, 3rd ed. Chicago: AHIMA.

Centers for Medicare and Medicaid Services. 2010. National health expenditure data. https://www.cms.gov/NationalHealthExpendData.

DeNavas-Walt, C., B. Proctor, and J. Smith. 2010. *US Census Bureau, Current Population Reports, P60-238, Income, Poverty, and Health Insurance Coverage in the United States: 2009.* Washington, DC: US Government Printing Office. http://www.census.gov/prod/2010pubs/p60-238.pdf.

Fox, W., and J. Pickering. 2008. Hospital and physician cost shift: Payment level comparison of Medicare, Medicaid and commercial payers. Milliman technical report to the American Hospital Association. http://publications.milliman.com/research/health-rr/pdfs/hospital-physician-cost-shift-RR12-01-08.pdf.

IRS. 2010a. Exemption Requirements—Section 501(c)(3) Organizations. http://www.irs.gov/charities/charitable/article/0,,id=96099,00.html.

IRS. 2010b. IRS Form 990. http://www.irs.gov/pub/irs-pdf/i990sh.pdf.

IRS. 2010c. IRS Form 990, Schedule H. http://www.irs.gov/pub/irs-tege/highlights_schedule_h.pdf.

Martinez, M.E., and R.A. Cohen. 2010. Health insurance coverage: Early release of estimates from the National Health Interview Survey, January–June 2010. National Center for Health Statistics. http://www.cdc.gov/nchs/nhis.htm.

Organisation for Economic Co-operation and Development. n.d. StatExtracts. http://stats.oecd.org/Index.aspx?DataSetCode=DECOMP.

Reid Hatton, Melinda. 2008. AHA comments on Draft Form 990, Schedule H and selected other instructions. http://www.aha.org/aha/letter/2008/080515-cl-irs-990.pdf.

Sisko, A., C. Truffer, S. Smith, S. Keehan, J. Cylus, J. Poisal, and J. Lizonitz. 2009. Health spending projections through 2018: Recession effects add uncertainty to the outlook. *Health Affairs (Project Hope)* 28(2):w346–w357.

Williams, Jeni. 2008. Schedule H: What hospitals should do to prepare: Schedule H of the new Form 990 requires detailed reporting of the community benefit hospitals provide, beginning with tax year 2009. Is your organization ready? *Healthcare Financial Management* 62(3):50–54.

Appendix 1.1: IRS Form 990 Schedule H

SCHEDULE H (Form 990)	**Hospitals**	OMB No. 1545-0047
Department of the Treasury Internal Revenue Service	► Complete if the organization answered "Yes" to Form 990, Part IV, question 20. ► Attach to Form 990. ► See separate instructions.	20**10** Open to Public Inspection

Name of the organization | Employer identification number

Part I Financial Assistance and Certain Other Community Benefits at Cost

		Yes	No
1a	Did the organization have a financial assistance policy during the tax year? If "No," skip to question 6a .	1a	
b	If "Yes," was it a written policy?	1b	
2	If the organization had multiple hospital facilities, indicate which of the following best describes application of the financial assistance policy to its various hospital facilities during the tax year.		

☐ Applied uniformly to all hospital facilities ☐ Applied uniformly to most hospital facilities
☐ Generally tailored to individual hospital facilities

3 Answer the following based on the financial assistance eligibility criteria that applied to the largest number of the organization's patients during the tax year.

a	Did the organization use Federal Poverty Guidelines (FPG) to determine eligibility for providing *free* care to low income individuals? If "Yes," indicate which of the following was the FPG family income limit for eligibility for free care: . .	3a	

☐ 100% ☐ 150% ☐ 200% ☐ Other _____ %

b	Did the organization use FPG to determine eligibility for providing *discounted* care to low income individuals? If "Yes," indicate which of the following was the family income limit for eligibility for discounted care:	3b	

☐ 200% ☐ 250% ☐ 300% ☐ 350% ☐ 400% ☐ Other _____ %

c If the organization did not use FPG to determine eligibility, describe in Part VI the income based criteria for determining eligibility for free or discounted care. Include in the description whether the organization used an asset test or other threshold, regardless of income, to determine eligibility for free or discounted care.

4	Did the organization's financial assistance policy that applied to the largest number of its patients during the tax year provide for free or discounted care to the "medically indigent"?	4	
5a	Did the organization budget amounts for free or discounted care provided under its financial assistance policy during the tax year?	5a	
b	If "Yes," did the organization's financial assistance expenses exceed the budgeted amount?	5b	
c	If "Yes" to line 5b, as a result of budget considerations, was the organization unable to provide free or discounted care to a patient who was eligible for free or discounted care?	5c	
6a	Did the organization prepare a community benefit report during the tax year?	6a	
b	If "Yes," did the organization make it available to the public?	6b	

Complete the following table using the worksheets provided in the Schedule H instructions. Do not submit these worksheets with the Schedule H.

7 Financial Assistance and Certain Other Community Benefits at Cost

Financial Assistance and Means-Tested Government Programs	(a) Number of activities or programs (optional)	(b) Persons served (optional)	(c) Total community benefit expense	(d) Direct offsetting revenue	(e) Net community benefit expense	(f) Percent of total expense
a Financial Assistance at cost (from Worksheets 1 and 2) . .						
b Unreimbursed Medicaid (from Worksheet 3, column a) . . .						
c Unreimbursed costs—other means-tested government programs (from Worksheet 3, column b)						
d **Total** Financial Assistance and Means-Tested Government Programs						
Other Benefits						
e Community health improvement services and community benefit operations (from Worksheet 4) .						
f Health professions education (from Worksheet 5)						
g Subsidized health services (from Worksheet 6)						
h Research (from Worksheet 7) .						
i Cash and in-kind contributions to community groups (from Worksheet 8)						
j **Total.** Other Benefits						
k **Total.** Add lines 7d and 7j . .						

For Paperwork Reduction Act Notice, see the Instructions for Form 990.　　Cat. No. 50192T　　Schedule H (Form 990) 2010

Schedule H (Form 990) 2010   Page **2**

Part II **Community Building Activities** Complete this table if the organization conducted any community building activities during the tax year, and describe in Part VI how its community building activities promoted the health of the communities it serves.

		(a) Number of activities or programs (optional)	(b) Persons served (optional)	(c) Total community building expense	(d) Direct offsetting revenue	(e) Net community building expense	(f) Percent of total expense
1	Physical improvements and housing						
2	Economic development						
3	Community support						
4	Environmental improvements						
5	Leadership development and training for community members						
6	Coalition building						
7	Community health improvement advocacy						
8	Workforce development						
9	Other						
10	Total						

Part III **Bad Debt, Medicare, & Collection Practices**

Section A. Bad Debt Expense

			Yes	No
1	Did the organization report bad debt expense in accordance with Healthcare Financial Management Association Statement No. 15?	1		
2	Enter the amount of the organization's bad debt expense (at cost)	**2**		
3	Enter the estimated amount of the organization's bad debt expense (at cost) attributable to patients eligible under the organization's financial assistance policy	**3**		
4	Provide in Part VI the text of the footnote to the organization's financial statements that describes bad debt expense. In addition, describe the costing methodology used in determining the amounts reported on lines 2 and 3, and rationale for including a portion of bad debt amounts as community benefit.			

Section B. Medicare

5	Enter total revenue received from Medicare (including DSH and IME)	**5**		
6	Enter Medicare allowable costs of care relating to payments on line 5	**6**		
7	Subtract line 6 from line 5. This is the surplus (or shortfall)	**7**		
8	Describe in Part VI the extent to which any shortfall reported in line 7 should be treated as community benefit. Also describe in Part VI the costing methodology or source used to determine the amount reported on line 6. Check the box that describes the method used: ☐ Cost accounting system ☐ Cost to charge ratio ☐ Other			

Section C. Collection Practices

9a	Did the organization have a written debt collection policy during the tax year?	9a		
b	If "Yes," did the organization's collection policy that applied to the largest number of its patients during the tax year contain provisions on the collection practices to be followed for patients who are known to qualify for financial assistance? Describe in Part VI	9b		

Part IV **Management Companies and Joint Ventures**

	(a) Name of entity	(b) Description of primary activity of entity	(c) Organization's profit % or stock ownership %	(d) Officers, directors, trustees, or key employees' profit % or stock ownership %	(e) Physicians' profit % or stock ownership %
1					
2					
3					
4					
5					
6					
7					
8					
9					
10					
11					
12					
13					

Schedule H (Form 990) 2010

Schedule H (Form 990) 2010   Page **3**

Part V	**Facility Information**

Section A. Hospital Facilities

(list in order of size, measured by total revenue per facility, from largest to smallest)

How many hospital facilities did the organization operate during the tax year? _____

Name and address	Licensed hospital	General medical & surgical	Children's hospital	Teaching hospital	Critical access hospital	Research facility	ER-24 hours	ER-other	Other (describe)
1									
2									
3									
4									
5									
6									
7									
8									
9									
10									
11									
12									
13									
14									
15									
16									

Schedule H (Form 990) 2010

Schedule H (Form 990) 2010   Page **4**

Part V   **Facility Information** *(continued)*

Section B. Facility Policies and Practices

(Complete a separate Section B for each of the hospital facilities listed in Part V, Section A)

Name of Hospital Facility: _____

Line Number of Hospital Facility (from Schedule H, Part V, Section A): _____

		Yes	No
Community Health Needs Assessment (Lines 1 through 7 are optional for 2010)			
1	During the tax year or any prior tax year, did the hospital facility conduct a community health needs assessment (Needs Assessment)? If "No," skip to line 8 . . . . **1**		
	If "Yes," indicate what the Needs Assessment describes (check all that apply):		
a	☐ A definition of the community served by the hospital facility		
b	☐ Demographics of the community		
c	☐ Existing health care facilities and resources within the community that are available to respond to the health needs of the community		
d	☐ How data was obtained		
e	☐ The health needs of the community		
f	☐ Primary and chronic disease needs and other health issues of uninsured persons, low-income persons, and minority groups		
g	☐ The process for identifying and prioritizing community health needs and services to meet the community health needs		
h	☐ The process for consulting with persons representing the community's interests		
i	☐ Information gaps that limit the hospital facility's ability to assess all of the community's health needs		
j	☐ Other (describe in Part VI)		
2	Indicate the tax year the hospital facility last conducted a Needs Assessment: 20 __ __		
3	In conducting its most recent Needs Assessment, did the hospital facility take into account input from persons who represent the community served by the hospital facility? If "Yes," describe in Part VI how the hospital facility took into account input from persons who represent the community, and identify the persons the hospital facility consulted **3**		
4	Was the hospital facility's Needs Assessment conducted with one or more other hospital facilities? If "Yes," list the other hospital facilities in Part VI **4**		
5	Did the hospital facility make its Needs Assessment widely available to the public? **5**		
	If "Yes," indicate how the Needs Assessment was made widely available (check all that apply):		
a	☐ Hospital facility's website		
b	☐ Available upon request from the hospital facility		
c	☐ Other (describe in Part VI)		
6	If the hospital facility addressed needs identified in its most recently conducted Needs Assessment, indicate how (check all that apply):		
a	☐ Adoption of an implementation strategy to address the health needs of the hospital facility's community		
b	☐ Execution of the implementation strategy		
c	☐ Participation in the development of a community-wide community benefit plan		
d	☐ Participation in the execution of a community-wide community benefit plan		
e	☐ Inclusion of a community benefit section in operational plans		
f	☐ Adoption of a budget for provision of services that address the needs identified in the Needs Assessment		
g	☐ Prioritization of health needs in its community		
h	☐ Prioritization of services that the hospital facility will undertake to meet health needs in its community		
i	☐ Other (describe in Part VI)		
7	Did the hospital facility address all of the needs identified in its most recently conducted Needs Assessment? If "No," explain in Part VI which needs it has not addressed and the reasons why it has not addressed such needs **7**		
Financial Assistance Policy			
	Did the hospital facility have in place during the tax year a written financial assistance policy that:		
8	Explained eligibility criteria for financial assistance, and whether such assistance includes free or discounted care? **8**		
9	Used federal poverty guidelines (FPG) to determine eligibility for providing *free* care to low income individuals? **9**		
	If "Yes," indicate the FPG family income limit for eligibility for free care: __ __ __ %		

Schedule H (Form 990) 2010

Part V   **Facility Information** *(continued)*

			Yes	No

10   Used FPG to determine eligibility for providing *discounted* care to low income individuals? **10**
    If "Yes," indicate the FPG family income limit for eligibility for discounted care: _ _ _ %
11   Explained the basis for calculating amounts charged to patients? **11**
    If "Yes," indicate the factors used in determining such amounts (check all that apply):
    a ☐ Income level
    b ☐ Asset level
    c ☐ Medical indigency
    d ☐ Insurance status
    e ☐ Uninsured discount
    f ☐ Medicaid/Medicare
    g ☐ State regulation
    h ☐ Other (describe in Part VI)
12   Explained the method for applying for financial assistance? **12**
13   Included measures to publicize the policy within the community served by the hospital facility? **13**
    If "Yes," indicate how the hospital facility publicized the policy (check all that apply):
    a ☐ The policy was posted on the hospital facility's website
    b ☐ The policy was attached to billing invoices
    c ☐ The policy was posted in the hospital facility's emergency rooms or waiting rooms
    d ☐ The policy was posted in the hospital facility's admissions offices
    e ☐ The policy was provided, in writing, to patients on admission to the hospital facility
    f ☐ The policy was available on request
    g ☐ Other (describe in Part VI)

Billing and Collections

14   Did the hospital facility have in place during the tax year a separate billing and collections policy, or a written financial assistance policy that explained actions the hospital facility may take upon non-payment? . . . **14**
15   Check all of the following collection actions against a patient that were permitted under the hospital facility's policies at any time during the tax year:
    a ☐ Reporting to credit agency
    b ☐ Lawsuits
    c ☐ Liens on residences
    d ☐ Body attachments
    e ☐ Other actions (describe in Part VI)
16   Did the hospital facility engage in or authorize a third party to perform any of the following collection actions during the tax year? **16**
    If "Yes," check all collection actions in which the hospital facility or a third party engaged (check all that apply):
    a ☐ Reporting to credit agency
    b ☐ Lawsuits
    c ☐ Liens on residences
    d ☐ Body attachments
    e ☐ Other actions (describe in Part VI)
17   Indicate which actions the hospital facility took before initiating any of the collection actions checked in line 16 (check all that apply):
    a ☐ Notified patients of the financial assistance policy on admission
    b ☐ Notified patients of the financial assistance policy prior to discharge
    c ☐ Notified patients of the financial assistance policy in communications with the patients regarding the patients' bills
    d ☐ Documented its determination of whether a patient who applied for financial assistance under the financial assistance policy qualified for financial assistance
    e ☐ Other (describe in Part VI)

Schedule H (Form 990) 2010   Page **6**

Part V   **Facility Information** *(continued)*

Policy Relating to Emergency Medical Care

		Yes	No
18	Did the hospital facility have in place during the tax year a written policy relating to emergency medical care that requires the hospital facility to provide, without discrimination, care for emergency medical conditions to individuals regardless of their eligibility under the hospital facility's financial assistance policy? **18**		

If "No," indicate the reasons why (check all that apply):

a ☐ The hospital facility did not provide care for any emergency medical conditions

b ☐ The hospital facility did not have a policy relating to emergency medical care

c ☐ The hospital facility limited who was eligible to receive care for emergency medical conditions (describe in Part VI)

d ☐ Other (describe in Part VI)

Charges for Medical Care

19 Indicate how the hospital facility determined the amounts billed to individuals who did not have insurance covering emergency or other medically necessary care (check all that apply):

a ☐ The hospital facility used the lowest negotiated commercial insurance rate for those services at the hospital facility

b ☐ The hospital facility used the average of the three lowest negotiated commercial insurance rates for those services at the hospital facility

c ☐ The hospital facility used the Medicare rate for those services

d ☐ Other (describe in Part VI)

		Yes	No
20	Did the hospital facility charge any of its patients who were eligible for assistance under the hospital facility's financial assistance policy, and to whom the hospital facility provided emergency or other medically necessary services, more than the amounts generally billed to individuals who had insurance covering such care? **20**		
	If "Yes," explain in Part VI.		
21	Did the hospital facility charge any of its patients an amount equal to the gross charge for any service provided to that patient? **21**		
	If "Yes," explain in Part VI.		

Schedule H (Form 990) 2010

Part V   **Facility Information** *(continued)*

Section C. Other Facilities That Are Not Licensed, Registered, or Similarly Recognized as a Hospital Facility
(list in order of size, measured by total revenue per facility, from largest to smallest)

How many non-hospital facilities did the organization operate during the tax year? _____

Name and address	Type of Facility (describe)
1	
2	
3	
4	
5	
6	
7	
8	
9	
10	

Part VI Supplemental Information

Complete this part to provide the following information.

1 **Required descriptions.** Provide the descriptions required for Part I, lines 3c, 6a, and 7; Part II; Part III, lines 4, 8, and 9b; and Part V, Section B, lines 1j, 3, 4, 5c, 6i, 7, 11h, 13g, 15e, 16e, 17e, 18d, 19d, 20, and 21.

2 **Needs assessment.** Describe how the organization assesses the health care needs of the communities it serves, in addition to any needs assessments reported in Part V, Section B.

3 **Patient education of eligibility for assistance.** Describe how the organization informs and educates patients and persons who may be billed for patient care about their eligibility for assistance under federal, state, or local government programs or under the organization's financial assistance policy.

4 **Community information.** Describe the community the organization serves, taking into account the geographic area and demographic constituents it serves.

5 **Promotion of community health.** Provide any other information important to describing how the organization's hospital facilities or other health care facilities further its exempt purpose by promoting the health of the community (e.g., open medical staff, community board, use of surplus funds, etc.).

6 **Affiliated health care system.** If the organization is part of an affiliated health care system, describe the respective roles of the organization and its affiliates in promoting the health of the communities served.

7 **State filing of community benefit report.** If applicable, identify all states with which the organization, or a related organization, files a community benefit report.

Understanding Financial Statements

CHAPTER TWO

Learning Objectives

➥ Understand the distinction between financial and managerial accounting
➥ Identify cash-based versus accrual-based accounting
➥ Identify and interpret the four basic components of a financial statement

Key Terms

Accounts payable
Accounts receivable
Accrual-based accounting
Accrued expenses
Assets
Balance sheet
Board of directors
Cash-based accounting
Contractual allowance
Current assets
Depreciation
Double-entry bookkeeping system
Equity
Equity statement
Expenses
Financial accounting
Financial statement
Generally accepted accounting
    principles (GAAP)
Income
Income statement
Inventory
Liabilities
Long-term assets
Long-term liabilities
Managerial accounting

Matching
Net assets
Net patient service revenue
Nonoperating activities
Nonoperating gains and losses
Nonoperating revenue and
    expenses
Operating activities
Operating expenses
Operating income
Permanently restricted net assets
Prepaid expenses
Profit and loss statement
Restricted net assets
Retained earnings
Revenue
Short-term investments
Statement of activities
Statement of cash flow
Statement of net assets
Statement of revenue and expenses
Statement of shareholder equity
Temporarily restricted net assets
Third-party payer settlements
Transactions
Unrestricted net assets

Accounting Review

Healthcare organization **financial statements** have four basic components. Before reviewing the contents of the financial statements, it is necessary to have an understanding of basic accounting concepts and vocabulary. This text does not include a comprehensive review of accounting principles but instead reviews just the basic concepts. There are two functional categories recognized in accounting: financial and managerial practices. The method of recognizing revenue and expenses is segmented into cash-based accounting and accrual-based accounting.

Financial Accounting versus Managerial Accounting

Accounting may be segmented into two functional categories. **Financial accounting** is the task of recording and preparing financial information for an audience that often includes users outside of the organization. Financial information is communicated to that audience via the financial statements. The guidelines for financial accounting are the **generally accepted accounting principles** (GAAP). Accounting and finance professionals may refer to GAAP (pronounced "gap") when determining how a figure should be represented on the financial statement. The GAAP guidelines ensure that there is comparability among financial statements for different organizations and across time periods. Accurate financial performance benchmarking would not be feasible without a common vocabulary and definitions among financial statements. Table 2.1 lists other sources of financial reporting standards.

Table 2.1   Sources of accounting and reporting standards

Organization	Description
Financial Accounting Standards Board (FASB)	Independent organization that maintains GAAP
Securities and Exchange Commission (SEC)	Establishes accounting standards for publicly traded companies
Government Accounting Standards Board (GASB)	Establishes accounting standards for state, local, and federal governmental agencies
Public Company Accounting Oversight Board (PCAOB)	Established by Congress to oversee the audits of public companies
Other comprehensive basis of accounting (OCBOA)	An alternative to GAAP; allows for case-based accounting
Generally accepted accounting principles (GAPP)	A collection of accounting rules that guides the reporting of financial statements; maintained by the FASB

Managerial accounting focuses on financial information for internal audiences. The information conveyed to that audience includes reports that measure performance versus budget, cost control information, and other key performance indicators. The reports are distributed internally to department managers to assess their performance and guide decision making.

Cash versus Accrual Accounting

There are two basic methods of accounting: cash-based and accrual-based. The distinction between these two methods is the timing used to record **income** and **expenses.** In an organization that uses a **cash-based accounting** method, income is recorded or recognized on the date it is received. Similarly, expenses are recognized on the date the expense is actually paid. In an **accrual-based accounting** system, income is recognized when a service is provided and an invoice is issued for payment. Expenses in an accrual-based system are recognized when the expense is incurred.

The difference between the two accounting methods is best understood via an example. It will be helpful to review some terms before presenting the example. **Accounts receivable** are monies owed to the firm for services that have been provided. In the healthcare setting, a patient may come in for an office visit and the physician will deliver services. If the patient has health insurance, then the physician will not receive payment immediately. The physician's practice will create an accounts receivable entry for the amount of payment expected from the insurance company. **Accounts payable** are invoices the firm is obligated to pay but will pay at a later date. The same physician's office pays $5,000 per month to lease office space. The rent is paid at the end of the month, but the practice likely creates an accounts payable entry for the amount of the rent at the beginning of the month.

The example outlined in table 2.2 will help explain the difference between these two accounting methods. In this example, a physician's office is providing flu vaccines to both insured and self-pay patients during a flu shot clinic. The physician pays the supplier of the vaccine at the end of the flu season, November 30, based on the number of doses delivered. The physician is supplied with 25 doses at $10 each on October 1. A flu clinic is held on October 8. Vaccines are provided to 10 self-pay patients and 15 insured patients. The self-pay patients pay for their vaccines at the time of service. The insured patients pay nothing at the time of service. The physician must wait to be reimbursed by the insurance companies providing coverage to the insured patients.

Table 2.2   Cash versus accrual accounting example—flu shot clinic

Date	Transaction	#	Unit Cost	Total	Accrual Transaction Type: Amount	Cash Transaction Type: Amount
1-Oct	Flu vaccine delivered to office	25	$10	$250	Accounts payable: $250	None
8-Oct	Self-pay patients receive vaccine	10	$15	$150	Revenue: $150	Revenue: $150
8-Oct	Insured patients receive vaccine	15	$15	$225	Accounts receivable: $225	None
October profit					= (−$250 + $150 + $225 = $125)	= $150
8-Nov	Insurance payment received	15	$15	$225	None	Revenue: $225
30-Nov	Flu vaccine provider paid	25	$10	$250	None	Expense: $250
November profit					= 0	= −$25
Total profit for October/November					= $125	= $125

Table 2.2 shows a timeline of the various transactions for the flu shot clinic. Notice that when the shots are delivered to patients on October 8 there is a difference in both the revenues and expenses recognized. Under accrual-based accounting, revenue is recognized for both the self-pay patients (cash) and the insured patients (accounts receivable for amount to be paid). Under cash-based accounting, only the cash received from the self-pay patients is recorded as revenue. In terms of expenses, the cost of the vaccines delivered is recognized on the date of receipt at the clinic and as an account payable under accrual-based accounting. No expenses are recognized in October under cash-based accounting. At the end of October, it appears that the clinic was more profitable under cash-based accounting: $150 versus $125 profit under the accrual method. This situation reverses in November when under cash-based accounting the $225 is actually received as payment for the insured patients and the vaccine supplier is paid $250 for the 25 doses dispensed. At the end of the two months, the profit is the same under both accounting systems.

Financial reports are a snapshot in time. The difference between the two bases is essentially the timing with which transactions are recorded. If the October financial statement were important to the physician for external reporting either to investors or for securing a loan, the cash-based accounting might be more favorable in this case. Organizations may not switch between accounting bases and should therefore choose carefully from the outset.

Accrual-based accounting tends to even out fluctuations in revenue and expenses that occur in cash-based accounting. Accrual-based accounting also demonstrates an accounting concept called **matching.** The matching principle states that the expenses incurred in generating revenue should be matched with the corresponding revenues created (Hart 2006, 157). Cash-based accounting tends to be more intuitive because it is based on the actual movement of money but does not include the reporting of future financial obligations. There is no right or wrong basis of accounting. It is important that a firm be consistent in the accounting basis implemented to ensure that financial reports are comparable across periods.

Healthcare providers have a large number of accounts and transactions occurring simultaneously. Since insurance payments are often delayed by 30 days or more and supplies are not paid for on the date of delivery, accrual-based accounting is generally used. The advantage of the accrual method for healthcare entities is that it records a transaction when the service is rendered and therefore gives a more realistic picture of the level and intensity of the provider's operations. Accrual-based accounting is required by GAAP.

Basic Accounting Equation

The basic accounting equation defines the relationship between an entity's assets and liabilities. **Assets** are items with a cash value that an organization owns. **Liabilities** represent money to be paid by the organization. This equation is the basis for the **double-entry bookkeeping system** that is used to record financial **transactions** in accounting systems. Each asset or input of value must have a corresponding liability or output of value in order for the equation to remain in balance. Liabilities and **equity** are both types of financial obiligations or outputs of value for an organization. In a corporation, equity is the amount of investment from shareholders or the owner of the company and any profits that are retained by the company. In not-for-profit entities, equity may come through grants, charitable contributions, or government support. Equity in not-for-profit entities also includes **retained earnings.**

In reporting financial results, balancing the basic accounting equation does not ensure that there have not been any accounting errors. If the equation does not balance, then there is definitely an accounting error that must be corrected

Figure 2.1   Basic accounting equation

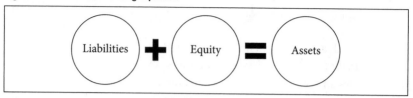

before reporting. The equation, depicted in figure 2.1, serves as a check and balance for the most basic types of transaction entry errors.

Financial Statements

According to GAAP, an organization should compile four basic financial reports:

1. Balance sheet
2. Income statement
3. Statement of changes in net assets or equity statement
4. Statement of cash flow

In practice, the compilation of these four statements or reports is referred to as the financial statements. Financial statements typically have footnotes that explain any unusual circumstances and may clarify the method used to account for those circumstances. For instance, footnotes may explain accounting of any mergers and acquisitions, the method used to value investments, or assumptions made in the estimation of any figures. Figures that may require an estimate include allowances for doubtful accounts or the value of inventory at the close of the accounting period. Appendix 3.1 presents a full set of financial statements for an example hospital, including footnotes.

Many hospitals must submit their financial statements to state government agencies. Those submitted financial statements may be made available to the public via a website or special request. Hospital websites may also include a recent audited financial statement for public review. The financial statements are the primary mode of communicating the financial health of an organization to the public.

Financial statements may be prepared on a monthly or quarterly basis but are typically reported outside of the organization only on an annual basis. A healthcare entity's financial statement may be prepared or audited by a third party at the completion of a fiscal year. An audited financial statement must be prepared using GAAP guidelines. The reported values are validated by examining evidence to support the figures and assertions made in the financial statements. The requirements for the audit and release of healthcare entity financial statements are regulated at the state level.

Financial statements are both a financial and managerial accounting tool. From the financial accounting perspective, it is important that the statement include enough detailed information to allow the financial position or performance of the organization to be assessed by an external reviewer. For managerial accounting purposes, the financial statement allows a global comparison of financial performance from year to year that may be used to identify areas for improvement.

Balance Sheet

The **balance sheet** is a representation of the basic accounting equation depicted in figure 2.1. It provides information about an organization's assets, liabilities, and equity at a snapshot in time. The balance sheet may also be called the statement of financial position or **statement of net assets**.

Figure 2.2 contains an example of a hospital balance sheet. The values displayed in the balance sheet are scaled to $1,000 increments. In other words, the $932 listed as the value for "cash and cash equivalents" is actually $932,000. Since the figures in the typical hospital financial statement may range from thousands to millions of dollars, it is common to see the values scaled to thousands of dollars. Here, the "$(000)" at the top of the column is a signal that the reporting unit is in thousands of dollars. Financial statements should have some indication of the scale either in the heading of the value column or in the footnotes. Figure 2.2 includes a reference column that displays a label for each row in the balance sheet. These references are used to show the relationship between the various components of the report. This example includes the most common elements of a hospital balance sheet. Individual hospitals may report more or less detail as deemed appropriate by their management staff and **board of directors.**

The major headings in the balance sheet (assets, liabilities, and **net assets**) correspond to the components of the basic accounting equation. Notice that the total assets ($28,835,000) are equal to the sum of the liabilities and net assets ($28,835,000). The assets and liabilities for Memorial Hospital are divided into current and long-term.

Figure 2.2   Memorial Hospital balance sheet

Memorial Hospital Balance Sheet—2010 Fiscal Year		
	$(000)	**Reference**
Assets		
Current assets		
Cash and cash equivalents	$932	a
Short-term investments	$2,410	b
Patient accounts receivable, less estimated doubtful accounts and allowances $2,167,000	$5,663	c
Accounts receivable, other	$376	d
Estimated third-party settlements	$249	e
Inventories	$479	f
Prepaid expenses	$239	g
Total current assets	**$10,348**	**h = sum a to g**
Long-term assets		
Property and equipment	$33,684	i
Construction in progress	$30	j
Less accumulated depreciation	$(15,227)	k
Total long-term assets	**$18,487**	**l = i + j + k**
Total assets	**$28,835**	**m = h + l**
Liabilities and net assets		
Current liabilities		
Accounts payable	$264	n
Accrued expenses	$586	o
Total liabilities	**$850**	**p = n + o**
Net assets		
Unrestricted	$27,985	q
Total liabilities and net assets	**$28,835**	**r = p + q**

Assets

Assets are items that an organization owns that have a value and may be converted to cash or are highly liquid. Items that are prepaid are also considered assets (such as advertising, insurance, and legal fees). Common assets that may be found in a healthcare organization are as follows:

- **Current assets** (typically convert to cash in one year or less)
  - Cash (such as bank accounts and short-term CDs)
  - Inventory (such as pharmaceuticals and supplies)
  - **Prepaid expenses** (such as rent and insurance)
  - Accounts receivable
- **Long-term assets** (require longer than one year to convert to cash)
  - Investments such as long-term bonds
  - Buildings
  - Property and equipment (such as land and automobiles)

In the example balance sheet in figure 2.2, the largest single current asset is patient accounts receivable at $5,663,000. This figure represents payments that are expected but have not yet been received for care that was provided during the fiscal year. The amount recorded on the balance sheet represents the amount that Memorial Hospital expects to collect in the next 12 months. In this example, the item includes a notation that $2,167,000 was deducted due to doubtful accounts and allowances. Amounts deducted for doubtful accounts may also be referred to as bad debt. See chapter 1 for more information about bad debt. Patient accounts receivable is reported as net or the amount that the hospital expects to actually collect. This figure should be net of any bad debt, charity care, or contractual allowances for third-party payments. **Contractual allowances** are the difference between the amount charged for services to a patient and the amount the provider expects to collect from the payer. The contractual allowance may be as high as 50–60 percent for some government payers. Contractual allowances for private payers are typically lower than for government payers, because their payment rates are more generous. The proper estimation of the value of allowances and doubtful accounts is critical in reporting an accurate balance sheet. The methodology used to derive this figure is heavily scrutinized by auditors during their review. If the contractual allowances or bad debt are underestimated, then the patient accounts receivable may be overvalued. This results in an overstatement of the organization's assets.

The **short-term investments** listed in the current assets section of the balance sheet are those that will likely be held for less than 12 months. These are typically short-term bonds or stocks that can be converted to cash quickly.

Third-party payer settlements may be positive or negative values. They are amounts that payers may have prepaid or owe for services provided to their subscribers. For instance, a major payer may pay Memorial Hospital a fixed installment of $100,000 per month for services provided to its subscribers during a contract year. At the end of the contract year, the amount owed to the hospital and paid by the payer are reconciled and a settlement is made to ensure that the balance owed is zero at the commencement of the next contract year. In this case, it appears that payers underpaid for services during the year and owe Memorial Hospital a settlement of $249,000.

For a healthcare entity, **inventory** represents drugs, supplies, and equipment that are on hand for patient treatment. Most unused items in inventory are used in less than a year from purchase and are therefore considered a current asset. Estimation of the value of inventory may be accomplished using a number of methods. If the entity has software that tracks inventory, then estimating the value of items in inventory is relatively simple. There are multiple methods used to place a value on the inventory. Some entities use a first in, first out (FIFO) method and some use a last in, first out (LIFO) method. The detailed calculation of the value of inventory is beyond the scope of this text but may be found in a number of online and text resources.

Prepaid expenses include insurance premiums, leased equipment, and other payments that are made in advance of the date the service is actually provided to the entity. For instance, a hospital pays the premium for its liability insurance policy on January 1. If the hospital's fiscal year ended on June 30, then six months or one-half of the premium for the liability insurance policy would be recognized as a prepaid expense. Insurance policies of all types are prepaid. No insurance company would sell insurance to a customer after they incurred a loss.

Long-term assets include items of value that cannot be converted to cash in the short term, typically defined as a period of longer than 12 months. This includes categories like property, buildings, and construction in progress. Long-term assets are offset somewhat by accumulated depreciation. The value of long-term assets is reduced by depreciation each year. **Depreciation** is the decrease in value of the asset. Accumulated depreciation is the total amount that an asset has depreciated since purchase. Items such as buildings, medical equipment, and computer equipment may be depreciated. Not all long-term assets are depreciated; land is an example of a long-term asset that is not depreciated.

The most straightforward method of calculating depreciation is the straight-line method. Depreciation can be calculated over what is called the useful life

Table 2.3   Straight-line depreciation example

Year	Value	Depreciation	Accumulated Depreciation
0 (purchased)	$1,000	—	—
1	$800	$200	$200
2	$600	$200	$400
3	$400	$200	$600
4	$200	$200	$800
5 (end of useful life)	—	$200	$1,000

of an item. The IRS defines useful life as "an estimate of how long an item of property can be expected to be usable in trade or business or to produce income" (IRS 2011). Suppose a computer that cost $1,000 has a useful life of five years and at the end of that life it has no value. Table 2.3 demonstrates that the depreciation on that computer would be $200 per year ($1,000/5). The accumulated depreciation after three years would be $600 ($200 × 3). Many items such as automobiles do not depreciate according to a straight-line schedule. Modified accelerated cost recovery system (MACRS) includes two methods of depreciation that are not based on straight-line calculations. The first is the general depreciation system (GDS). The second is the alternative depreciation system (ADS). These are both examples of declining balance depreciation. GDS allows for faster depreciation and more depreciation each year of the useful life of the item. ADS allows for a longer depreciation period and a higher value for the item. Examples of these methods are beyond the scope of this text. The IRS website (www.irs.gov) presents excellent examples of each method. The IRS has strict guidelines on depreciation methods and the items that may be depreciated.

Liabilities

Liabilities are items that the healthcare entity is obligated to pay that are the result of past transactions. Liabilities are typically classified as either current or long term. Current liabilities are due within one year of the balance sheet date. **Long-term liabilities** have a due date longer than one year after the ending date of the report. Common liabilities found on a healthcare balance sheet are as follows:

- Current liabilities (due within one year)
  - Accounts payable
  - Short-term loans
  - Accrued payroll

- Long-term liabilities (due date more than one year from period end)
  - Long-term debt (mortgages, etc.)
  - Capital lease obligations

The current liabilities section of Memorial Hospital's balance sheet shows both accounts payable and **accrued expenses.** Accounts payable are amounts that the entity is obligated to pay. Since the item appears in the current liabilities section, this figure represents amounts that are due in less than one year. Memorial Hospital may owe vendors for various medical supplies and pharmaceuticals that they have received. Monies owed to those vendors are examples of short-term accounts payable that may be incurred by a hospital. Utilities, rent, and payroll taxes are examples of accrued expenses. Accrued expenses are typically periodic in nature; the entity knows that they will occur and they are regularly scheduled events. An accrued expense is the opposite of a prepaid expense. For an accrued expense, the funds are earmarked or put aside for the expense, but they physically remain in the provider's bank account. Prepaid expenses are paid before their due date and therefore the funds are no longer present in the provider's account.

Equity (Net Assets)

Equity or net assets are the fund balance or cash reserves for a not-for-profit entity. In for-profit corporations, net assets are the shareholder equity or value. In not-for-profit organizations, the net assets are segmented into **unrestricted, permanently restricted,** and **temporarily restricted.** In the example balance sheet, Memorial Hospital recorded only unrestricted net assets. If a donor made a contribution to a not-for-profit hospital for a specific purpose (building a children's play area or funding research for a particular disease), then those net assets would be recorded as **restricted.** Lane et al. offer the following definitions of net assets for a not-for-profit organization in *A Community Leader's Guide to Hospital Finance* (Lane et al. 2001):

Permanently restricted net assets
Includes funds permanently restricted by donor or grantor stipulations

Temporarily restricted net assets
Includes funds temporarily restricted by donor or grantor stipulations
Includes funds called for a specific purpose; property, plant, and replacement; or endowment funds

Unrestricted net assets
Includes all net assets that are not temporarily or permanently restricted by donor or grantor

The classification of net assets for a not-for-profit is dependent on any conditions placed on the contribution by the donor. The donor may be an individual, fund, or government granting agency. For example, a donor may leave a sum of money to a hospital for the purpose of improving its pediatric patient play area. If the donation was made for that express purpose, it is referred to as a directed contribution and is classified in the permanently restricted net assets section of the balance sheet. If that same donor also included a statement that the donation may be used for other purposes if the hospital no longer treats pediatric patients, then the donation would be classified as temporarily restricted net assets since there are conditions that may remove the restrictions.

Income Statement

The **income statement** or **statement of activities** provides detail on the types of **revenue** and expenses resulting from primary business operations and other activities. The income statement measures the financial performance of an organization during the reporting period by tracking the revenues and expenses for both operating and **nonoperating activities.** The income statement may also be referred to as a **profit and loss statement** or **statement of revenue and expenses.** The balance sheet is a report that reflects the basic accounting equation. Similarly, the income statement reports the **operating income** for an entity as displayed in figure 2.3. While the balance sheet is a report that reflects the basic accounting equation at a specific point in time, the income statement represents the revenue and expenses experienced during the reporting period.

A positive operating income is certainly desirable for a healthcare facility. Our example facility, Memorial Hospital, has an operating loss of more than $1.7 million as displayed in figure 2.4. The loss is offset somewhat by a nonoperating gain from investment income and contributions.

Operating Revenues

For healthcare organizations, revenues and expenses related to treating patients are recorded in the operating portions of the income statement. The largest source of operating revenue at Memorial Hospital is net patient service revenues. **Net patient service revenue** is the gross patient revenue or total

Figure 2.3   Operating income formula

Operating income = Operating revenue – Operating expenses

Figure 2.4   Memorial Hospital income statement

Memorial Hospital Income Statement—January 1, 2010 to December 31, 2010		
	$(000)	Reference
Operating revenues		
Net patient service revenues (net of provision for bad debts)	$24,980	a
Other operating revenues	$557	b
Total operating revenues	**$25,537**	**c = a + b**
Operating expenses		
Personnel	$16,953	d
Supplies	$2,637	e
Purchased services	$3,171	f
Professional fees	$891	g
Other	$1,608	h
Depreciation	$2,015	i
Total operating expenses	**$27,275**	**j = sum d to i**
Loss from operations	**$(1,738)**	**k = c + j**
Nonoperating revenues (expenses)		
Interest expense	$(160)	l
Investment income	$1,052	m
Total nonoperating revenues (expenses)	**$892**	**n = l + m**
Deficiency of revenues under expenses before contributions	**$(846)**	**o = k + n**
Contributions	$521	p
Decrease in net assets	**$(325)**	**q = o + p**
Net assets, beginning of the year	**$28,310**	**r**
Net assets, end of the year	**$27,985**	**s = q + r**

amount charged to patients minus any discounts that the facility may negotiate with third-party payers. For instance, if a patient were charged $10,000 for services provided by Memorial Hospital and that patient were covered by a plan that agreed to pay the hospital 65 percent of charges, then that patient would contribute $6,500 to the net patient service revenue for the year. The discount from billed charges, $3,500 in this example, is called a contractual allowance. It represents the amount of the total charge that the hospital will not collect due to a contractual arrangement with the third-party payer. The footnotes to the financial statements often list the amount of patient service revenue from major payers such as Medicare, Medicaid, and large insurance firms.

Other operating revenues may include tuition for healthcare-related educational programs, grants, or hospital gift shop or cafeteria revenue. Memorial Hospital recorded $557,000 in other operating revenues, which is a relatively small percentage of the total operating revenues for the facility (2 percent).

Operating Expenses

Operating expenses include expenses that are required to deliver care to patients or operate the facility. Personnel expenses represent the largest operating expense at Memorial Hospital. This is typical of most healthcare entities. Purchased services are portions of the facility operations that are outsourced to an outside company and not provided by employees. Some examples of purchased services may be temporary nursing staff, documentation management, and coding or information technology.

The depreciation figure found in the operating expenses portion of the income statement represents the depreciation expensed during the reporting year. Recall that the balance sheet includes the accumulated depreciation that represents all of the depreciation taken during the life of items still in use and subject to depreciation at the facility. The concepts of depreciation discussed earlier still apply, but the depreciation reported as an operating expense is only for the reporting year and reflects the impact of depreciation on the facility's operating income for the reporting period.

Nonoperating Revenues (Expenses)

Nonoperating revenues and expenses represent revenue received for activities that are not related to healthcare. Some income statements use the term **nonoperating gains and losses** instead of revenues and expenses. The most common entries in this portion of the income statement are investment revenue and expense. Many healthcare facilities have large endowments due to donations and income from previous years' operations. Those endowments are invested and the returns and expenses on those investments are recorded as nonoperating revenue and expenses. Previous period income is reinvested into the facility for not-for-profit entities and may be distributed to shareholders or owners in the case of a for-profit entity.

In our example income statement, figure 2.4, the nonoperating revenues and expenses are reported in one section of the report. They may be broken out or combined at the discretion of the staff and board of the facility. Contributions are also considered nonoperating revenues. Any gains or losses from property, building, or equipment sales would also be categorized as nonoperating revenue. In the example of Memorial Hospital, the nonoperating revenue and expenses are due to interest expense and investment income. The investment income is likely due to income earned on the investment of the hospital's endowment funds.

The classification of revenues into operating and nonoperating revenue is not always clear-cut. Assumptions and the basis for decisions regarding the classification of revenue as operating and nonoperating are often found in the footnotes to the financial statement.

Statement of Change in Net Assets or Equity Statement

The **equity statement** details the changes in the equity found on the balance sheet either year-to-date or from one year to the next. In for-profit organizations, this report is referred to as the **statement of shareholder equity.** The change in net assets may also be called the "change in unrestricted fund balance" in not-for-profit facilities. In a for-profit entity this figure would be labeled as profit or loss. The change in net assets is the overall impact of the reporting period activities on the financial position of the facility. For our example facility, the statement of change in net assets is integrated into the income statement in figure 2.4. Although this information is a required component of financial statements according to GAAP, it is often combined with the income statement in not-for-profit entities.

Statement of Cash Flow

The **statement of cash flow** reports the flow of cash into and out of an entity during the reporting period. Figures from the balance sheet and income statement are related, showing their impact on the cash position of the entity. The statement of cash flow is also used to measure the liquidity of an organization or the ability of the organization to pay its bills, meet payroll, and stay in business in the short term.

Since the majority of healthcare entities use accrual-based accounting, the balance sheet and income statement do not give a picture of the cash position of the entity. Accounts receivable is recognized as an asset on the balance sheet, but that asset may or may not be available as cash for the organization to use in the short term. Depreciation is recognized as an expense on the income statement, but the cash required to pay for the depreciating asset may have been expended in a previous period. This shift in the timing of transactions makes it difficult to assess the cash position of an organization based on the balance sheet and income statement alone. The statement of cash flow fills this void.

Cash Flow from Operating and Nonoperating Activities

The first portion of the statement of cash flow measures the cash from **operating activities** recognized during the reporting period. Figure 2.5 shows the statement of cash flow for Memorial Hospital. The largest source of incoming cash for Memorial Hospital was receipts from and on behalf of patients. This figure represents cash actually received to reimburse Memorial Hospital for patient care. This includes payments received during the reporting period for care provided in previous periods and prepayments for services that may be provided in later periods. The "Payments to suppliers and contractors" figure represents the amount actually expended to pay invoices during the reporting period. Payments to employees represent the single largest cash expense during the reporting period. The cash from operating activities netted a positive $2.24 million for Memorial Hospital.

The remaining portions of the statement of cash flow enumerate the cash from nonoperating activities, including cash from the following:

- Noncapital financing activities
- Capital and related financing activities
- Investing activities

Loan payments reduced the cash for the reporting period, while the sale of investments increased the cash. Memorial Hospital ended the year with an increase in cash and cash equivalents of $869,000. This result must be reconciled against the negative change in net assets reported on the income statement. Figure 2.6 shows the second part of the statement of cash flow that will step through that reconciliation.

Reconciliation to the Balance Sheet

Recall that the cash and cash equivalents reported on the balance sheet in figure 2.2, line a, was $932,000. That is the same figure reported as the cash at the end of the year on the statement of cash flow (figure 2.5, line q) and the starting point for the reconciliation (figure 2.6, line r). The adjustments to reconcile the operating income will show how an operating income of –$1.74 million can result from $2.24 million in net operating cash.

Figure 2.5   Memorial Hospital statement of cash flow—Part 1

Memorial Hospital Statement of Cash Flow—January 1, 2010 to December 31, 2010		
	$(000)	Reference
Cash flows from operating activities		
Receipts from and on behalf of patients	$21,856	a
Payments to suppliers and contractors	$(8,371)	b
Payments to employees	$(12,404)	c
Other receipts and payments, net	$1,159	d
Net cash provided by operating activities	$2,240	e = sum a to d
Cash flows from noncapital financing activities		
Noncapital grants and contributions	$521	f
Cash flows from capital and related financing activities		
Purchase of capital assets	$(1,212)	g
Proceeds from loans	$2,629	h
Principal paid on loans	$(4,794)	i
Interest paid on loans	$(160)	j
Net cash used by capital and related financing activities	$(3,537)	k = sum g to j
Cash flows from investing activities		
Investment fees	$(5)	l
Sales of investments	$1,650	m
Net cash provided by investing activities	$1,645	n = l + m
Net increase in cash and cash equivalents	$869	o = e + f + k + n
Cash and cash equivalents, beginning of the year	$63	p
Cash and cash equivalents, end of the year	$932	q = p + k + f + e + n

The first adjustment in figure 2.6 is for depreciation during the year. Recall that depreciation is the decrease in the value of a capital asset like an MRI machine or other equipment. The depreciation expense does not represent an actual cash transaction, so that is added back into the equation. The provision for bad debts represents an adjustment to the expected income from patient services (the first line in the income statement). Since the cash for these services was not received during the reporting period, there is no cash expense associated with that transaction, and that figure is also added back to the operating income.

Figure 2.6   Memorial Hospital statement of cash flow—Part 2

	$(000)	Reference
Reconciliation of cash and cash equivalents to the Statement of Net Assets		
Cash and cash equivalents in current assets	$932	r = a from balance sheet
Restricted cash and cash equivalents	—	s
Total cash and cash equivalents	**$932**	**t = r + s**
Reconciliation of operating income to net cash used by		
Operating loss	$(1,738)	u = k from income statement
Adjustments to reconcile operating income to net cash flows used in operating activities		
Depreciation	$2,015	v = i from income statement
Provision for bad debts	$5,174	w
(Increase) decrease in current assets		
Patient accounts receivable	$(3,428)	x
Supplies and other current assets	$818	y
Estimated third-party payer settlements	$249	z
Decrease in current liabilities		
Accounts payable and accrued expenses	$(850)	aa
Net cash provided in operating activities	**$2,240**	**bb = u + v + w + x + y + z + aa**

The next set of adjustments in the reconciliation has to do with changes in the current assets. The patient accounts receivable balance increased in value in comparison to the previous year. An increase in the value of the accounts receivable during the year should be realized as a reduction in the actual cash receipts from patients or third-party payers. The operating income should be reduced by this amount. The supplies, other current assets, and estimated **third-party payer settlements** all decreased in value in comparison to the previous year and therefore should be added back into the calculation since these two transaction types represent an increase in cash. The change in current liabilities was a decrease in the accounts payable and accrued expenses. This means that the entity expended cash to pay the liabilities and therefore this is represented as a decrease in the cash position.

The final net cash provided in operating activities for Memorial Hospital is $2.24 million. This value matches row e in Figure 2.5. This reconciliation is necessary to ensure that the balance sheet, income statement, and statement of cash flow are all in sync.

Notes to the Financial Statement

Financial statements typically include a number of notes following the four basic reports. The notes include valuable information regarding the assumptions used in compiling the information in the reports as well as detailed calculations for figures. The notes will state if the organization uses cash or accrual accounting. They may include information about depreciation, debt financing terms, and payer mix or collection rates.

The following is an example of the topics explained in the notes of hospital financial statements (State of Indiana n.d.):

- *Nature of operations*—statement of for-profit/not-for-profit status, ownership, and service area
- *Summary of significant accounting policies*—definitions of terms like cash equivalents, details on investment policy, depreciation method, charity care, handling of contributions, and malpractice costs
- *Net patient service revenue*—may include proportion of care provided to Medicare and Medicaid patients and some general description of the commercial third-party payer terms
- *Concentration of credit risk*—description of the mix of patient accounts receivable amounts and any extension of credit to patients or third-party payers
- *Investments and investment return*—categories of investments and the return, investment fees, and impact of investment return on net assets
- *Property, plant, and equipment*—property, plant, and equipment (PPE) broken out into categories such as land, improvements, buildings, and equipment; may also include useful life and accumulated depreciation
- *Long-term debt*—a description of any bond offerings by the organization, long-term lease obligations, and any restructuring of debt that may have occurred during the reporting period
- *Related party transactions*—transactions between any related foundations or other entities

The notes appended to each financial statement are organization-specific and can prove to be valuable to an understanding of the context of values reported on in the financial statement.

Summary

The four components of an entity's financial statement represent the external view of its financial health. The balance sheet is a report of the financial position of an organization as a snapshot in time. The income statement presents information about the operations of the organization. The statement of change in net assets presents changes in net assets from one period to the next. Finally, the statement of cash flow makes the connection between cash flow and the balance sheet. All four reports give a different perspective in measuring financial performance and must be analyzed together for a full understanding of the finances of an organization.

CHECK YOUR UNDERSTANDING

1. Managerial accounting focuses on financial reporting for internal audiences. (True/False)
2. The balance sheet reports the results of the operations of an organization. (True/False)
3. Depreciation is considered to be a cash transaction. (True/False)
4. The basic accounting equation states: Net Assets = Assets + Liabilities. (True/False)
5. Most healthcare facilities use cash-based accounting. (True/False)
6. Which of the following would be considered short-term assets?
    a. Cash and cash equivalents
    b. 60-month CD
    c. MRI machine
    d. 10-year loan
7. If a hospital bed costs $5,000 and has a useful life of 10 years, then the annual depreciation using the straight-line method is:
    a. $50
    b. $500
    c. $10
    d. $2,500
8. A contractual allowance is the difference between the gross charge and:
    a. The expected payment for services
    b. The cost of services
    c. The accounts receivable amount
    d. The copayment

9. Short-term liabilities are due:
   a. Within 10 years
   b. Within 5 years
   c. Within 1 year
   d. Currently
10. Which of the following expenses are considered operational?
    a. Inventory
    b. Investment fees
    c. Granted funds
    d. Investment losses

References

Hart, Leita. 2006. *Accounting Demystified*. New York: McGraw Hill.

IRS. 2011. Publication 946: How to Depreciate Property. http://www.irs.gov/pub/irs-pdf/p946.pdf.

Lane, S., E. Longstreth, and V. Nixon. 2001. *A Community Leader's Guide to Hospital Finance: Evaluating How a Hospital Gets and Spends Its Money*. Boston: The Access Project.

State of Indiana. n.d. 2009 Hospital Audited Financial Statements. http://www.in.gov/isdh/24801.htm.

Financial Performance Measurement

Learning Objectives

⇒ Explore the motivation for measuring financial performance
⇒ Calculate key financial ratios
⇒ Understand the relationships between the financial ratios
⇒ Analyze the financial position of a facility based on financial statement data

Key Terms

Asset management
Average age of plant
Capitalization ratios
Common size
Coverage ratios
Critical access hospitals (CAHs)
Current ratio
Days cash on hand
Days in patient accounts receivable
   (DPAR)
Debt performance
Debt ratio
Debt to equity ratio
Earnings before interest and taxes
   (EBIT)
Financial ratios

Fixed asset turnover
Horizontal analysis
Hospital Cost Reporting
   Information System (HCRIS)
Liquidity
Medicare Cost Report
Operating margin
Profitability
Quick ratio
Return on assets (ROA)
Return on equity (ROE)
Times interest earned (TIE) ratio
Total asset turnover (TAT) ratio
Total margin (TM)
Trend analysis
Vertical analysis

The component reports of a healthcare firm's financial statements contain valuable information that may be used to assess the firm's financial performance. The balance sheet and income statement present a picture of the financial health of an organization as a snapshot in time. The statement of cash flow and changes in net assets statement complete that picture by showing where changes occurred during the fiscal period and give insight into the cause of changes in the financial position.

The real analytic power in the financial statements can be leveraged by strategically examining how the values are related and benchmarking those values against competitor facilities. Examining trends over time can give insight for strategic planning and help the board of directors understand the performance of a facility. Comparisons to industry standards or even internal year-to-year comparisons must be performed using techniques that allow comparability among facilities or periods of time.

Common Size Financial Statements

The balance sheet and income statement are used to report the financial position of a firm to the outside world. The information contained in those reports also provides a tool for analyzing the financial success or failure of the firm. Comparisons of data elements over time or in relationship to a peer group or competitor can identify areas for improvement or areas where the firm excels. To make these comparisons, the values in the financial statements must be standardized so that comparison from year to year or facility to facility is based on a **common size.** The net income for a hospital may increase by $1 million from one year to the next, but we cannot determine if that increase is due purely to a growth in the number of patients treated or to an increase in financial performance. A common size income statement makes the year-to-year figures more comparable.

A common size analysis of the income statement requires dividing each element by the total operating revenues (Gapenski 2006, 483). Each figure is then reported as a percentage of total operating revenues. Operating revenue serves as an overall measure of the size of the entity's operating activities. Dividing each figure by the operating revenue allows the comparison of organizations of different sizes. For instance, comparing the operating expenses for a 200-bed hospital and a 500-bed hospital would not be a fair comparison. The 500-bed hospital likely treats significantly more patients and would therefore incur more operating expenses. A common size income statement would standardize the operating expense as a percentage of the operating revenue and allow an apples-to-apples comparison of the two hospitals.

In a common size analysis of the balance sheet, each element is divided by the total assets. Each figure reported is a percentage of the total assets. Total assets is a measure of the overall size of an entity that is appropriate for use in standardizing the balance sheet. If a physician practice recently expanded, then the value of the net assets for the current year will not be comparable to that of the previous year. The common size balance sheet normalizes for the change in the overall size of the practice and may be used to compare the performance between the two years.

The common size statements described here are sometimes referred to as vertical common size. Each column of data is divided by the same figure. Columns of data are vertical and therefore the term **vertical analysis** is used to describe this type of analysis.

Figure 3.1 shows the balance sheet reported and common size values for Regional Hospital for 2009 and 2008. The first two columns represent the reported figures and the last two columns represent the reported figures divided by the total assets, or $13,611,266 for 2009 and $12,149,169 for 2008.

Figure 3.1   Regional Hospital balance sheet

	Reported Values ($)		Common Size (%)	
	2009	2008	2009	2008
Assets				
Current assets				
Cash and cash equivalents	3,199,568	1,739,826	23.5	14.3
Patient accounts receivable, net of estimated uncollectibles of $1,880,369 and $1,795,057 in 2009 and 2008, respectively	3,534,735	2,770,972	26.0	22.8
Estimated third-party settlements	—	111,971	0.0	0.9
Supplies and other current assets	806,432	866,696	5.9	7.1
Total current assets	7,540,735	5,489,465	55.4	45.2
Noncurrent cash				
Restricted by contributors and grantors	809,491	640,080	5.9	5.3
Total noncurrent cash and investments	809,491	640,080	5.9	5.3
Capital assets				
Land and construction in progress	884,936	713,688	6.5	5.9
Depreciable capital assets, net	4,266,520	5,161,352	31.3	42.5
Total capital assets	5,151,456	5,875,040	37.8	48.4
Other assets	109,584	144,584	0.8	1.2
Total assets	**13,611,266**	**12,149,169**	**100.0**	**100.0**

(continued)

Figure 3.1   Regional Hospital balance sheet *(continued)*

	Reported Values ($)		Common Size (%)	
	2009	2008	2009	2008
Liabilities				
Current liabilities				
Current maturities of capital leases	288,305	386,894	2.1	3.2
Accounts payable and accrued expenses	564,458	397,412	4.1	3.3
Accrued salaries and related liabilities	913,372	1,058,539	6.7	8.7
Estimated third-party settlements	688,000	—	5.1	0.0
Other current liabilities	201,331	133,492	1.5	1.1
Total current liabilities	2,655,466	1,976,337	19.5	16.3
Long-term liabilities				
Capital leases	470,937	670,689	3.5	5.5
Other long-term liabilities	99,167	134,167	0.7	1.1
Total long-term liabilities	570,104	804,856	4.2	6.6
Total liabilities	**3,225,570**	**2,781,193**	**23.7**	**22.9**
Net assets				
Unrestricted	5,273,575	4,038,876	38.7	33.2
Invested in capital assets, net of related debt	4,293,047	4,683,290	31.5	38.5
Restricted				
Expendable for capital acquisitions	740,539	577,536	5.4	4.8
Expendable for specific op. activities	78,535	68,274	0.6	0.6
Total net assets	**10,385,696**	**9,367,976**	**76.3**	**77.1**
Total liabilities and net assets	**13,611,266**	**12,149,169**	**100.0**	**100.0**

Source: The Indiana State Department of Health (ISDH) requires hospitals operating in the state to submit a copy of their audited financial statements on an annual basis. The statements are posted on the website (http://www.in.gov/isdh). The hospital's name was changed for this publication.

Notice that the balance sheet follows the basic accounting equation Assets = Net Assets + Liabilities. The common size percentages allow a comparison between the 2008 and 2009 performance for Regional Hospital even though the total assets grew during the same period by nearly $1.5 million or 12 percent.

The mix of assets at Regional Hospital changed significantly from 2008 to 2009. In 2008, current assets made up 45.2 percent and capital assets made up

48.4 percent of total assets. In 2009, 55.4 percent of the total assets were current and 37.8 percent were in the capital category. The increase in total assets was due to the combination of cash increasing from $1.74 million in 2008 to $3.20 million in 2009 and accounts receivable increasing from $2.77 million in 2008 to $3.53 million in 2009. These two indicators are positive and show that the cash position of the facility is improving year over year even after adjusting for the increase in total assets. The increase in total assets must be due to a decrease in total liabilities or an increase in the net assets per the basic accounting equation. Further analysis of the income statement will show the root cause of this shift.

The common size income statement for Regional Hospital appears in figure 3.2. The common size percentages are the values divided by the operating revenue. For 2008, the denominator for the vertical common size percentage is $20,148,474; for 2009, the denominator for the vertical common size percentage is $20,550,695. The common size percentages are presented in the last two columns of figure 3.2.

Regional Hospital experienced a significant increase in net assets between 2008 and 2009. The common size income statement may be used to investigate the factors that contributed to that increase. The net patient service revenue increased from 2008 to 2009, but the common size percentages show that increase was minor when standardized by the operating revenue. The most significant changes appear in salary and benefits and other nonoperating revenue (expense). The decrease in salary and benefits was accompanied by an increase in professional fees. This may be indicative of the outsourcing of some functions. An explanation of this change is likely in the notes to the Regional Hospital financial statements.

The strength of common size analysis is that changes in the mix of liabilities, assets, and net assets in the balance sheet may be identified quickly. In the case of Regional Hospital, there is little change in the total liabilities, but the mix of liabilities changed significantly from 2008 to 2009. Current liabilities increased while long-term liabilities decreased. This could be due to timing. Recall that current or short-term liabilities are due within 12 months, while long-term liabilities are obligations that have a due date of more than 12 months after the reporting period. This may be illustrated by comparing the capital lease long-term liabilities for 2008 and 2009. If no new equipment was leased during 2008, then the outstanding balance on the leases in place would have decreased as the end of the lease neared. This trend may be identified quickly using the common size percentages.

Figure 3.2   Regional Hospital income statement

	Reported Values ($)		Common Size (%)	
	2009	2008	2009	2008
Operating revenue				
Net patient service revenue	19,879,358	19,378,966	96.7	96.2
Other	671,337	769,508	3.3	3.8
Total operating revenue	20,550,695	20,148,474	100.0	100.0
Operating expenses				
Salaries and benefits	10,936,559	11,536,019	53.2	57.3
Medical professional fees	737,359	715,652	3.6	3.6
Other professional fees	1,934,956	1,694,130	9.4	8.4
Supplies and drugs	3,021,130	2,960,692	14.7	14.7
Rent	144,644	177,666	0.7	0.9
Insurance	298,533	280,873	1.5	1.4
Depreciation and amortization	1,335,081	1,243,393	6.5	6.2
Other	1,280,605	1,359,251	6.2	6.7
Total operating expenses	19,688,867	19,967,676	95.8	99.1
Operating income	861,828	180,798	4.2	0.9
Nonoperating revenue (expense)				
Investment income	66,778	46,935	0.3	0.2
Interest expense	−42,184	−48,036	−0.2	−0.2
Other	131,298	−150,828	0.6	−0.7
Total nonoperating revenue (expense)	155,892	−151,929	0.8	−0.8
Change in net assets	1,017,720	28,869	5.0	0.1
Net assets, beginning of the year	**9,367,976**	**9,339,107**	45.6	46.4
Net assets, end of the year	**10,385,696**	**9,367,976**	50.5	46.5

Source: The Indiana State Department of Health (ISDH) requires hospitals operating in the state to submit a copy of their audited financial statements on an annual basis. The statements are posted on the website (http://www.in.gov/isdh). The hospital's name was changed for this publication.

On the income statement, common size analysis shows changes in the mix of revenue and expenses. Regional Hospital experienced an increase in net income. By using the common-size analysis, the source of that shift can be tracked to changes in expenses. Operating expenses were 99.1 percent of operating revenue in 2008 and 95.8 percent of operating revenue in 2009. A decrease in the salary and benefit expense can be identified as the key driver of the expense decrease. Note that salary and benefits represented 57.3 percent of operating revenue in 2008 and 53.2 percent of operating revenue in 2009.

One of the weaknesses of common size analysis is that changes in the standardizing factor are not measured. In the balance sheet, we cannot readily see the change in assets from year to year. In the income statement, the change in operating revenue is not calculated. It is useful to combine common size analysis with other financial statement analysis strategies such as trend analysis.

Trend Analysis

Trend analysis is another tool that transforms the figures on the financial statements into statistics that may be used to measure performance for the same facility over the course of time. The percentage change for each data element is presented to assist in understanding where the most significant shifts in values occur. Trend analysis is sometimes referred to as **horizontal analysis.** The percentage change is calculated across the rows of the statement. Rows of data are horizontal in nature, hence the term horizontal analysis.

In calculating a percentage change, it is important to define the base or denominator in the calculation. By convention, the percentage change is calculated as the difference between the new value and the old value, divided by the old value. In the sample balance sheet displayed in figure 3.3, the percentage change is calculated as follows:

$$\text{Percentage change 2008 to 2009} = \frac{(2009 \text{ value} - 2008 \text{ value})}{2008 \text{ value}}$$

Our previous common size analysis of this balance sheet did not include a measurement of the growth in total assets, but that figure was computed and displayed in the trend analysis report. The 12 percent growth in total assets is driven by both the 10.9 percent increase in net assets and a 16 percent growth in liabilities.

The growth in current assets as a percentage of total assets was identified in reviewing the common size percentages. In the trend report, we can see that this was due to an 83.9 percent increase in cash and cash equivalents. A significant year-over-year increase in unrestricted net assets (30.6 percent), accounts payable (42 percent), and current liabilities due to third-party settlements (100 percent) are all presented clearly in the trend report.

Figure 3.3   Regional Hospital balance sheet

| | Reported Values ($) | | Trend |
	2009	2008	(% change)
Assets			
Current assets			
Cash and cash equivalents	3,199,568	1,739,826	83.9
Patient accounts receivable, net of estimated uncollectibles of $1,880,369 and $1,795,057 in 2009 and 2008, respectively	3,534,735	2,770,972	27.6
Estimated third-party settlements	—	111,971	−100.0
Supplies and other current assets	806,432	866,696	−7.0
Total current assets	7,540,735	5,489,465	37.4
Noncurrent cash			
Restricted by contributors and grantors	809,491	640,080	26.5
Total noncurrent cash and investments	809,491	640,080	26.5
Capital assets			
Land and construction in progress	884,936	713,688	24.0
Depreciable capital assets, net	4,266,520	5,161,352	−17.3
Total capital assets	5,151,456	5,875,040	−12.3
Other assets	109,584	144,584	−24.2
Total assets	**13,611,266**	**12,149,169**	**12.0**
Liabilities			
Current liabilities			
Current maturities of capital leases	288,305	386,894	−25.5
Accounts payable and accrued expenses	564,458	397,412	42.0
Accrued salaries and related liabilities	913,372	1,058,539	−13.7
Estimated third-party settlements	688,000	—	100.0
Other current liabilities	201,331	133,492	50.8
Total current liabilities	2,655,466	1,976,337	34.4
Long-term liabilities			
Capital leases	470,937	670,689	−29.8
Other long-term liabilities	99,167	134,167	−26.1
Total long-term liabilities	570,104	804,856	−29.2
Total liabilities	**3,225,570**	**2,781,193**	**16.0**

Figure 3.3   Regional Hospital balance sheet *(continued)*

	Reported Values ($)		Trend
	2009	2008	(% change)
Net assets			
Unrestricted	5,273,575	4,038,876	30.6
Invested in capital assets, net of related debt	4,293,047	4,683,290	−8.3
Restricted			
Expendable for capital acquisitions	740,539	577,536	28.2
Expendable for specific op. activities	78,535	68,274	15.0
Total net assets	**10,385,696**	**9,367,976**	**10.9**
Total liabilities and net assets	**13,611,266**	**12,149,169**	**12.0**

Source: The Indiana State Department of Health (ISDH) requires hospitals operating in the state to submit a copy of their audited financial statements on an annual basis. The statements are posted on the website (http://www.in.gov/isdh). The hospital's name was changed for this publication.

The trend analysis of the income statement is presented in figure 3.4. The 10.9 percent increase in net assets noted in the trend analysis of the balance sheet for Regional Hospital was driven by a 2.6 percent increase in net patient service revenue and a 1.4 percent decrease in total operating expenses from 2008 to 2009. The reduction in operating expenses can be traced directly to a 5.2 percent decrease in salaries and benefits, since that category makes up over one-half of the operating expenses.

Notice that when a value changes from positive to negative or vice versa, the trend percentage is listed as N/A or not applicable. For example, the other non-operating revenue (expense) and the total nonoperating revenue (expense) both change from negative values in 2008 to positive values in 2009. The traditional calculation for percentage change would yield a negative number for both of these value, but clearly there was an increase from 2008 to 2009. The calculated values are replaced with N/A to avoid any confusion for the reader of the trend analysis.

A common size presentation of the cash flow statement is not typically presented because it is difficult to choose an appropriate denominator for the standardization. A trend analysis of the cash flow is useful in showing year-over-year changes in the components. The 2008 and 2009 cash flow statement for Regional Hospital is presented in figure 3.5.

Recall that one of the drivers in the change in total assets was growth in cash and cash equivalents. From the trend analysis of the cash flow statement, it appears that this was not due to an increase in cash received from patients or

Figure 3.4   Regional Hospital income statement

	Reported Values ($)		Trend
	2009	2008	(% change)
Operating revenue			
Net patient service revenue	19,879,358	19,378,966	2.6
Other	671,337	769,508	−12.8
Total operating revenue	20,550,695	20,148,474	2.0
Operating expenses			
Salaries and benefits	10,936,559	11,536,019	−5.2
Medical professional fees	737,359	715,652	3.0
Other professional fees	1,934,956	1,694,130	14.2
Supplies and drugs	3,021,130	2,960,692	2.0
Rent	144,644	177,666	−18.6
Insurance	298,533	280,873	6.3
Depreciation and amortization	1,335,081	1,243,393	7.4
Other	1,280,605	1,359,251	−5.8
Total operating expenses	19,688,867	19,967,676	−1.4
Operating income	861,828	180,798	376.7
Nonoperating revenue (expense)			
Investment income	66,778	46,935	42.3
Interest expense	−42,184	−48,036	−12.2
Other	131,298	−150,828	−187.1
Total nonoperating revenue (expense)	155,892	−151,929	−202.6
Change in net assets	1,017,720	28,869	3425.3
Net assets, beginning of the year	**9,367,976**	**9,339,107**	0.3
Net assets, end of the year	**10,385,696**	**9,367,976**	10.9

Source: The Indiana State Department of Health (ISDH) requires hospitals operating in the state to submit a copy of their audited financial statements on an annual basis. The statements are posted on the website (http://www.in.gov/isdh). The hospital's name was changed for this publication.

third-party payers. Instead, it was due primarily to reductions in salaries and cash payments to vendors for goods and services.

The 376.7 percent change in operating income is due to a decrease in the provision for bad debt and a large increase in estimated third-party settlements. This is important information for future budgeting and planning at Regional Hospital. Third-party settlements are difficult to predict and are typically due

Figure 3.5 Regional Hospital cash flow statement

	Reported Values ($)		Trend
	2009	**2008**	**(% change)**
Operating activities			
Cash received from patients and third-party payers	19,915,566	20,363,530	−2.2
Cash paid to employees for salaries and benefits	(11,081,726)	(11,349,910)	−2.4
Cash paid to vendors for goods and services	(7,166,776)	(7,724,464)	−7.2
Other operating receipts, net	671,212	1,015,964	−33.9
Net cash from operating activities	2,338,276	2,305,120	1.4
Capital and related financing activities			
Acquisition and construction of capital assets	(477,992)	(401,572)	19.0
Proceeds from sale of capital assets	3,980	—	N/A
Interest paid on long-term debt	(42,184)	(48,036)	−12.2
Payments on line of credit	—	(150,000)	N/A
Proceeds on long-term debt	—	125,000	N/A
Principal payments on long-term debt	(391,003)	(352,225)	11.0
Net cash from capital and related financing activities	(907,199)	(826,833)	9.7
Investing activities			
Investment and other nonoperating income	198,076	(103,893)	N/A
Net cash from investing activities	198,076	(103,893)	N/A
Net change in cash and cash equivalents	1,629,153	1,374,394	18.5
Cash and cash equivalents, beginning of year	2,379,906	1,005,512	136.7
Cash and cash equivalents, end of year	4,009,059	2,379,906	68.5
Reconciliation of cash and cash equivalents to the balance sheets			
Cash and cash equivalents			
In current assets	3,199,568	1,739,826	83.9
In noncurrent cash and investments	809,491	640,080	26.5
Total cash and cash equivalents	4,009,059	2,379,906	68.5
Reconciliation of operating loss to net cash from operating activities			
Operating income	861,828	180,798	376.7

(continued)

Figure 3.5   Regional Hospital cash flow statement *(continued)*

	Reported Values		Trend
	2009	2008	(% change)
Adjustments to reconcile operating income to net cash from operating activities			
Depreciation and amortization	1,335,081	1,243,393	7.4
(Gain) loss on disposal of capital assets	(125)	246,456	N/A
Provision for bad debt	1,281,107	1,402,017	−8.6
Changes in assets and liabilities			
Patient accounts receivable	(2,044,870)	(717,771)	184.9
Estimated third-party settlements	799,971	300,318	166.4
Supplies and other current assets	60,264	(221,648)	N/A
Other assets	(9,698)	7,760	N/A
Accounts payable and accrued expenses	167,046	(364,752)	N/A
Other current liabilities	67,839	77,440	−12.4
Accrued salaries and related liabilities	(145,167)	186,109	N/A
Other long-term liabilities	(35,000)	(35,000)	0.0
Net cash flows from operating activities	2,338,276	2,305,120	1.4

Source: The Indiana State Department of Health (ISDH) requires hospitals operating in the state to submit a copy of their audited financial statements on an annual basis. The statements are posted on the website (http://www.in.gov/isdh). The hospital's name was changed for this publication.

to unusual events such as a malpractice claim or a settlement with a third-party payer that was not paying according to their contract.

A trend analysis or horizontal analysis of the financial statements can highlight significant shifts in financial statistics from year to year. One weakness of trend analysis is that it does not allow for the direct comparison of two facilities. Common size analysis is better suited for that purpose. The strength of trend analysis is that the reported statistics with the largest relative changes are readily identified for further review.

Ratio Analysis

Financial ratios are used to analyze the relationships between data elements found on the financial statements. Common size and trend analysis are both special cases of ratio analysis. The ratios in both techniques are formulated by dividing the values on the financial statements by a consistent value either horizontally or vertically to allow a standardized comparison within the statement. Financial ratios that allow standardized comparisons across the balance sheet, income statement, and cash flow statement are used to understand the relationship between the figures and how changes impact the overall financial performance of an organization.

Financial ratios are typically segmented into categories that represent the aspect of financial performance that is measured. The number of categories and specific ratios used are somewhat dependent on the type of organization being assessed. The categories of ratios that apply to the healthcare setting are:

1. **Profitability** ratios
2. **Liquidity** ratios
3. **Debt performance** ratios
4. **Asset management** ratios

The formula for calculating the ratio, the financial statement report where the ratio components may be located, the interpretation of the value, and an example using the Regional Hospital financial statements is presented in the following sections for the most common ratios in each of these categories.

Profitability Ratios

Profitability is a standard measure of the overall performance of any type of firm. Even though most healthcare providers are not-for-profit entities, profitability is critically important. In the January 7, 1998, issue of the *Wall Street Journal*, Sister Irene Kraus, former president of the Daughters of Charity National Health System, famously stated, "No margin, no mission" (Langley 1998). Although this quote was much maligned at the time and the Daughters of Charity were referred to as the "Daughters of Currency" in the press, Sister Kraus made an excellent point. Profit or a positive net income is essential to allow the acquisition of new technology and the replacement of equipment that has reached the end of its useful life as much for a not-for-profit facility as a for-profit one. Her assertion was that executive leadership at not-for-profit hospitals should not be ashamed of taking in more revenue than expenses.

Each of the following profitability ratios follows the same pattern. The numerator is a measure of profit or net income. The denominator is a measure of the size of the business. This allows the level of profitability to be compared across providers or across years for a particular provider.

Total Margin

$$\text{Total Margin} = \frac{\text{Net Income}}{\text{Total Revenues}}$$

Net income and total revenues are both located on the income statement. Net income may also be referred to as the change in net assets. The total revenues in this ratio represent both the operating and nonoperating revenues. The **total margin** (TM) is a measurement of the overall profitability of a firm. The TM may be interpreted as the proportion of the revenue that is retained by the facility. The TM is typically reported as a percentage. A high value is better for this ratio. The TMs for Regional Hospital for 2008 and 2009 are as follows:

$$2008 \text{ Total Margin} = \frac{28,869}{20,148,474 - 151,929} \times 100 = 0.1\%$$

$$2009 \text{ Total Margin} = \frac{1,017,720}{20,550,695 - 155,892} \times 100 = 4.9\%$$

Return on Assets

$$\text{Return on Assets} = \frac{\text{Net Income}}{\text{Total Assets}}$$

Return on assets (ROA) combines figures from the income statement and balance sheet. Net income may be found on the income statement. The value of total assets is located on the balance sheet. The ROA is also an overall measurement of financial performance. The ROA is a measurement of how productively the facility is using its assets (Gapenski 2006, 472). The ratio measures the net income produced by a dollar of total assets. A higher value is indicative of a better-performing facility. The ROA is reported as a percentage. The ROAs for Regional Hospital for 2008 and 2009 are as follows:

$$2008 \text{ Return on Assets} = \frac{28,869}{12,149,169} \times 100 = 0.2\%$$

$$2009 \text{ Return on Assets} = \frac{1,017,720}{13,611,266} \times 100 = 7.5\%$$

Return on Equity

$$\text{Return on Equity} = \frac{\text{Net Income}}{\text{Total Equity}}$$

Net income may be found on the income statement. The value of total equity is located on the balance sheet. Recall that equity is another term for net assets. Equity is a term typically used in the for-profit setting. The **return on equity** (ROE) is also an overall measurement of financial performance. The ROE is a measurement of how well a not-for-profit facility is using its capital (Gapenski 2006, 472.). A higher value is indicative of a better-performing facility. The ROE is reported as a percentage. The ROEs for Regional Hospital for 2008 and 2009 are as follows:

$$2008 \text{ Return on Equity} = \frac{28,869}{9,367,976} \times 100 = 0.3\%$$

$$2009 \text{ Return on Equity} = \frac{1,017,720}{10,385,696} \times 100 = 9.8\%$$

Operating Margin

$$\text{Operating Margin} = \frac{\text{Operating Income}}{\text{Operating Revenues}}$$

All of the components of the **operating margin** (OM) may be found on the income statement. The OM measures the level of profitability experienced in a firm's operations. For a healthcare entity, *operations* is defined as primarily patient care. The OM may be interpreted as the percentage of each dollar in operating revenue that is retained by the facility. A higher value is indicative of a better-performing facility. The OM is reported as a percentage. The OMs for Regional Hospital for 2008 and 2009 are as follows:

$$2008 \text{ Operating Margin} = \frac{180,798}{20,148,474} \times 100 = 0.9\%$$

$$2009 \text{ Operating Margin} = \frac{861,828}{20,550,695} \times 100 = 4.2\%$$

Liquidity Ratios

Liquidity ratios measure the ability of a company to meet its current obligations or debt. Liquidity ratios come primarily from balance sheet figures. Therefore, they measure the ability of a firm to pay its short-term debt at a particular point in time. These ratios may be used to judge the creditworthiness of a firm for short-term loans.

The numerator in liquidity ratios is current assets or some subset of current assets. The denominator is a size measurement of the facility's liabilities.

Current Ratio

$$\text{Current Ratio} = \frac{\text{Total Current Assets}}{\text{Total Current Liabilities}}$$

The values required to calculate the **current ratio** (CR) are all found on the balance sheet. The CR measures the short-term or current assets that are available to cover short-term liabilities. If the CR value is larger than 1, then the facility has enough readily available assets to cover its short-term liabilities. A higher value is better in most cases. A value that is too high compared to norms for the healthcare industry may indicate that a facility is not efficiently using its assets. The CR is typically reported as a decimal ratio and not a percentage. The CRs for Regional Hospital for 2008 and 2009 are as follows:

$$2008 \text{ Current Ratio} = \frac{5,489,465}{1,976,337} = 2.78$$

$$2009 \text{ Current Ratio} = \frac{7,540,735}{2,655,466} = 2.84$$

Quick Ratio

$$\text{Quick Ratio} =$$

$$\frac{\text{Cash \& Cash Equivalents} + \text{Short–Term Investments} + \text{Accounts Receivable}}{\text{Total Current Liabilities}}$$

The components of the **quick ratio** (QR) may be found on the balance sheet. The interpretation of the QR is basically the same as for the CR. The difference between the two is that the QR is a more conservative measure of liquidity. The numerator is stricter in that only the most quickly accessible current assets are included. Items such as supplies and inventory that are more difficult to convert to cash are not included. Therefore, the QR is always less than or equal to the CR. The QR is called the acid test in some texts. As with the CR, a higher QR value indicates a stronger ability to meet short-term liabilities. A value extremely high compared to industry norms may indicate an inefficient use of assets. The QR is reported as a decimal and not a percentage. The QRs for Regional Hospital for 2008 and 2009 are as follows:

$$2008 \text{ Quick Ratio} = \frac{1,739,826 + 2,770,972 + 111,971}{1,976,337} = 2.34$$

$$2009 \text{ Quick Ratio} = \frac{3,199,568 + 3,534,735}{2,655,466} = 2.54$$

Note: The estimated third-party settlements figure listed in the current assets portion of the 2008 balance sheet should be considered an additional accounts receivable figure and is therefore included in the numerator of the quick ratio.

Days Cash on Hand

$$\text{Days Cash on Hand} = \frac{\text{Unrestricted Cash \& Cash Equivalents}}{(\text{Operating Expense} - \text{Depreciation and Amortization})/\text{Number of Days in Period}}$$

Days cash on hand (DCOH) combines figures from the balance sheet and income statement. Unrestricted cash and cash equivalents are reported on the balance sheet. The operating expense and depreciation figures are listed on the income statement. If the financial statements are based on a full year, then the number of days in the period is 365. The denominator in the DCOH ratio is the daily cash expense for operating the facility. Depreciation and amortization are excluded from the expense because they are not cash expenses. DCOH may be interpreted as the number of days the facility could stay in operation if it stopped collecting cash. It measures the adequacy of the firm's cash reserves. A higher value is generally better, as long as the value is not extremely high compared to industry norms. A value that is too high could be indicative of a facility that is not investing its cash in improving and updating services. The DCOH is reported in days. The DCOH values for Regional Hospital for 2008 and 2009 are as follows:

$$2008 \text{ Days Cash on Hand} = \frac{1,739,826}{(19,647,676 - 1,243,393)/365}$$

$$= \frac{1,739,826}{50,423} = 34.5 \text{ days}$$

$$2009 \text{ Days Cash on Hand} = \frac{3,199,568}{(19,688,867 - 1,335,081)/365}$$

$$= \frac{3,199,568}{50,284} = 63.6 \text{ days}$$

Note: The order of operation in the calculation of DCOH requires careful attention. Calculating the denominator first and then inserting that value in the ratio formula will help avoid any errors.

Debt Performance Ratios

Debt performance ratios are used to judge the creditworthiness of a firm. Favorable values for debt performance ratios indicate that a facility is less likely to default on a loan. The ratios presented in this section are used to determine bond ratings and other factors that can impact the cost for a facility to access capital.

Two types of debt ratios are presented here. The first are **capitalization ratios** that depend on balance sheet data and measure the proportion of the assets that were funded by debt. The second are **coverage ratios** that depend on income statement data. They measure the ability of the facility to pay debt based on its current level of income (Gapenski 2006, 474).

Debt Ratio

$$\text{Debt Ratio} = \frac{\text{Total Liabilities}}{\text{Total Assets}}$$

The components of the **debt ratio** (DR) are found on the balance sheet. The DR is a comparison of a facility's total debt to its total assets. It is used to determine how heavily in debt or leveraged a firm is at the time of the financial reporting. A lower value means that a facility has the capacity to take on more debt; a high value may mean that the facility will have difficulty paying off its debt. Lending institutions review the DR as one measure of an organization's creditworthiness. The DR is reported as a percentage. The DR values for Regional Hospital for 2008 and 2009 are as follows:

$$2008 \,\text{Debt Ratio} = \frac{2,781,193}{9,367,976} = 29.7\%$$

$$2009 \,\text{Debt Ratio} = \frac{3,225,570}{10,385,696} = 31.0\%$$

Debt to Equity Ratio

$$\text{Debt to Equity Ratio} = \frac{\text{Total Liabilities}}{\text{Total Equity}}$$

The two figures required to calculate the **debt to equity ratio** (DER), total liabilities and total equity, are both found on the balance sheet. Total equity may be called total net assets on not-for-profit entity balance sheets. In for-profit firms, the DER measures the investment in the firm by lenders and suppliers versus the investment by shareholders. In not-for-profit facilities, the DER measures the amount of debt compared to the amount collected via charitable contributions and grants. A low DER implies that a facility has the capacity to take on more debt if needed. A high value may cause creditors to avoid lending capital to the firm. The DER is reported as a percentage. The DER values for Regional Hospital are as follows:

$$2008 \text{ Debt to Equity Ratio} = \frac{2,781,193}{9,367,976} \times 100 = 29.7\%$$

$$2009 \text{ Debt to Equity Ratio} = \frac{3,225,570}{10,385,696} \times 100 = 31.1\%$$

Times Interest Earned Ratio

$$\text{Times Interest Earned} = \frac{\text{Earnings Before Interest and Taxes (EBIT)}}{\text{Interest Expense}}$$

Earnings before interest and taxes (EBIT) is the net income plus interest or taxes paid during the year. Net income, taxes, and interest expense all appear on the income statement. For not-for-profit entities, the taxes would be entered into the formula as zero. The **times interest earned** (TIE) **ratio** measures the amount of income that is available to pay interest on debt (Gapenski 2006, 474). A larger value is desirable for this ratio. The TIE ratio should be compared to industry norms to judge performance. The TIE is reported as a decimal. The TIE values for Regional Hospital for 2008 and 2009 are as follows:

$$2008 \text{ Times Interest Earned} = \frac{28,869 + 48,036}{48,036} = 1.6 \text{ times}$$

$$2009 \text{ Times Interest Earned} = \frac{1,017,700 + 42,184}{42,184} = 25.1 \text{ times}$$

Note: The interest expense is reported as a negative value on the Regional Hospital income statement. It is common for the nonoperating revenues and expenses to be reported in a combined section of the income statement. When values are reported in a combined section, the sign on the expense items is negative. The sign should be switched to positive for the purposes of calculating the TIE ratio.

Asset Management Ratios

Asset management ratios are also known as activity ratios. These ratios measure how effective a facility is in utilizing its assets to improve the facility's financial health. The denominator in these ratios is typically the total or net fixed assets. The numerator is a measurement of the size of the business by either revenues or level of accounts receivable. The exception to this pattern is the average age of plant. That ratio measures the age of the facility's fixed assets to assess the need for replacement.

Fixed Asset Turnover

$$\text{Fixed Asset Turnover} = \frac{\text{Total Operating Revenues}}{\text{Net Fixed Assets}}$$

The total operating revenues are reported on the income statement. The value for net fixed assets is found on the balance sheet. Net fixed assets may be titled as net capital assets or net plant and equipment (Zelman et al. 2009). **Fixed asset turnover** (FAT) measures the amount of revenue produced by each dollar of fixed assets or property and equipment. The denominator is the net fixed assets or the value of the assets after depreciation. A large value indicates more efficient use of fixed assets. FAT is reported as a decimal value. The FAT ratios for Regional Hospital for 2008 and 2009 are as follows:

$$2008 \text{ Fixed Asset Turnover} = \frac{20,148,474}{5,875,040} = 3.4$$

$$2009 \text{ Fixed Asset Turnover} = \frac{20,550,695}{5,151,456} = 4.0$$

Total Asset Turnover

$$\text{Total Asset Turnover} = \frac{\text{Total Operating Revenues}}{\text{Total Assets}}$$

Total operating revenues are reported on the income statement and total assets may be found on the balance sheet. **Total asset turnover** (TAT) is used to measure the turnover or utilization of a facility's assets (Gapenski 2006, 478). Because the denominator for TAT is total assets, TAT cannot be a smaller value than FAT for the same financial reporting period. A higher value indicates that a facility is efficiently using its assets to produce revenue. A low value may identify an issue with a particular type of asset. For instance, a large amount of inventory (pharmacy or supplies) may yield a TAT lower than industry norms.

The TAT is reported as a decimal. The TATs for Regional Hospital in 2008 and 2009 are as follows:

$$2008 \text{ Total Asset Turnover} = \frac{20,148,474}{12,149,169} = 1.7$$

$$2009 \text{ Total Asset Turnover} = \frac{20,550,695}{13,611,266} = 1.5$$

Days in Patient Accounts Receivable

Days in Patient Accounts Receivable =

$$\frac{\text{Net Patient Accounts Receivable}}{\text{Net Patient Service Revenue/Number of days in period}}$$

Net patient accounts receivable is reported on the balance sheet. Net patient service revenue is reported on the income statement. **Days in patient accounts receivable** (DPAR) is sometimes categorized as a liquidity ratio and may be referred to as days in receivables, average collection period, and days' sales outstanding (Gapenski 2006, 478). DPAR measures the average number of days that the facility takes to collect for services provided to patients. A lower number for DPAR indicates that the facility is collecting cash for services rendered more quickly. A DPAR that is significantly lower than industry norms may indicate that the facility is very efficient in collecting payments or that the volume of patient services is decreasing over time. DPAR is reported in days. The values for DPAR for Regional Hospital in 2008 and 2009 are as follows:

$$2008 \text{ Days in Patient Accounts Receivable} = \frac{2,770,972}{19,378,966/365}$$

$$= \frac{2,770,972}{53,093} = 52.2 \text{ days}$$

$$2009 \text{ Days in Patient Accounts Receivable} = \frac{3,534,735}{19,879,358/365}$$

$$= \frac{3,534,735}{54,464} = 64.9 \text{ days}$$

Note: The order of operation in the calculation of DPAR requires careful attention. Calculation of the denominator first and then inserting that value in the ratio formula will help avoid any errors.

Average Age of Plant

$$\text{Average Age of Plant} = \frac{\text{Accumulated Depreciation}}{\text{Depreciation Expense}}$$

Accumulated depreciation is typically located on the balance sheet but may be presented in the notes to the financial statement. Accumulated depreciation is the amount of depreciation taken from the time that capital items still in service were purchased. Depreciation expense may be found on the income statement. The **average age of plant** (AAP) is an estimate of the number of years that capital items have been depreciated. A large value for AAP indicates that the facility should be preparing for replacement of equipment that is nearing the end of its useful life. AAP is reported in years.

The calculation of AAP for Regional Hospital requires the value of accumulated depreciation as reported in the notes to the financial statement. The relevant note appears in figure 3.6.

$$2008 \text{ Average Age of Plant} = \frac{12.5}{1.2} = 10.4 \text{ years}$$

$$2009 \text{ Average Age of Plant} = \frac{13.8}{1.3} = 10.6 \text{ years}$$

Figure 3.6   Capital assets and debt administration

Capital Assets

As of September 30, 2009 and 2008, the Hospital had $5.1 million invested in capital assets. Capital assets are comprised of the following as of September 30, 2009 and 2008.

	2009 ($ millions)	2008 ($ millions)
Land	0.2	0.2
Land improvements	0.3	0.3
Buildings	7.4	7.4
Equipment	10.3	10.0
Construction in process	0.7	0.5
Total	18.9	18.4
Less accumulated depreciation	13.8	12.5
Net capital assets	5.1	5.9

Note: Changes in capital assets are reflected in the notes to the financial statements.

Sources of Industry Standard Data

A complete assessment of a facility's performance should include comparisons to industry norms. For hospitals, the comparative data may be calculated using **Medicare Cost Reports.** Each hospital participating in Medicare must submit a cost report on an annual basis. Cost reports are stored in the **Hospital Cost Reporting Information System** (HCRIS) and may be downloaded from the CMS website free of charge. Worksheet G of the cost report includes information found on the balance sheet. Worksheet G-3 includes information found on the income statement. There is no cash flow statement included in the cost report worksheets. The contents of Worksheets G and G-3 may be found in Appendix 3.2.

The link to download Medicare Cost Report data is http://www.cms.gov/CostReports/02_HospitalCostReport.asp#TopOfPage. The data are updated on a quarterly basis and may be analyzed using a database program or SAS. The files are too large to analyze using traditional spreadsheet programs. A number of maps from the various cost report worksheets to financial ratios appear in the healthcare finance literature (Schuhmann 2008; Pink et al. 2005).

The Flex Monitoring Team (FMT), a consortium of the Universities of Minnesota, Southern Maine, and North Carolina, was formed to monitor the performance of **critical access hospitals** (CAHs). CAHs are paid for services provided to Medicare patients via a cost-based system. Other acute-care hospitals are paid by Medicare via various prospective payment systems. The FMT developed a mapping from the Medicare Cost Report to various financial ratios. The FMT also provides guidance on how to address data anomalies that may be present in cost report data. Since facilities may be part of larger entities such as systems or universities, the reporting of equity, fund balances, and some other figures may appear to be out of reasonable range.

A data file containing selected cost report elements accompanies this text and may be useful in practicing application of some of the analysis techniques presented in this chapter. Guidance for mapping cost report data elements to ratio components is based on industry standards, the FMT recommendations, and information from Schuhmann's 2008 article from *Healthcare Financial Management.* Although cost report data are audited, care should be taken when calculating ratios to be sure that the values are reasonable. This may be accomplished by referencing standard financial analysis texts.

Other sources of comparative data include trade journals and state departments of health. A number of health finance consulting firms also market and sell hospital benchmarking reports. Nonhospital financial benchmarks are more difficult to find but may be available in trade journals or from specialized consulting firms.

Case Study: Regional Hospital Ratio Analysis

A summary of the ratios calculated in the previous sections is presented in table 3.1, along with benchmark values from 2009 Medicare Cost Reports. Regional Hospital improved all four of the profitability ratios from 2008 to 2009. The CR and QR both improved slightly, but the significant change in liquidity is illustrated with a nearly 30-day change in DCOH. From the trend analysis of the balance sheet and income statement, we know that Regional Hospital was able to increase their cash and cash equivalents by 83.9 percent while slightly decreasing their operating expense. These are the two figures used to calculate DCOH that are driving the change.

Table 3.1   Regional Hospital summary of ratios

Regional Hospital Ratio	2009	2008	Acute Care Hospital Median from 2009 Medicare Cost Report Data
Profitability Ratios			
Total Margin (TM)	4.9%	0.1%	1.5%
Return on Assets (ROA)	7.5%	0.2%	4.1%
Return on Equity (ROE)	9.8%	0.3%	N/A
Operating Margin (OM)	4.2%	0.9%	−0.2%
Liquidity Ratios			
Current Ratio (CR)	2.84	2.78	2.0
Quick Ratio (QR)	2.54	2.34	1.5
Days Cash on Hand (DCOH)	63.6 days	33.9 days	20.8 days
Debt Performance Ratios			
Debt Ratio (DR)	23.7%	22.9%	50.7%
Debt to Equity Ratio (DER)	31.1%	29.7%	75.9%
Times Interest Earned (TIE)	25.1	1.6	N/A
Asset Management Ratios			
Fixed Asset Turnover (FAT)	4.0	3.4	2.4
Total Asset Turnover (TAT)	1.5	1.7	1.0
Days in Patient Accounts Receivable (DPAR)	64.9 days	52.2 days	46.4 days
Average Age of Plant (AAP)	10.6 years	10.4 years	N/A

Source: Acute Care Hospital Medians from 2009 submitted Medicare Cost Reports.

In the debt performance ratio category, the DR and DER did not show significant change from 2008 to 2009, but the TIE increased dramatically. Recall that the numerator in TIE is net income or change in net assets. From the trend analysis, we know that the net income increased from $29,000 to $1 million from 2008 to 2009. The increase in net income was driven by a 2 percent increase in operating revenue and a 1.4 percent decrease in operating expenses.

The performance of Regional Hospital in the asset management ratio category was mixed. The FAT increased slightly due to a decrease in net fixed assets. This is driven by annual depreciation without any newly purchased capital items. The change in total assets from 2008 to 2009 was a slight increase but resulted in a small decrease in TAT when combined with a decrease in operating revenue. The DPAR increased by 12.7 days or 24 percent. This is a significant increase in DPAR that is due to an increase in patient accounts receivable. This should be investigated further to determine if the increase in accounts receivable is due to an increase in patient volume or a decrease in payment collections.

Regional Hospital improved its performance in many of the financial ratios. The combination of the common size and trend financial statements with the ratio analysis gives a full picture of the financial performance of Regional Hospital from year to year.

Summary

Financial statements provide a picture of a facility's financial position. To measure the financial performance of a facility, the financial statement must be transformed into standardized values. Three strategies are typically used to normalize or standardize the financial statement values. First, vertical or common size analysis may be used to standardize the balance sheet by dividing each value by total assets. The income statement may be converted to common size by dividing by the total revenues. A common size balance sheet or income statement may be used to compare a facility's performance across time or against peer facility financial statements.

The second strategy for standardizing financial statements is trend analysis. Horizontal or trend analysis may be used to compare a facility's performance over time. Finally, ratio analysis is used in a number of industries including healthcare to compare an entity's performance both over time and versus a competitor or industry standard.

Table 3.2 presents a summary of the ratios discussed in this chapter. The general performance guide gives only directional guidance regarding the type of values that are considered better performing. All values should be benchmarked against industry norms when possible.

Table 3.2   Summary of ratios in chapter 3

Ratio	Numerator	Denominator	General Performance Guide (within Industry Norms)
Profitability Ratios			
Total Margin	Net Income	Total Revenues	Higher value = better performance
Return on Assets	Net Income	Total Assets	Higher value = better performance
Return on Equity	Net Income	Total Equity	Higher value = better performance
Operating Margin	Operating Income	Operating Revenues	Higher value = better performance
Liquidity Ratios			
Current Ratio	Total Current Assets	Total Current Liabilities	Higher value = better performance
Quick Ratio	Cash & Cash Equivalents + Short-Term Investments + Accounts Receivable	Total Current Liabilities	Higher value = better performance
Days Cash on Hand	Unrestricted Cash & Cash Equivalents	Operating Expenses per Day Less Depreciation	Higher value = better performance
Debt Performance Ratios			
Debt Ratio	Total Liabilities	Total Assets	Lower value = better performance
Debt to Equity Ratio	Total Liabilities	Total Equity	Lower value = better performance
Times Interest Earned	EBIT	Interest Expense	Higher value = better performance
Asset Management Ratios			
Fixed Asset Turnover	Total Operating Revenues	Net Fixed Assets	Higher value = better performance
Total Asset Turnover	Total Operating Revenues	Total Assets	Higher value = better performance
Days in Patient Accounts Receivable	Net Patient Accounts Receivable	Net Patient Service Revenue per Day	Lower value = better performance
Average Age of Plant	Accumulated Depreciation	Depreciation Expense	Lower value = better performance

An analysis of these standardized financial statements allows an understanding of the areas where a facility excels and areas for improvement.

Exercise: Financial Statement Scavenger Hunt

The notes to a financial statement hold a wealth of information about the financial performance of a facility. Appendix 3.1 includes the entire financial statement for Regional Hospital. The balance sheet, income statement, and statement of cash flows were all used as examples in this chapter. This scavenger hunt is designed to help you understand the contents of the notes and how they may be used in analyzing the financial position of a facility.

1. Find the details behind the calculation of net capital assets.
   a. Did Regional Hospital make any significant capital purchases during 2008?
   b. What was the reason for the decrease in the net capital assets additions between 2008 and 2009?
2. What major payers are active at Regional Hospital?
3. How much did Regional Hospital spend on advertising in 2008 and 2009?
4. What percentage of gross patient service revenue came from the outpatient setting? Did this figure increase or decrease from 2008 to 2009?
5. How much patient service revenue was excluded from the financial statement due to the hospital's charity care policy?

CHECK YOUR UNDERSTANDING

1. Common size analysis is the practice of averaging financial statement data over two or more years. (True/False)
2. Financial ratios allow comparisons of financial statement results among facilities. (True/False)
3. Depreciation is excluded from the daily operating expense when calculating the days cash on hand. (True/False)
4. The current ratio is always a smaller value than the quick ratio. (True/False)
5. Not-for-profit entities should not have a positive operating margin. (True/False)
6. The return on assets is a measure of:
   a. The ability of a facility to pay its short-term obligations
   b. Overall profitability
   c. The amount of short-term assets available
   d. The size of a facility

7. Which of the following is *not* a measure of liquidity?
   a. Days cash on hand
   b. Quick ratio
   c. Current ratio
   d. Fixed asset turnover
8. The days in patient accounts receivable increased from one period to the next for a hospital. Which of the following events may have caused that change?
   a. Total assets increased
   b. Current liabilities increased
   c. Net patient service revenue decreased
   d. Depreciation decreased
9. Which of the following relationships is true?
   a. Operating margin is always less than total margin.
   b. Fixed asset turnover is always less than total asset turnover.
   c. Days cash on hand is always more than days in patient accounts receivable.
   d. Relationships depend on the financial results of the facility.
10. Which of the following is a measure of the overall profitability of a facility?
    a. Fixed asset turnover
    b. Total margin
    c. Days cash on hand
    d. Current ratio

References

Gapenski, L.C. 2006. *Understanding Healthcare Financial Management,* 5th ed. Chicago: Health Administration Press.

State of Indiana. n.d. 2009 Hospital Audited Financial Statements. http://www.in.gov/isdh/24801.htm.

Langley, M. 1998. Nun's zeal for profits shapes hospital chain, wins Wall Street fans. *Wall Street Journal,* January 7: A1.

Pink, G.H., G.M. Holmes, C. D'Alpe, L.A. Strunk, P. McGee, and R.T. Slifkin. 2005. Flex Monitoring Team Briefing Paper no. 7: Financial indicators for critical access hospitals. Minneapolis: Flex.

Schuhmann, T. 2008. Hospital financial performance: Trends to watch: Financial indicators derived from Medicare cost report data are reliable tools for assessing the effectiveness of a hospital's operations. *Healthcare Financial Management,* July 2008: I–VII.

Zelman, W., A. McCue, and N. Glick. 2009. *Financial Management of Health Care Organizations,* 3rd ed. Malden, MA: Blackwell.

Appendix 3.1: 2009 Regional Hospital Financial Statement

MANAGEMENT'S DISCUSSION AND ANALYSIS (UNAUDITED)
SEPTEMBER 30, 2009 AND 2008

Summarized Financial Statement Information

The Hospital's net assets are the difference between its assets and liabilities. The following information documents in summary the net assets and the changes in net assets related to activities of the Hospital as of September 30, 2009 and 2008 and for the years then ended.

	2009 (millions)	2008 (millions)
Current assets	$ 7.5	$ 5.5
Non-current cash and investments	0.8	0.6
Capital assets and other assets	5.3	6.0
Total assets	$ 13.6	$ 12.1
Current liabilities	$ 2.6	$ 2.0
Long-term debt and capital leases, net	0.6	0.8
Total liabilities	$ 3.2	$ 2.8
Net assets		
Invested in capital assets, net of related debt	$ 4.3	$ 4.7
Restricted expendable	0.8	0.6
Unrestricted	5.3	4.0
	$ 10.4	$ 9.3

	2009 (millions)	2008 (millions)
Revenue		
Net patient service revenue	$ 19.9	$ 19.4
Other revenue	0.7	0.8
Total operating revenue	20.6	20.2
Expenses		
Salaries and benefits	10.9	11.5
Medical professional fees	0.7	0.7
Other professional fees	1.9	1.7
Medical supplies and drugs	3.0	3.0
Rent	0.2	0.2
Insurance	0.3	0.3
Depreciation and amortization	1.3	1.2
Other	1.3	1.4
Total operating expenses	19.6	20.0
Operating income	1.0	0.2
Nonoperating revenue (expense)	0.1	(0.2)
Change in assets	$ 1.1	$ 0.0

MANAGEMENT'S DISCUSSION AND ANALYSIS
SEPTEMBER 30, 2009 AND 2008

Economic Factors

The local economy is feeling the effects as evidenced in layoffs in the major manufacturers within the community we serve. Management anticipates ER volumes to increase marginally as the community foregoes family physician visits for budgetary purposes. Self-pay as well as Medicaid volumes are expected to rise creating additional cash flow challenges for the future. Being a Critical Access Hospital (CAH), we are reimbursed the cost of providing inpatient and outpatient services to Medicare patients, which is approximately 50% of the Hospital's revenue.

BALANCE SHEETS
SEPTEMBER 30, 2009 AND 2008

ASSETS

	2009	2008
Current assets		
Cash and cash equivalents	$ 3,199,568	$ 1,739,826
Patient accounts receivable, net of estimated uncollectibles of $1,880,369 and $1,795,057 in 2009 and 2008, respectively	3,534,735	2,770,972
Estimated third party settlements	-0-	111,971
Supplies and other current assets	806,432	866,696
Total current assets	7,540,735	5,489,465
Noncurrent cash		
Restricted by contributors and grantors	809,491	640,080
Total noncurrent cash and investments	809,491	640,080
Capital assets		
Land and construction in progress	884,936	713,688
Depreciable capital assets, net	4,266,520	5,161,352
Total capital assets	5,151,456	5,875,040
Other assets	109,584	144,584
Total assets	$ 13,611,266	$ 12,149,169

LIABILITIES AND NET ASSETS

	2009	2008
Current liabilities		
Current maturities of capital leases	$ 288,305	$ 386,894
Accounts payable and accrued expenses	564,458	397,412
Accrued salaries and related liabilities	913,372	1,058,539
Estimated third party settlements	688,000	-0-
Other current liabilities	201,331	133,492
Total current liabilities	2,655,466	1,976,337
Long-term liabilities		
Capital leases	470,937	670,689
Other long-term liabilities	99,167	134,167
Total long-term liabilities	570,104	804,856
Total liabilities	3,225,570	2,781,193
Net assets		
Unrestricted	5,273,575	4,038,876
Invested in capital assets, net of related debt	4,293,047	4,683,290
Restricted		
Expendable for capital acquisitions	740,539	577,536
Expendable for specific operating activities	78,535	68,274
Total net assets	10,385,696	9,367,976
Total liabilities and net assets	$ 13,611,266	$ 12,149,169

See accompanying notes to financial statements.

STATEMENTS OF REVENUES, EXPENSES AND CHANGES IN NET ASSETS
YEARS ENDED SEPTEMBER 30, 2009 AND 2008

	2009	2008
Revenues		
Net patient service revenue	$ 19,879,358	$ 19,378,966
Other	671,337	769,508
Total operating revenue	20,550,695	20,148,474
Expenses		
Salaries and benefits	10,936,559	11,536,019
Medical professional fees	737,359	715,652
Other professional fees	1,934,956	1,694,130
Supplies and drugs	3,021,130	2,960,692
Rent	144,644	177,666
Insurance	298,533	280,873
Depreciation and amortization	1,335,081	1,243,393
Other	1,280,605	1,359,251
Total operating expenses	19,688,867	19,967,676
Operating income	861,828	180,798
Nonoperating revenue (expense)		
Investment income	66,778	46,935
Interest expense	(42,184)	(48,036)
Other	131,298	(150,828)
Total nonoperating revenue (expense)	155,892	(151,929)
Change in net assets	1,017,720	28,869
Net assets, beginning of year	9,367,976	9,339,107
Net assets, end of year	$ 10,385,696	$ 9,367,976

See accompanying notes to financial statements.

STATEMENTS OF CASH FLOWS
YEARS ENDED SEPTEMBER 30, 2009 AND 2008

	2009	2008
Operating activities		
Cash received from patients and third party payors	$ 19,915,566	$ 20,363,530
Cash paid to employees for salaries and benefits	(11,081,726)	(11,349,910)
Cash paid to vendors for goods and services	(7,166,776)	(7,724,464)
Other operating receipts, net	671,212	1,015,964
Net cash from operating activities	2,338,276	2,305,120
Capital and related financing activities		
Acquisition and construction of capital assets	(477,992)	(401,572)
Proceeds from sale of capital assets	3,980	-0-
Interest paid on long-term debt	(42,184)	(48,036)
Payments on line of credit	-0-	(150,000)
Proceeds on long-term debt	-0-	125,000
Principal payments on long-term debt	(391,003)	(352,225)
Net cash from capital and related financing activities	(907,199)	(826,833)
Investing activities		
Investment and other nonoperating income	198,076	(103,893)
Net cash from investing activities	198,076	(103,893)
Net change in cash and cash equivalents	1,629,153	1,374,394
Cash and cash equivalents, beginning of year	2,379,906	1,005,512
Cash and cash equivalents, end of year	$ 4,009,059	$ 2,379,906
Reconciliation of cash and cash equivalents to the balance sheets		
Cash and cash equivalents		
In current assets	$ 3,199,568	$ 1,739,826
In noncurrent cash and investments	809,491	640,080
Total cash and cash equivalents	$ 4,009,059	$ 2,379,906

See accompanying notes to financial statements.

STATEMENTS OF CASH FLOWS
YEARS ENDED SEPTEMBER 30, 2009 AND 2008

	2009	2008
Reconciliation of operating loss		
to net cash from operating activities		
Operating income	$ 861,828	$ 180,798
Adjustments to reconcile operating income		
to net cash from operating activities:		
Depreciation and amortization	1,335,081	1,243,393
(Gain) loss on disposal of capital assets	(125)	246,456
Provision for bad debt	1,281,107	1,402,017
Changes in assets and liabilities		
Patient accounts receivable	(2,044,870)	(717,771)
Estimated third-party settlements	799,971	300,318
Supplies and other current assets	60,264	(221,648)
Other assets	(9,698)	7,760
Accounts payable and accrued expenses	167,046	(364,752)
Other current liabilities	67,839	77,440
Accrued salaries and related liabilities	(145,167)	186,109
Other long-term liabilities	(35,000)	(35,000)
Net cash flows from operating activities	$ 2,338,276	$ 2,305,120

Property was acquired under capital leases in the amount of $92,662 and $1,042,780 for 2009 and 2008, respectively.

See accompanying notes to financial statements.

NOTES TO FINANCIAL STATEMENTS
SEPTEMBER 30, 2009 AND 2008

1. SIGNIFICANT ACCOUNTING POLICIES

Reporting Entity

██████████ Hospital (the Hospital) is a county owned facility and operates under the Indiana County Hospital Law, Indiana Code 16-22. The Hospital provides short-term inpatient and outpatient health care.

The Board of County Commissioners ██████████ appoints the Governing Board of the Hospital (Board) and a financial benefit/burden relationship exists between the County and the Hospital. For these reasons, the Hospital is considered a component unit of ██████████

The accompanying financial statements present the activities of the Hospital (primary government). There are no significant component units which require inclusion.

Use of Estimates

The preparation of financial statements in conformity with generally accepted accounting principles requires management to make estimates and assumptions that affect the reported amounts of assets and liabilities and disclosures of contingent assets and liabilities at the date of the financial statements and the reported amounts of revenues and expenses during the reporting period. Actual results could differ from those estimates.

Enterprise Fund Accounting

The Hospital uses enterprise fund accounting. Revenues and expenses are recognized on the accrual basis using the economic resources measurement focus. Based on Governmental Accounting Standards Board (GASB) Statement No. 20, Accounting and Financial Reporting for Proprietary Funds and Other Governmental Entities That Use Proprietary Fund Accounting, as amended, the Hospital has elected to apply the provisions of all relevant pronouncements of the Financial Accounting Standards Board (FASB), including those issued after November 30, 1989, that do not conflict with or contradict GASB pronouncements.

Cash and Cash Equivalents

Cash and cash equivalents include demand deposits and investments in highly liquid debt instruments with an original maturity date of three months or less. The Hospital maintains its cash in accounts, which at times, may exceed federally insured limits. The Hospital has not experienced any losses in such accounts. The Hospital believes that it is not exposed to any significant credit risk on cash and cash equivalents. Cash paid for interest in 2009 and 2008 was $42,184 and $48,036, respectively.

NOTES TO FINANCIAL STATEMENTS
SEPTEMBER 30, 2009 AND 2008

Noncurrent Cash

Internally designated – Funded Depreciation – Amounts transferred from the Operating Fund by the Hospital Board of Trustees through funding depreciation expense. Such amounts are to be used for equipment and building, remodeling, repairing, replacing or making additions to the Hospital buildings as authorized by IC 16-22-3-13.

Restricted by contributors and grantors – Amounts include cash from three funds that are restricted for specific operating purposes either by the donor or funding source. The funds include Sweet Beginnings, Building and Donated, and Cumulative Building Fund.

Capital Assets

Capital assets, which include land, land improvements, buildings and improvements, and equipment, are reported at historical cost. Contributed or donated assets are reported at estimated fair value at the time received. Capital assets under capital lease obligations are amortized on the straight-line method over the shorter period of the lease term or the estimated useful life of the equipment. Such amortization is included in depreciation and amortization in the financial statements.

Capitalization thresholds (the dollar values above which asset acquisitions are added to the capital asset accounts), depreciation methods and estimated useful lives of capital assets reported in the financial statements are as follows:

Description	Capitalization Threshold		Depreciation Method	Estimated Useful Life
Land improvements	$	2,000	Straight line	*
Buildings and fixed equipment	$	2,000	Straight line	*
Major movable and minor equipment	$	2,000	Straight line	*

* Based on the most current edition of the American Hospital Association's (AHA's) Estimated Useful Lives of Depreciable Hospital Assets, for each individual capital asset.

For depreciated assets, the cost of normal maintenance and repairs that do not add to the value of the asset or materially extend assets lives are not capitalized.

NOTES TO FINANCIAL STATEMENTS
SEPTEMBER 30, 2009 AND 2008

Costs of Borrowing

Except for capital assets acquired through gifts, contributions, or capital grants, interest cost on borrowed funds during the period of construction of capital assets is capitalized as a component of the cost of acquiring those assets. No interest was capitalized during either 2009 or 2008.

Grants and Contributions

From time to time, the Hospital receives grants from ███████████ and the State of Indiana as well as contributions from individuals and private organizations. Revenues from grants and contributions (including contributions of capital assets) are recognized when all eligibility requirements, including time requirements are met. Grants and contributions may be restricted for either specific operating purposes or for capital purposes. Amounts that are unrestricted or that are restricted to a specific operating purpose are reported as nonoperating revenues. Amounts restricted to capital acquisitions are reported after nonoperating revenues and expenses.

Restricted Resources

When the Hospital has both restricted and unrestricted resources available to finance a particular program, it is the Hospital's policy to use restricted resources before unrestricted resources.

Net Assets

Net assets of the Hospital are classified in three components.

Net assets invested in capital assets net of related debt consist of capital assets net of accumulated depreciation and reduced by the current balances of any outstanding borrowings used to finance the purchase or construction of those assets.

Restricted expendable net assets are net assets that must be used for a particular purpose, as specified by creditors, grantors, or contributors external to the Hospital.

Unrestricted net assets are remaining net assets that do not meet the definition of invested in capital assets net of related debt or restricted.

NOTES TO FINANCIAL STATEMENTS
SEPTEMBER 30, 2009 AND 2008

Operating Revenues and Expenses

The Hospital's statement of revenues, expenses and changes in net assets distinguishes between operating and nonoperating revenues and expenses. Operating revenues result from exchange transactions associated with providing health care services, the Hospital's principal activity. Nonoperating revenues include contributions received for purposes other than capital asset acquisition, and other nonoperating activities and are reported as nonoperating revenues. Operating expenses are all expenses incurred to provide health care services, other than financing costs.

Estimated Third-Party Settlements

Regulations in effect require annual retroactive settlements for third-party settlements based upon cost reports filed by the Hospital. These retroactive settlements are estimated and recorded in the accompanying financial statements. Changes in these estimates are reflected in the year in which they occur. Net patient service revenues in the accompanying statements of revenues, expenses and changes in net assets were increased by approximately $278,000 during 2009, to reflect changes in the estimated settlements for certain prior years. Net patient service revenues in the accompanying statements of revenues, expenses and changes in net assets were increased by approximately $376,000 during 2008, to reflect changes in the estimated settlements for certain prior years.

Patient Accounts Receivable, Revenues and Operating Expenses

Net patient service revenues are reported at the estimated net realizable amounts from patients, third-party payors, and others for services rendered, including estimated adjustments under reimbursement agreements. Retroactive adjustments are accrued on an estimated basis in the period the related services are rendered and adjusted in future periods, as final settlements are determined.

The Hospital is a provider of services to patients entitled to coverage under Medicare. The Hospital was granted Critical Access Status by Medicare. The Hospital is paid for Medicare services based upon a cost reimbursement methodology. The Hospital is reimbursed for cost reimbursable items at a tentative rate, with final settlement determined after submission of annual cost reports.

Final determination of amounts earned is subject to review by the fiscal intermediary. Medicare reports have been settled through 2007. Management believes adequate provision has been made in the financial statements for any adjustments.

NOTES TO FINANCIAL STATEMENTS
SEPTEMBER 30, 2009 AND 2008

Management estimates an allowance for doubtful accounts receivable based on an evaluation of historical losses, current economic conditions, and other factors unique to the Hospital's patient base.

Revenue from Medicare and Medicaid programs account for approximately 41 percent and 6 percent, respectively, of the Hospital's net patient service revenue for the fiscal year ended 2009, and 35 percent and 6 percent, respectively, of the Hospital's net patient revenue for the fiscal year ended 2008.

Charity Care

The Hospital provides care to patients who meet certain criteria under its charity care policy without charge or at amounts less than its established rates. Amounts deemed to be charity care are not reported as revenues.

Advertising Costs

The Hospital expenses advertising costs as they are incurred. Advertising expense for the years ended September 30, 2009 and 2008 was $130,601 and $120,439, respectively.

Compensated Absences

Sick Time – Hospital employees earn sick leave at various rates per pay period. Unused sick leave may be accumulated to a maximum of ninety-six hours. Accumulated sick leave over ninety-six hours is paid to employees through cash payments upon proper notice of termination or upon request of the employee to be included on the last pay of each calendar year.

Paid Time Off – Hospital employees earn paid time off at various rates per pay period based upon their classification and their number of years of service. Paid time off may be accumulated to a maximum of 136 to 216 hours based on their number of years of service. Accumulated paid time off is paid to employees through cash payments upon proper notice of termination. Paid time off and sick leave are accrued when incurred and reported as a liability.

Risk Management

The Hospital is exposed to various risks of loss from torts; theft of, damage to, and destruction of assets; business interruption; errors and omissions; employee injuries and illnesses; natural disasters; medical malpractice; and employee health, dental, and accident benefits. Commercial insurance coverage is purchased for claims arising from such matters. Settled claims have not exceeded this commercial coverage in any of the three preceding years.

NOTES TO FINANCIAL STATEMENTS
SEPTEMBER 30, 2009 AND 2008

Income Taxes

The Hospital is a governmental instrumentality organized under Title 16, Article 12, of the Indiana statutes. The Hospital is exempt from federal income tax under Section 115 of the Internal Revenue Code of 1986 as a not-for-profit organization under Section 501(c)(3).

Accounting for Uncertainty in Income Taxes

The Income Tax Topic of the FASB ASC clarifies accounting principles generally accepted in the United States of America for recognition, measurement, presentation and disclosure relating to uncertain tax positions. It applies to business enterprises, not-for-profit entities, and pass-through entities, such as S corporations and limited liability companies. As permitted, the Hospital elected to defer application until issuance of its September 30, 2010 financial statements. For financial statements covering periods prior to fiscal year 2010, the Hospital evaluates uncertain tax positions in accordance with existing accounting principles generally accepted in the United States of America and makes such accruals and disclosures as might be required thereunder.

Fair Value Measurements

The Fair Value Measurements and Disclosures topic of the FASB Accounting Standards Codification requires certain disclosures regarding the fair value of financial instruments. The Hospital partially adopted the provisions of the topic for fiscal year 2009, but will delay adoption related to non-financial assets and non-financial liabilities. Companies are permitted to partially defer the effective date for non-financial assets and non-financial liabilities, except for items that are recognized or disclosed at fair value in the financial statements on a recurring basis, until fiscal year 2010. When fully adopted, the Hospital will apply the provisions to certain nonfinancial assets and liabilities and is currently evaluating the impact of the full adoption of this statement on the financial statements.

When fully adopted, the Hospital will apply the provisions of the topic to certain non-financial assets and liabilities and is currently evaluating the impact of the full adoption of this statement on the financial statements.

NOTES TO FINANCIAL STATEMENTS
SEPTEMBER 30, 2009 AND 2008

Minimum Revenue Guarantees

The Minimum Revenue Guarantee Granted to a Business or Its Owners topic of the FASB Accounting Standards Codification was amended and is effective as of January 1, 2006. This topic amended Guarantor's Accounting and Disclosure Requirements for Guarantees, including indirect Guarantees and Indebtedness of Others topic. The amended topic requires a guarantor to recognize, at the inception of a guarantee, a liability for the fair value of the obligation undertaken in issuing the guarantee. This topic is effective for new minimum revenue guarantees issued or modified on or after January 1, 2006.

The Hospital adopted this topic as required for all new minimum revenue guarantees issued or modified on or after January 1, 2006. For periods ending before January 1, 2006, the Hospital did not report the fair value of its obligations under physician revenue guarantee agreements. However, under the topic as amended, the Hospital is required to report the liability for these physician revenue guarantees on its balance sheets at fair value and amortize the related prepaid physician recruitment expense over the period of the physician's contractual commitment to practice in the local community.

Subsequent Events

The Hospital evaluated events or transactions occurring subsequent to the balance sheet date for recognition and disclosure in the accompanying financial statements through the date the financial statements are available to be issued which is February 5, 2010.

2. CHARITY CARE

Charges excluded from patient service revenue under the Hospital's charity care policy were $312,889 and $345,912 for 2009 and 2008, respectively.

3. DEPOSITS

Deposits with financial institutions in the State of Indiana at year-end were entirely insured by the Federal Depository Insurance Corporation or by the Indiana Public Deposit Insurance Fund. This includes any deposit accounts issued or offered by a qualifying financial institution.

NOTES TO FINANCIAL STATEMENTS
SEPTEMBER 30, 2009 AND 2008

The Hospital's deposits are generally are reported at cost, as discussed in Note 1. As of September 30, 2009 and 2008, the Hospital had the following deposits and maturities, all of which were held in the Hospital's name by custodial banks that are agents of the Hospital:

September 30, 2009

| | Carrying Amount | Deposit Maturities (in years) | | | |
		Less than 1	1-5	6-10	More than 10
Cash and cash equivalents	$ 4,009,059	$ 4,009,059	$ -0-	$ -0-	$ -0-

September 30, 2008

| | Carrying Amount | Deposit Maturities (in years) | | | |
		Less than 1	1-5	6-10	More than 10
Cash and cash equivalents	$ 2,379,906	$ 2,379,906	$ -0-	$ -0-	$ -0-

Interest rate risk – The Hospital does not have a formal investment policy that limits investment maturities as a means of managing its exposure to fair value losses arising from changing interest rates.

Credit risk – Statutes authorize the Hospital to invest in interest bearing deposit accounts, passbook savings accounts, certificates of deposit, money market accounts, mutual funds, pooled fund investments, securities backed by the full faith and credit of the United States Treasury and repurchase agreements. The statutes require that repurchase agreements be fully collateralized by U.S. Government or U.S. Government Agency obligations.

Concentration of credit risk – The Hospital places no limit on the amount it may invest in any one issuer. The Hospital believes that it is not exposed to any significant credit risk on investments.

Deposits consist of the following as of September 30, 2009 and 2008:

	2009	2008
Cash and cash equivalents	$ 4,009,059	$ 2,379,906
Included in the following balance sheet		
Cash and cash equivalents	$ 3,199,568	$ 1,739,826
Restricted by contributors and grantors	809,491	640,080
	$ 4,009,059	$ 2,379,906

NOTES TO FINANCIAL STATEMENTS
SEPTEMBER 30, 2009 AND 2008

4. ACCOUNTS RECEIVABLE AND PAYABLE

Patient accounts receivable and accounts payable (including accrued expenses) reported as current assets and liabilities by the Hospital at year-end consisted of the following amounts at September 30, 2009 and 2008:

	2009	2008
Patient accounts receivable		
Receivable from patients and their insurance carriers	$4,360,007	$4,134,179
Receivable from Medicare	1,734,706	1,611,199
Receivable from Medicaid	1,163,333	1,131,480
Total patient accounts receivable	7,258,046	6,876,858
Less allowance for contractual agreements		
and uncollectible amounts	3,723,311	4,105,886
Patient accounts receivable, net	$3,534,735	$2,770,972
Accounts payable and accrued expenses		
Payable to employees (including payroll taxes)	$ 738,858	$ 733,539
Payable to suppliers	564,458	397,412
Accrued employee health benefit claims	174,514	325,000
Total accounts payable and accrued expenses	$1,477,830	$1,455,951

5. CAPITAL ASSETS

Capital asset activity for 2009 and 2008 is as follows:

	Balance September 30, 2008	Additions	Retirements	Transfers	Balance September 30, 2009
Land	$ 189,325	$ -0-	$ -0-	$ -0-	$ 189,325
Land improvements	281,113	-0-	-0-	-0-	281,113
Buildings and fixtures	7,401,988	1,555	(1,555)	-0-	7,401,988
Fixed equipment	3,565,295	53,034	-0-	641	3,618,970
Moveable equipment	6,388,122	341,898	(2,300)	2,278	6,729,998
Construction in process	524,364	174,167	-0-	(2,919)	695,612
Total	18,350,207	570,654	(3,855)	-0-	18,917,006
Accumulated depreciation	12,475,167	1,290,383	-0-	-0-	13,765,550
Net capital assets	$ 5,875,040	$ (719,729)	$ (3,855)	$ -0-	$ 5,151,456

NOTES TO FINANCIAL STATEMENTS
SEPTEMBER 30, 2009 AND 2008

	Balance September 30, 2007	Additions	Retirements	Transfers	Balance September 30, 2008
Land	$ 189,325	$ -0-	$ -0-	$ -0-	$ 189,325
Land improvements	281,113	-0-	-0-	-0-	281,113
Buildings and fixtures	7,394,995	6,993	-0-	-0-	7,401,988
Fixed equipment	3,565,295	-0-	-0-	-0-	3,565,295
Moveable equipment	6,039,163	993,657	(671,082)	26,384	6,388,122
Construction in process	283,528	267,220	-0-	(26,384)	524,364
Total	17,753,419	1,267,870	(671,082)	-0-	18,350,207
Accumulated depreciation	11,683,637	1,216,153	(424,623)	-0-	12,475,167
Net capital assets	$ 6,069,782	$ 51,717	$ (246,459)	$ -0-	$ 5,875,040

6. PHYSICIAN RELOCATION AGREEMENTS AND OTHER MINIMUM REVENUE GUARANTEES

Consistent with the Hospital's policy on physician relocation and recruitment, the Hospital provides income guarantee agreements to certain physicians who agree to relocate to the community to fill a need in the Hospital's service area and commit to remain in practice there. Annually, under such agreements, the Hospital is required to make payments to the physicians in excess of the amounts they earn in their practice up to the amount of the income guarantee. Such payments are recoverable from the physicians if they do not fulfill their commitment period to the community, which is typically five years. The Hospital also provides minimum revenue collection guarantees to Hospital-based physician groups providing certain services at the Hospital with terms of one year. At September 30, 2009 and 2008, the maximum potential amount of future payments under these guarantees was approximately $99,000, which is included in the assets and liabilities in the Balance Sheets.

7. LINE OF CREDIT

The Hospital had an $800,000 line of credit, which expired on August 28, 2008. Interest was due monthly at 6.25%.

NOTES TO FINANCIAL STATEMENTS
SEPTEMBER 30, 2009 AND 2008

8. LONG-TERM DEBT AND OTHER NONCURRENT LIABILITIES

A schedule of changes in the Hospital's noncurrent liabilities for the years ended September 30, 2009 and 2008, was as follows:

	Balance September 30, 2008	Additions	Reductions	Balance September 30, 2009	Current portion	Long-term portion
Notes Payable and Capital Leases:						
Notes Payable	$ 131,117	$ -0-	$ (131,117)	$ -0-	$ -0-	$ -0-
Capital Leases	926,466	92,662	(259,886)	759,242	288,305	470,937
Total Long-Term Debt	1,057,583	92,662	(391,003)	759,242	288,305	470,937
Other Liabilities	134,167	-0-	(35,000)	99,167	-0-	99,167
Total Noncurrent liabilities	$ 1,191,750	$ 92,662	$ (426,003)	$ 858,409	$ 288,305	$ 570,104

	Balance September 30, 2007	Additions	Reductions	Balance September 30, 2008	Current portion	Long-term portion
Notes Payable and Capital Leases:						
Notes Payable	$ 139,437	$ 125,000	$ (133,320)	$ 131,117	$ 131,117	$ -0-
Capital Leases	279,076	1,042,784	(395,394)	926,466	255,777	670,689
Total Long-Term Debt	418,513	1,167,784	(528,714)	1,057,583	386,894	670,689
Other Liabilities	169,167	-0-	(35,000)	134,167	-0-	134,167
Total Noncurrent liabilities	$ 587,680	$ 1,167,784	$ (563,714)	$ 1,191,750	$ 386,894	$ 804,856

Long-Term Debt

The Hospital obtained an unsecured note payable during 2008. Payments, including interest at prime plus 2.25%, of $10,831 were due monthly through April 2009. The Hospital also has a note payable, secured by computer equipment. Payments, including interest at an annual rate of 4.75%, of $7,266 were due monthly through May 2009. These notes were paid in full during fiscal year 2009.

The Hospital has also entered into various capital leases at varying rates of imputed interest from 2.8% to 6.9%, collateralized by leased equipment.

Scheduled principal and interest repayments on capital lease obligations are as follows:

Year ending September 30,	Principal	Interest
2010	$ 288,305	$ 28,993
2011	255,231	20,221
2012	177,003	6,615
2013	38,703	279
	$ 759,242	$ 56,108

The following is an analysis of the leased assets included in property and equipment as of September 30:

	2009	2008
Equipment	$ 979,321	$ 1,083,296
Accumulated depreciation	406,019	317,879
	$ 573,302	$ 765,417

9.   PATIENT SERVICE REVENUE

Patient service revenue for the years ended September 30, 2009 and 2008 consists of the following:

	2009	2008
Inpatient services	$ 12,490,602	$ 10,400,782
Outpatient services	25,904,418	24,297,052
Gross patient service revenue	38,395,020	34,697,834
Contractual allowances	(16,921,666)	(13,570,939)
Charity care	(312,889)	(345,912)
Bad debt	(1,281,107)	(1,402,017)
Deductions from revenue	(18,515,662)	(15,318,868)
Net patient service revenue	$ 19,879,358	$ 19,378,966

NOTES TO FINANCIAL STATEMENTS
SEPTEMBER 30, 2009 AND 2008

10.   EMPLOYEE HEALTH PLAN

The Hospital has established a risk financing fund for risks associated with medical benefits to employees and dependents. The risk financing fund is accounted for in the Operating Fund where assets are set aside and a liability is accrued for claim settlements. An excess policy through commercial insurance covers individual claims in excess of $100,000 per year.

Claim expenditures and liabilities of the fund are reported when it is probable that a loss has occurred and the amount of the loss can be reasonable estimated. These losses include an estimate of claims that have been incurred but not reported (IBNR). Claim liabilities are calculated considering the effect of inflation, recent claim settlement trends, including frequency and amounts of payouts, and other economic and social factors.

Health insurance expense for the years ended September 30, 2009 and 2008, was approximately $2,047,000 and $2,434,000 respectively.

11.   MEDICAL MALPRACTICE

The Indiana Medical Malpractice Act, IC 27-12 (the Act), provides a recovery for an occurrence of malpractice and for any injury or death of a patient due to an act of malpractice in excess of certain thresholds. The Act requires the Hospital to maintain medical malpractice liability insurance on a per occurrence basis and in the annual aggregate.

12.   CONCENTRATIONS OF CREDIT RISK

The Hospital grants credit without collateral to its patients, most of whom are local residents and are insured under third-party payor agreements. Accounts receivable and revenues from self-pay and third-party payors were as follows:

	Receivables		Revenue	
	2009	2008	2009	2008
Medicare and Medicaid	41%	41%	62%	61%
Blue Cross	10%	9%	18%	15%
Commercial and other payors	16%	14%	15%	17%
Self-pay payors	33%	36%	5%	7%
	100%	100%	100%	100%

NOTES TO FINANCIAL STATEMENTS
SEPTEMBER 30, 2009 AND 2008

13. COMMITMENTS AND CONTINGENCIES

The Hospital is involved in litigation and regulatory investigations arising in the course of business. After consultation with legal counsel, management estimates that these matters will be resolved without material adverse effect on the Hospital's future financial position or results from operations.

Appendix 3.2: Medicare Cost Report

3690 (Cont.)	FORM CMS-2552-96				06-03
BALANCE SHEET (If you are nonproprietary and do not maintain fund-type accounting records, complete the General Fund column only)		PROVIDER NO.:	PERIOD: FROM _____ TO _____	WORKSHEET G	
Assets (Omit cents)	General Fund	Specific Purpose Fund	Endowment Fund	Plant Fund	
	1	2	3	4	
CURRENT ASSETS					
1 Cash on hand and in banks					1
2 Temporary investments					2
3 Notes receivable					3
4 Accounts receivable					4
5 Other receivables					5
6 Allowances for uncollectible notes and accounts receivable					6
7 Inventory					7
8 Prepaid expenses					8
9 Other current assets					9
10 Due from other funds					10
11 Total current assets (sum of lines 1-10)					11
FIXED ASSETS					
12 Land					12
13 Land improvements					13
13.01 Accumulated depreciation					13.01
14 Buildings					14
14.01 Accumulated depreciation					14.01
15 Leasehold improvements					15
15.01 Accumulated depreciation					15.01
16 Fixed equipment					16
16.01 Accumulated depreciation					16.01
17 Automobiles and trucks					17
17.01 Accumulated depreciation					17.01
18 Major movable equipment					18
18.01 Accumulated depreciation					18.01
19 Minor equipment depreciable					19
19.01 Accumulated depreciation					19.01
20 Minor equipment-nondepreciable					20
21 Total fixed assets (sum of lines 12-20)					21
OTHER ASSETS					
22 Investments					22
23 Deposits on leases					23
24 Due from owners/officers					24
25 Other assets					25
26 Total other assets (sum of lines 22-25)					26
27 Total assets (sum of lines 11, 21, and 26)					27

FORM CMS-2552-96 (6/2003) (INSTRUCTIONS FOR THIS WORKSHEET ARE PUBLISHED IN CMS PUB. 15-II, SECTION 3640)

10-96	FORM CMS-2552-96			3690 (Cont.)

BALANCE SHEET	PROVIDER NO.:	PERIOD:	WORKSHEET G
(If you are nonproprietary and do not maintain fund-type accounting records, complete the General Fund column only)		FROM _____ TO	(CONT.)

Liabilities and Fund Balances (Omit cents)	General Fund	Specific Purpose Fund	Endowment Fund	Plant Fund	
	1	2	3	4	
CURRENT LIABILITIES					
28 Accounts payable					28
29 Salaries, wages, and fees payable					29
30 Payroll taxes payable					30
31 Notes and loans payable (short term)					31
32 Deferred income					32
33 Accelerated payments					33
34 Due to other funds					34
35 Other current liabilities					35
36 Total current liabilities (sum of lines 28 thru 35)					36
LONG TERM LIABILITIES					
37 Mortgage payable					37
38 Notes payable					38
39 Unsecured loans					39
40 Loans from owners .01 Prior to 7/1/66					40.01
.02 On or after 7/1/66					40.02
41 Other long term liabilities					41
42 Total long term liabilities (sum of lines 37 thru 41)					42
43 Total liabilities (sum of lines 36 and 42)					43
CAPITAL ACCOUNTS					
44 General fund balance					44
45 Specific purpose fund					45
46 Donor created - endowment fund balance - restricted					46
47 Donor created - endowment fund balance - unrestricted					47
48 Governing body created - endowment fund balance					48
49 Plant fund balance - invested in plant					49
50 Plant fund balance - reserve for plant improvement, replacement, and expansion					50
51 Total fund balances (sum of lines 44 thru 50)					51
52 Total liabilities and fund balances (sum of lines 43 and 51)					52

FORM CMS-2552-96 (6/2003) (INSTRUCTIONS FOR THIS WORKSHEET ARE PUBLISHED IN CMS PUB. 15-II, SECTION 3640)

10-96

FORM CMS-2552-96

3690 (Cont.)

STATEMENT OF CHANGES IN FUND BALANCES

PROVIDER NO.:

PERIOD:
FROM _____
TO _____

WORKSHEET G-1

	GENERAL FUND	SPECIFIC PURPOSE FUND	ENDOWMENT FUND	PLANT FUND	
	1	2	3	4	5	6	7	8	
1 Fund balances at beginning of period					1
2 Net income (loss) (from Wkst. G-3, line 31)					2
3 Total (sum of line 1 and line 2)					3
4 Additions (credit adjustments) (specify)					4
5					5
6					6
7					7
8					8
9					9
10 Total additions (sum of lines 4-9)					10
11 Subtotal (line 3 plus line 10)					11
12 Deductions (debit adjustments) (specify)					12
13					13
14					14
15					15
16					16
17					17
18 Total deductions (sum of lines 12-17)					18
19 Fund balance at end of period per balance sheet (line 11 minus line 18)					19

FORM CMS-2552-96 (9/96) (INSTRUCTIONS FOR THIS WORKSHEET ARE PUBLISHED IN CMS PUB. 15-II, SECTION 3640)

Rev. 1

36-602

FORM CMS-2552-96

STATEMENT OF PATIENT REVENUES AND OPERATING REVENUES	PROVIDER NO.:	PERIOD: FROM ___ TO ___	WORKSHEET G-2, PARTS I & II

PART I - PATIENT REVENUES

	REVENUE CENTER	INPATIENT	OUTPATIENT	TOTAL	
		1	2	3	
	GENERAL INPATIENT ROUTINE CARE SERVICES				
1	Hospital				1
2	Subprovider				2
4	Swing bed - SNF				4
5	Swing bed - NF				5
6	Skilled nursing facility				6
7	Nursing facility				7
8	Other long term care				8
9	Total general inpatient care services (sum of lines 1-8)				9
	INTENSIVE CARE TYPE INPATIENT HOSPITAL SERVICES				
10	Intensive care unit				10
11	Coronary care unit				11
12	Burn intensive care unit				12
13	Surgical intensive care unit				13
14	Other special care (specify)				14
15	Total intensive care type inpatient hospital services (sum of lines 10-14)				15
16	Total inpatient routine care services (sum of lines 9 and 15)				16
17	Ancillary services				17
18	Outpatient services				18
19	Home health agency				19
20	Ambulance				20
21	Outpatient rehabilitation providers				21
22	ASC				22
23	Hospice				23
24					24
25	Total patient revenues (sum of lines 16-24) (transfer column 3 to Wkst. G-3, line 1)				25

PART II - OPERATING EXPENSES

		1	2	
26	Operating expenses (per Wkst. A, column 3, line 101)			26
27	Add (specify)			27
28				28
29				29
30				30
31				31
32				32
33	Total additions (sum of lines 27-32)			33
34	Deduct (specify)			34
35				35
36				36
37				37
38				38
39	Total deductions (sum of lines 34-38)			39
40	Total operating expenses (sum of lines 26 and 33 minus line 39) (transfer to Wkst. G-3, line 4)			40

FORM CMS-2552-96 (9/96) (INSTRUCTIONS FOR THIS WORKSHEET ARE PUBLISHED IN CMS PUB. 15-II, SECTION 3640)

	3690 (Cont.)	FORM CMS-2552-96		10-96
	STATEMENT OF REVENUES AND EXPENSES	PROVIDER NO.:	PERIOD: FROM ___ TO ___	WORKSHEET G-3

	Description		
1	Total patient revenues (from Wkst. G-2, Part I, column 3, line 25)		1
2	Less contractual allowances and discounts on patients' accounts		2
3	Net patient revenues (line 1 minus line 2)		3
4	Less total operating expenses (from Wkst. G-2, Part II, line 40)		4
5	Net income from service to patients (line 3 minus line 4)		5
	OTHER INCOME		
6	Contributions, donations, bequests, etc		6
7	Income from investments		7
8	Revenues from telephone and telegraph service		8
9	Revenue from television and radio service		9
10	Purchase discounts		10
11	Rebates and refunds of expenses		11
12	Parking lot receipts		12
13	Revenue from laundry and linen service		13
14	Revenue from meals sold to employees and guests		14
15	Revenue from rental of living quarters		15
16	Revenue from sale of medical and surgical supplies to other than patients		16
17	Revenue from sale of drugs to other than patients		17
18	Revenue from sale of medical records and abstracts		18
19	Tuition (fees, sale of textbooks, uniforms, etc.)		19
20	Revenue from gifts, flowers, coffee shops, and canteen		20
21	Rental of vending machines		21
22	Rental of hospital space		22
23	Governmental appropriations		23
24	Other (specify)		24
25	Total other income (sum of lines 6-24)		25
26	Total (line 5 plus line 25)		26
27	Other expenses (specify)		27
28			28
29			29
30	Total other expenses (sum of lines 27-29)		30
31	Net income (or loss) for the period (line 26 minus line 30)		31

FORM CMS-2552-96 (9/96) (INSTRUCTIONS FOR THIS WORKSHEET ARE PUBLISHED IN CMS PUB. 15-II, SECTION 3640)

Budgets

Learning Objectives

→ Develop and implement budgets appropriate to the organization and situation
→ Explain the source of the revenue budget
→ Calculate factors that influence the expense budget
→ Explain the difference between expenses and costs
→ Explain the allocation of overhead costs to revenue-producing areas
→ Explain the relationship between the operating budget and the cash budget

Key Terms

Allocation

Benchmarking

Bill hold

Bottom-up

Budget cycle

Capital budget

Case-mix index

Cash budget

Cash flow

Charges

Claims correction

Controllability

Cost

Desired earnings

Desired rate of growth

Direct method allocation

Discharged and not final billed (DNFB)

Double step-down allocation

Exempt

Favorable variance

Fiscal year

Flexible budget

Labor pool

Market share

Nonexempt

Operating budget

Overhead

Permanent variance

Revenue cycle

Statistical budget

Step-down allocation

Temporary variance

Top-down

Traceability

Traditional budget

Unfavorable variance

Variability

Variance

Working capital

Zero-based budget

Measuring Management Financial Performance

Formal financial statements are useful in analyzing the financial performance of an organization. They can provide a window into the overall management of an organization and how that organization is working to achieve its mission. However, financial statements are intended primarily for users who want an overview—a "big picture" of the organization and its activities. Many of these users are external to the organization, such as lenders, investors, donors, and the general public. They do not assist managers in controlling their day-to-day activities, nor do they provide executive leadership with the level of detail needed to measure management performance. For controlling and measuring activities at the department level, a different type of reporting is required: the budget. The same transaction-level detail that is cumulated through financial accounting conventions into the organization's financial statements is also cumulated through managerial accounting conventions into the organization's management reporting. Managerial accounting is a branch of the accounting profession that focuses on measuring management performance and focuses primarily on the internal users of financial information. Managerial accounting helps managers develop their financial plans—their budgets—and monitor their success at controlling their compliance with them.

Operating Budget

A budget is a plan. A financial budget is a financial plan. There are different types of financial plans that fit different organizations and situations. For department-management purposes, an **operating budget** defines the routine revenue and expenses that the department estimates for the coming period. The operating budget may also contain infrequent or nonroutine, low-dollar items. For example, routine items in the health information management (HIM) department operating budget include paper and other general office supplies. Nonroutine items may include replacement of staplers or hole punchers.

The purpose of the operating budget is to communicate financial expectations between the organization's executive team and the management team. The executive team defines the strategic goals of the organization and projects or estimates its view of the next financial period. The executive team communicates these goals and projections to the management team, which in turn develops its own estimates of its contribution (revenue) and resource utilization (expenses) needed to achieve the goals. The management team then communicates its estimates to the executive team for approval.

Budget Cycle

The **budget cycle** consists of the period beginning with the executive team's strategic planning for the coming periods and projects and ends with the final analysis of the completed period's or project's results. The cycle-ending activities of one period typically overlap the beginning of the subsequent period. Each component of the cycle has a specific purpose and activities that should take place. Figures 4.1 and 4.2 illustrate the operating budget cycle and timeline.

A **fiscal year** is the organization's 12-month period that encompasses a single business cycle. For federal tax purposes, the organization's year end must be specified at inception. Occasionally, organizations do change their fiscal year, but changes are not routine and not typically repeated. Generally, organizations use the calendar year—January 1 through December 31—for the fiscal year. The US government has a fiscal year of October 1 through September 30. Many academic institutions use August 1 through July 30, to coincide with the academic calendar.

Figure 4.1 Operating budget cycle

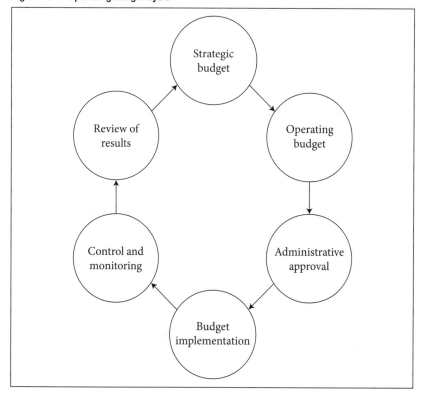

Figure 4.2   Budget cycle timeline

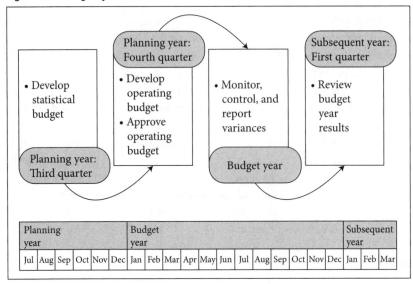

All budgets address either a specified period of time, usually a fiscal year, or a project, which can be for a single purchase or a multiyear activity. For budget purposes, the fiscal year is often segmented into equal periods, usually months, that coincide with financial reporting periods.

The executive team's strategic planning addresses the mission, goals, and vision of the organization. Part of strategic planning is to determine the overall budgetary assumptions for the coming fiscal year. These assumptions include **desired rate of growth, desired earnings,** and **market share.** Rate of growth can be expressed as the increase in equity or fund balance. Desired earnings is often described as a percentage: net income before taxes, divided by net service revenue. Market share is the percentage of available business that is captured by the organization. Market share can refer to particular service lines, such as neonatology, or to the organization's peer group as a whole (such as an acute care hospital versus all other acute care hospitals within a specified area). The collective strategic assumptions are the **statistical budget.** Department managers will use the statistical budget as their framework for developing their operating budgets and **capital budget.**

The operating budget is the plan for the coming fiscal year that describes the estimated results of activities in a particular department or program. The system by which an organization develops the operating budget depends on the nature of its activities. For example, a professional association or charitable organization may develop its budget along program lines. Once the programmatic budget is developed, it is then broken out or allocated to individual departments in order to assign financial responsibility to individual managers. Hospitals, on the other hand, generally develop operating budgets by department, since hospitals tend to be organized along service lines. The operating budget consists of estimated revenues and the estimated expenses needed to generate those revenues. Executive leadership uses the approved operating budget as a benchmark against which to measure departmental management performance.

The capital budget is defined by the organization as any project in which the purchases of depreciable assets exceed a specified dollar limit. (See chapter 2 for an explanation of depreciation.) Automobiles, major structural improvements, and diagnostic equipment are examples of depreciable assets that would be included in the capital budget. The evaluation of capital requests is discussed in chapter 8.

Budget Tools

Budgets tools include the systems and analytical tools used during the budget process. Operational budgets focus on the revenue and expenses of the organization. The organization's financial accounting system will generate the historical revenue and expenses for a department. The organization may use a separate managerial accounting system that will compare the financial accounting data with the same period's operational budget. This activity can also be done with spreadsheets.

Historical data are useful in determining the experience of the responsible area; however, that experience may not be consistent with the organization's goals and objectives going forward.

Although leadership has already developed expectations through the statistical budget, the responsible area may also need to obtain detailed data on the historical financial results of the area as well as on environmental issues, such as competitive market share in the service line.

Typically, the budget process for the responsible areas involves the completion of worksheets and questionnaires to help leadership understand the budget request. For example, if leadership projects a 3 percent increase in patient volume, the health information services department may project an increase in supply. On the budget worksheet, the manager of the department would have the opportunity to tie patient volume to the expense increase.

Management Reporting

During the budget cycle, the department manager will be expected to analyze the financial results of operations (the revenue and expenses) for the period against the budget. Typically a monthly activity, managers may be required to explain the difference between the budget (expected results) and the actual financial results. This difference is called the **variance.**

Budget variances are either positive or negative. The organization sets thresholds of tolerance, above or below which managers are required to explain. For example, an organization may set a 10 percent variance threshold. If the revenue for a particular month exceeds budget by more than 10 percent or falls short of budget by more than 10 percent, the manager will be required to explain the variance. If the variance is less than 10 percent, no explanation is needed. Variance thresholds may be expressed as percentages of budget or specific dollar limits. Chapter 5 includes a discussion of other methods to identify significant budget variances.

Revenue in excess of budget is a **favorable variance;** it is a better financial result than what was predicted. Revenue that falls short of budget is an **unfavorable variance.** Expenses have the opposite result. Lower expenses are favorable; higher expenses are unfavorable. Since expenses are often tied to volume and hence revenue, unfavorable expenses may be offset by favorable revenue. Thus, the revenue results become the explanation for the expense variance. Table 4.1 shows an example of a budget variance report with favorable and unfavorable variances and explanations.

Some variances occur because activity occurred in a particular month but was budgeted for a different month. For example, a new employee was budgeted to start in February but was not actually hired until March. This favorable

Table 4.1   Budget variance report—favorable and unfavorable variances

	March Actual	March Budget	YTD Actual	YTD Budget	March Variance	YTD Variance
Salaries	$230,000	$240,000	$710,000	$720,000	$10,000	$10,000
Benefits	$80,000	$82,000	$236,000	$238,000	$2,000	$2,000

In this report, there is a favorable variance in the March Actual Salaries and Benefits. This variance is also reflected in the year to date (YTD) columns. The manager will have to identify and explain the variances.

Example Explanation: *The favorable variance in March and YTD Salaries and Benefits is the result of the unanticipated resignation of the coding manager at the end of February.*

expense variance in February is a **permanent variance,** because the salary and benefits expense budgeted in February will never actually be spent. This permanent variance will be reported on every monthly variance report for the rest of the year if it exceeds the stated threshold. Other timing differences may be **temporary variances.** For example, an outpatient service department budgeted for 300 visits in March and 250 visits in April. The actual visits in March were 270 and in April were 304. Both variances are temporary. The surge in visits expected in March did not occur until April. March's unfavorable variance was therefore offset by April's favorable variance, as illustrated in table 4.2. Although the department manager may not know for sure on April 1 that the variance will resolve, the budget variance reports are frequently not distributed until after the financial month-end close—often midmonth—at which point the April surge would likely be at least projected.

If the variance is expected to resolve before the end of the fiscal year, then it is temporary. Otherwise, it is a permanent variance. A variance may be explained as temporary in October, but it becomes permanent if not resolved by the end of the fiscal year in December. So, the explanation changes as the actual results become known. Some variances offset each other, as illustrated previously. Another example of an offsetting variance is the use of a contracted employee to fill a vacant position during the hiring process. If a coder resigns effective March 1, the salary and benefits budget line will have a favorable variance at the end of March. However, the contracted services line will have an offsetting unfavorable variance. There may not have been any budget for contracted coding services in March at all. The two variances offset each other and the difference is permanent. Table 4.3 shows these offsetting variances.

Table 4.2   Budget variance report—permanent and temporary variances

	March Actual	March Budget	YTD Actual	YTD Budget	March Variance	YTD Variance
Salaries	$230,000	$240,000	$710,000	$720,000	$10,000	$10,000
Benefits	$80,000	$82,000	$236,000	$238,000	$2,000	$2,000
Supplies	$2,000	$4,000	$6,000	$8,000	$2,000	$2,000

In this report, the Supplies line has a favorable variance, but not the same type of variance seen in Salaries and Benefits.

Example Explanation: *The favorable variance in March and YTD Salaries and Benefits is the result of the unanticipated resignation of the coding manager at the end of February. This is a permanent variance in Salaries and Benefits. The favorable variance in March and YTD Supplies is the result of a timing difference in purchasing folders. The folders budgeted for March were not purchased until April. This is a temporary variance that will resolve in April.*

Table 4.3   Budget variance report—offsetting variances in the same month

	March Actual	March Budget	YTD Actual	YTD Budget	March Variance	YTD Variance
Salaries	$230,000	$240,000	$710,000	$720,000	$10,000	$10,000
Benefits	$80,000	$82,000	$236,000	$238,000	$2,000	$2,000
Contract services	$13,000	—	$13,000	—	($13,000)	($13,000)

In this report, there is a favorable variance in the March Actual Salaries and Benefits. This variance is also reflected in the YTD columns. There is also an unfavorable variance in Contract services. The manager will have to identify and explain the variances.

Example Explanation: *The favorable variance in March and YTD Salaries and Benefits is the result of the unanticipated resignation of the coding manager at the end of February. This is a permanent variance in Salaries and Benefits. The unfavorable variance in March and YTD Contract services is for the temporary staffing of the coding manager position. This unfavorable variance is permanent and is expected to increase until a replacement coding manager is hired. This unfavorable variance is partially offset by the permanent, favorable variances in Salaries and Benefits.*

Types of Budgets

Financial budgets can be developed in different ways, depending on the needs of the organization. A department with a well-established function and clearly identified goals may have little change in its budget from year to year. A new department or new project would have no historical information from which to create a budget and would have to depend on projections and other estimates. Thus, the type of budget used can vary even within an organization. Common types of budgets include the following:

- Traditional budget, with target percentage increases or decreases for the coming year
- Flexible budget, which varies depending on the actual volume experienced
- Zero-based budget, assuming that the service or department must justify its benefit with every budget cycle

Traditional

A **traditional budget** model is one in which the department is given a projected increase or decrease in expected revenue or expenses for the coming year, usually expressed as a percentage. This **top-down** process (flowing from the executive level down to the department or function) forces departments to conform their budgets to the executive team's expectations. While this may be a reasonable approach financially, it does have the potential to stifle creativity and to misallocate resources. For example, suppose all departments are given a target 3 percent increase in expenses. If the radiology department is experiencing a 5 percent increase in supply expenses, it will have to cut other expenses, perhaps salaries, in order to make up the difference. In that same organization, the HIM department might be rejoicing because it has just completed a system upgrade that will reduce expenses by 1 percent, thus giving it an actual increase of 4 percent.

A variation on the traditional budget model is a **bottom-up** approach. In this model, the department would develop its budget based on its own known contractual obligations and expectations. It would also include any new service lines or projects that it proposed undertaking. The departmental budgets would then be used to build the overall organizational budget. In reviewing such a budget proposal, the executive team reaps the benefit of the creativity and deep understanding of its management team and can choose to allocate resources with better information.

A traditional budget is fixed. The total expected revenue and expenses are the threshold against which the manager's performance is measured. Any variance in results would have to be explained, usually monthly. In departments whose financial results are tied to volume, a flexible budget may be more useful.

Flexible

A **flexible budget** varies with the volume experienced by the department. For example, if volume is 300 cases per month, the expenses will be $9,000; if volume is 350 cases, the expenses will be $10,500. Flexible budgeting is useful when the expenses are directly tied to volume. If expenses lag or precede volume, this method is not as useful. In the HIM department, expenses lag volume. In March, the census may be 250 patients per day, creating high volume for nursing and ancillary departments. However, as those patients are discharged and census is reduced, the volume shifts to HIM. Therefore, measurement of volume indicated from census or admissions is not as useful a predictor of resource utilization for HIM as measurement of volume by discharges. Over time, during the budget period such anomalies would offset each other, but the explanation of budget variance each month is time consuming.

Zero-Based

A **zero-based budget** is used for new projects and for service lines or projects that must be evaluated for continued existence. The budget does not begin with historical budget line evaluations. Rather, it begins with the evaluation of the success of the service line or project, whether it is meeting its goals and objectives, and a consideration of whether the service line or project continues to serve its purpose. This budget method is most appropriate for organizations whose work revolves around specific projects, such as charitable organizations, foundations, and professional associations. Zero-based budgeting may be applied simultaneously throughout the organization or periodically to individual projects or service lines.

Revenue Budget Development

The revenue budget inherently drives the rest of the operating budget. Realistic revenue expectations need to be matched with relevant expenses in order to arrive at an achievable goal. Revenue expectations consider volume and pricing.

Volume

Volume estimates for budget calculations are a function of existing market share and any projected increase or decrease due to external forces and changes in organizational priorities. For example, a physical therapy department may observe that its historical volume has remained static for the past two years, representing 35 percent of the existing market. The department manager has observed that a freestanding physical therapy facility is being opened within the catchment area. The new facility may have a direct impact on the current market share. The department manager must evaluate whether a significant decrease in market share is to be expected or whether the new facility will draw patients from a different pool.

Some departments, such as a clinic, would measure volume in terms of number of visits. The historical number of visits is known. There are also limitations on how many visits could be performed within the existing facility and with current staffing.

Other departments, such as laboratory and radiology, would estimate volume based on the procedures. As with estimating visits, the historical number of diagnostic and therapeutic procedures is known and the limitations of equipment, facility, and staffing alert management to potential overestimation of volume.

Other facility-specific factors may be involved in the estimation of volume, such as administration's service-line-specific growth targets. For example, leadership may decide that there is a need for increased pediatric services in the catchment area. In order to attract parents to expanded pediatric services, leadership may determine that expansion of neonatal/obstetrical services is required. Therefore, despite a 4 percent overall growth estimate, leadership may specify that neonatal and obstetrical services should grow 10 percent. Because growth is driven by many factors, there may be marketing as well as capital budget requirements to achieve and sustain desired growth.

Payer Mix

Payer mix is the percentage that each payer or type of payer contributes to the provider's total. This percentage can be calculated on total volume, gross charges, or expected reimbursement, for example. Payer mix will vary by service. Obstetrics will likely have a low volume of Medicare patients, whereas the volume of Medicare patients in geriatrics will be high. Payer mix is important in determining pricing.

Pricing

Once volume is determined, the pricing of services will play a role in determining revenue. Total revenue is the number of units times the price of the goods or services. Total revenue is then reduced by the discount negotiated with or imposed by specific payers to arrive at revenue, net of contractual allowance (see chapter 2). Prices, generally referred to as **charges,** are determined by a number of factors, not all of which relate to the underlying **cost** of providing the services.

Historical pricing involves increasing the existing price by a certain percentage. This increase may be in response to the rising prices of supplies or to inflation (see chapter 7). Price increases may be for all goods and services or they may target certain service lines. For new services or for services whose underlying costs have changed disproportionately, the price may be marked up a certain percentage over cost.

Pricing must also take reimbursement into consideration. For example, if the hospital has a contract with a payer that reimburses at 80 percent of charges and the hospital has priced services at a markup of 10 percent over cost, the hospital will lose money on every case. Further, the variation in pricing methodologies among multiple payers requires the hospital to consider the payer mix in determining pricing. Since hospitals must charge all payers the same price for services, but payers can negotiate for discounts, the rate and

Table 4.4   Impact of reimbursement methodologies on pricing

Lab Test			
Payer	Reimbursement Rate	Volume	Total Reimbursement
Medicare	$65.00	500	$32,500.00
Big managed care company	85% of charges	300	$23,314.65
Small managed care company	95% of charges	100	$8,685.85
Medicaid	$45.00	50	$2,240.00
Uncompensated care	$5.00	50	$250.00
Cost of lab test	$67.00	1,000	($67,000.00)
Price (charge)	$91.43		$0.50

In this example, the total cost of providing this lab test to 1,000 patients is $67,000. The Medicare and Medicaid reimbursement is known ($34,740), and the uncompensated care amount is estimated at $250.

In order to break even (reimbursement = cost) on this test, the price of the test must be $91.43.

complexity of discounts must be taken into consideration in the pricing structure. Table 4.4 illustrates this calculation.

Case-Mix Index

Case-mix index is the average weight of the diagnosis-related groups (DRGs) assigned to all of the cases in the period under review. It is used primarily in review of DRG-based payers to estimate reimbursement and to track and trend that reimbursement; however, it can also be used to track and trend the resource utilization of cases associated with non-DRG-based reimbursement. For budgetary purposes, trending changes in case mix can be used to predict the impact of a particular payer on revenue and expenses. For example, if the case-mix index for a particular payer is increasing but the volume is stable, the implied increase in intensity of services required by that payer's patients would necessitate a review of costs associated with those cases. Chapter 6 discusses contracts in detail.

The Medicare Inpatient Prospective Payment System (IPPS) is based on the Medicare Severity Diagnostic Related Group (MS-DRG) variation of DRGs. Reimbursement from Medicare can be projected by multiplying the target case-mix index by the hospital's blended rate, then by the projected volume (see figure 4.3). The blended rate is a composite of all the components of the IPPS payment to the hospital, including the cost-based rate, capital costs, regional variation, and graduate medical education. Other DRG-based payers may use DRGs to define a fee schedule. Rather than a case mix, then, a weighted average of the fees at predicted volumes per DRG would be used to predict the revenue from that payer.

Figure 4.3   Valuation of projected Medicare revenue—stroke program

MS-DRG	Description	Weight	Projected Volume	Weighted Volume
061	ACUTE ISCHEMIC STROKE W USE OF THROMBOLYTIC AGENT W MCC	2.9568	10	29.6
062	ACUTE ISCHEMIC STROKE W USE OF THROMBOLYTIC AGENT W CC	1.9479	150	292.2
063	ACUTE ISCHEMIC STROKE W USE OF THROMBOLYTIC AGENT W/O CC/MCC	1.5251	75	114.4
064	INTRACRANIAL HEMORRHAGE OR CEREBRAL INFARCTION W MCC	1.8674	12	22.4
065	INTRACRANIAL HEMORRHAGE OR CEREBRAL INFARCTION W CC	1.1667	130	151.7
066	INTRACRANIAL HEMORRHAGE OR CEREBRAL INFARCTION W/O CC/MCC	0.8198	60	49.2
067	NONSPECIFIC CVA & PRECEREBRAL OCCLUSION W/O INFARCT W MCC	1.4231	15	21.3
068	NONSPECIFIC CVA & PRECEREBRAL OCCLUSION W/O INFARCT W/O MCC	0.8751	40	35.0
069	TRANSIENT ISCHEMIA	0.7311	55	40.2
	Totals		547	756.0
	Case-mix index			1.3820
	Blended rate			$6,576.00
	Projected revenue			$4,971,219.44

Projected revenue = case-mix index × blended rate × total volume

Source: FY 2011 FR Table 5 Weights, Inpatient Prospective Payment System, Center for Medicare and Medicaid Services, July 8, 2010.

Reimbursement from non-DRG-based payers can be estimated based on the contracted rate for the services included in the contract, multiplied by the predicted volume.

Market Share

Many factors affect the market share enjoyed by a particular organization. Reputation, services, accessibility, and quality are some of those factors. For healthcare providers, the payment source is an increasingly important factor. If a provider does not have a contract with a particular payer, then patients insured by that payer are likely to seek services elsewhere.

The historical market share can be estimated by reviewing census and publicly available coded data for the hospital's catchment area. If vital statistics data indicate that there were 2,500 births in the area in a particular year and the hospital admitted 1,250 newborns, then the hospital can estimate a 50 percent market share. Much of this type of data is somewhat aged, sometimes by a number of years. Therefore, estimates may be inferred from related data. For example, looking at the population of women between the ages of 18 and 40, there may be a consistent relationship between the number of newborns and this population. Alternatively, there may have been an increase or decline in the general population of the area in recent years. Depending on the age stratification of the general population, one might infer an increase or decrease in a particular service, such as geriatrics.

Another way of looking at potential market share is to observe the competition. If the hospital offers bariatric surgery and the nearest competitor is 200 miles away, the hospital may infer a high market share in the catchment area. A hospital surrounded by independent imaging centers will have significant competition. Budgeting for significant growth of outpatient imaging services in such a highly competitive environment would not be realistic.

Potential market share is also a consideration in budgeting for new service lines. For example, a hospital that has a small inpatient rehabilitation department that primarily serves its orthopedic surgery patients may want to expand into offering outpatient rehabilitation services. Some considerations would include whether the hospital is losing surgery cases to nearby hospitals that offer outpatient rehabilitation, the availability of outpatient rehabilitation services in the hospital's catchment area, and the volume of cases that could be attracted independent of the postsurgical referrals.

Impact of Unreimbursed Services

Unreimbursed services consist of uncompensated (also known as charity) care, bad debt, and denials. Unreimbursed services must be considered in the operating budget as a reduction of total revenue.

Uncompensated care refers to the treatment of patients with no ability to pay but who have filed the appropriate applications to enable the provider to obtain payment from a state government source. State funding of uncompensated care varies and is not automatic. The funds must be available in the state's budget and the hospital must report its services according to state guidelines.

Bad debt refers to accounts receivable that will not be collected. The older the receivable, the less likely it is to be collected. Therefore, hospitals monitor aged receivables and collection activities closely. For financial statement purposes, bad debt is typically expensed periodically in order to accurately reflect the portion of reported revenue that will not be received and to avoid the variations in net income produced by writing off bad debt only when accounts become uncollectible.

Denials are refusals by the payer to reimburse for all or part of the services provided to a patient. The reasons for denials are numerous and include technical denials for failure to obtain preauthorization, lack of medical necessity for the service, and noncovered services. Although denials can be appealed, some percentage of them will ultimately be unreimbursed.

In general, the unreimbursed services would be estimated at the administrative level as an aggregate reduction in total budgeted revenue. However, department managers should be aware of these issues and their impact on revenue.

Cost of Producing Revenue

Up until now, we have been speaking in financial accounting terms. In financial accounting, an expense reflects the purchase of resources and is typically compared to the underlying revenue that was generated using those resources.

Cost, on the other hand, is a term that relates to the relationship between goods and services and the specific expenditures that contribute to producing them. In manufacturing or retail, we might refer in the income statement to cost of goods sold, reflecting the matching of various expenditures directly related to items that were sold during the period. To a healthcare provider, in a sense, cost of goods sold is reflected in the expenses charged against patient services revenue to derive net patient services revenue. However, those are aggregate numbers. In other words, they are all added together. But how does the provider know for sure which expenses to assign to patient service and which are unrelated? For that matter, how does a provider know that delivering a particular service will result in positive net revenue? It is through the identification and analysis of costs that these questions can be answered.

Think about an ice cream vendor. What should the price be for an ice cream cone? We know the wholesale price of the ice cream and the cones. But what about the refrigeration? Transportation to and from the sales site? The vendor's time? Carry that thinking forward into the acute care setting. How much does it cost the hospital to deliver room, board, and nursing care to a patient for one day? Clearly, some methodology must be developed in order to measure the components of those services and allocate them appropriately to patient care. Services like housekeeping and medical records are examples of costs that must be allocated.

If we know and understand the components of costs to deliver services, then we can exert control over those costs as much as possible. In an environment in which payers tend to dictate reimbursement, controlling costs is sometimes a provider's best tool for maintaining fiscal integrity. So, if the components of a surgical procedure (implants, for example) cost the hospital $15,000 and payers reimburse $12,000 for the procedure, then the hospital knows that it must negotiate with its vendors to lower costs or it will lose money on every case. A simplistic example, but a very real concern.

Expense versus Cost

Expense is a financial accounting term that refers to the use of resources that support the revenue earned during a period. Salaries, utilities, and depreciation are examples of expenses. Expenses reduce revenue on the statement of revenue and expenses (income statement) to arrive at net revenue, which contributes to retained earnings or fund balance. Cost is a managerial accounting term that expresses the specific resources used to produce a particular product or service.

Expenses are recognized in the financial statements when the resources are used. There is an actual journal entry that debits an expense account and credits another account, such as cash, inventory, accrued depreciation, or accounts payable. Table 4.5 illustrates this process.

Costs are not represented on financial statements, per se, because they are not transactions. For example, receipt of an invoice from the telephone company is an expense. When the invoice is received, a journal entry is made to debit

Table 4.5   Expenses versus costs

Financial Statement—Expenses		Management Reporting—Actual				
		Patient Care	HIM	Admin	Housekeeping	Facilities
Salaries & benefits	$225,000	$115,000	$25,000	$40,000	$20,000	$25,000
Contract services	$12,000	$6,000	$4,000	$1,000	—	$1,000
Telephone	$10,000	$8,000	$500	$500	$500	$500
Electricity	$45,000	$35,000	$5,000	$500	$200	$4,300
Office supplies	$2,000	$200	$1,000	$400	$200	$200
Medical devices	$100,000	$100,000	—	—	—	—
Total expenses	$394,000	$264,200	$35,500	$42,400	$20,900	$31,000
Expenses refer to financial accounting; costs refer to managerial accounting.						

telephone expense and credit accounts payable. When the invoice is paid, another entry is made to debit accounts payable and credit cash. In this manner, the telephone expense is reported in the correct period against revenue earned in that period, even though it is paid in a different period. However, the amount of the telephone bill also represents a cost to the departments that used the telephone in that period. There is no journal entry that expresses the departmental cost. That is why a managerial accounting system is needed: to identify which departments or other responsible area actually used the resource.

Cost Characteristics

Costs associated with a service can be expressed in terms of a variety of different characteristics. These characteristics determine which costs are to be included in the determination of the budget and against which management performance will be measured. Key characteristics of cost are **traceability, variability,** and **controllability.**

The cost characteristic of traceability refers to whether the cost is directly or indirectly traceable to the service. For example, pharmaceuticals administered to the patient are directly attributable to that patient's services. The reagents used in the laboratory to perform a test are directly attributable to that test.

Cost variability is expressed as the tendency of the cost to change with volume. A cost that does not change with volume is a fixed cost. An example of a fixed cost is the salary of an exempt staff person. Regardless of how many hours the person works or how much work the person accomplishes, the salary remains the same.

Whether a cost is fixed or variable has an impact on budget. For example, the contract price on an encoder used by the coders in an HIM department is typically a fixed cost. Regardless of the volume of cases processed during the contract period, the overall cost of encoding records will not change. However, the *per-unit* cost of processing decreases in a fixed cost when the volume increases.

Another characteristic of cost is controllability. The cost of heating and cooling the hospital is not generally within the control of the department manager. However, the cost of supplies is somewhat controllable. For example, the cost of copy paper—how much the hospital pays for a case of paper—is not typically negotiated by the individual departments. Also, the service-related use of the paper is tied to volume: the number of copies made for release of information, for example. The controllable portion of the cost is waste. Are unnecessary copies being made? Are other departments using the copier? Are individuals using the copier for personal reasons?

Cost Allocation

Determining the direct costs of treating a patient is fairly straightforward. The pharmaceutical administered to the patient can be traced to the invoice for the drug when it was purchased by the hospital. Similarly, the cost of individual supplies such as IV lines can be identified. However, it is not as easy or straightforward to determine the cost of cleaning a patient room, processing a medical record, or providing air-conditioning and light to the patient. These **overhead** costs are associated with delivering patient care but are not easily attributable to individual patient services.

Overhead costs not only are attributable to patient care but also are associated with other overhead areas. For example, housekeeping cleans patient rooms but also cleans the HIM department, administrative offices, and the housekeeping offices themselves. Identifying and associating all of the costs involved in providing services yields the most accurate calculation of net revenue from providing a particular service.

Not only must the costs themselves be identified, but the method of associating or allocating those costs must be determined. One could certainly follow a housekeeper around, doing time and motion studies and measuring cleaning products used. While that may be a strategy in the housekeeping department to identify process improvements and cost control opportunities, it is not practical for cost **allocation.**

For the purpose of cost allocation, each overhead department cost must be allocated according to a method that best serves the intention of the allocation. So, for the allocation of housekeeping costs, there are several choices: square footage and head count are two examples. Housekeeping costs may be allocated to the entire facility based on the square footage of facility space that is being cleaned. Another calculation might be the number of individuals working or being treated in the area being cleaned. The organization will choose the method of allocation that makes the most sense for its purposes.

Direct Method

The **direct method allocation** of cost is the simplest and also the least accurate. In this method, all overhead (non-patient-service) costs are distributed across all revenue-producing cost centers, according to the predetermined percentage described previously (see table 4.6, section A). In some small organizations or organizations with few staff on site, this may be an effective method of allocating costs. However, it is not appropriate for Medicare cost reporting and does not take into account the services provided to other non-revenue-producing departments.

Step-Down

Once the allocation strategy has been identified for each overhead department, the **step-down allocation** starts with the department that allocates to the greatest number of different other areas and works down to the revenue-producing areas, which likely do not need to be allocated to other departments (see table 4.6, section B). The advantage of this method is simplicity. It can be calculated in a simple spreadsheet and is easy to understand. This method is used for Medicare cost reporting. Step-down allocation does take into consideration the services of some overhead departments to each other. However, the calculation goes only from left to right and does not factor overhead contribution to earlier allocated departments. In the example in table 4.6, section B, note that administration allocates to housekeeping, but housekeeping does not allocate to administration. Further, if administration has not already absorbed all of the costs associated with it, then the allocation of housekeeping costs is not accurate. Administration may allocate based on personnel, but housekeeping may allocate based on square footage. Therefore, an additional calculation is necessary in order to allocate overhead more comprehensively.

Double Step-Down

The **double step-down allocation** method resolves the obvious problem identified in step-down allocation. The first step-down is performed in both directions, as illustrated in section C of table 4.6. This allocates costs to the departments on the right but also back to the departments on the left. After the first step-down, there are residual amounts left in all overhead departments. Thus, a second step-down is required in order to allocate out the residual amounts. Double step-down is still a fairly simple method of calculation. Once the methodology of allocation has been identified, the calculation can be laid out in a spreadsheet. Although somewhat tedious, it could also be done by hand if necessary. Although double step-down does at least partially resolve the issue of allocation of costs among overhead departments, it does not fully take into consideration all possible allocations, since the process is performed only twice. In other words, the first step-down goes in both directions, but the second step-down goes only from left to right. So there is still some further accuracy that could be obtained allocating in both directions more than once.

Table 4.6   Cost allocation

BASIS *Allocation of overhead costs*	Admin	HIM	Housekeeping	Facilities	Pharmacy	Lab	Radiology	Inpatient	Outpatient	
Admin	0%	10%	10%	15%	10%	10%	10%	20%	15%	100%
HIM	0%	0%	0%	0%	5%	5%	5%	65%	20%	100%
Housekeeping	10%	10%	0%	10%	10%	10%	10%	25%	15%	100%
Facilities	10%	5%	5%	0%	15%	15%	15%	20%	15%	100%

A *Direct method*	Admin	HIM	Housekeeping	Facilities	Pharmacy	Lab	Radiology	Inpatient	Outpatient	
Overhead	$35,500	$42,400	$20,900	$31,000						$129,800
Admin					$5,462	$5,462	$5,462	$10,923	$8,192	
HIM					$2,120	$2,120	$2,120	$27,560	$8,480	
Housekeeping					$2,986	$2,986	$2,986	$7,464	$4,479	
Facilities					$5,813	$5,813	$5,813	$7,750	$5,813	
Net effect					$16,380	$16,380	$16,380	$53,697	$26,963	$129,800

Column totals may reflect rounding of decimal places.

Table 4.6 Cost allocation *(continued)*

B Step-down method

	Admin	HIM	Housekeeping	Facilities	Pharmacy	Lab	Radiology	Inpatient	Outpatient	
Overhead	$35,500	$42,400	$20,900	$31,000						$129,800
Admin		$3,550	$3,550	$5,325	$3,550	$3,550	$3,550	$7,100	$5,325	
HIM			$0	$0	$2,298	$2,298	$2,298	$29,868	$9,190	
Housekeeping				$3,056	$3,056	$3,056	$3,056	$7,641	$4,584	
Facilities					$7,384	$7,384	$7,384	$9,845	$7,384	
Step-down allocation					$16,288	$16,288	$16,288	$54,453	$26,483	$129,800

C Double step-down method

First Step-Down	Admin	HIM	Housekeeping	Facilities	Pharmacy	Lab	Radiology	Inpatient	Outpatient	
Overhead	$35,500	$42,400	$20,900	$31,000						$129,800
Admin		$3,550	$3,550	$5,325	$3,550	$3,550	$3,550	$7,100	$5,325	
HIM	$0		$0	$0	$2,298	$2,298	$2,298	$29,868	$9,190	
Housekeeping	$2,445	$2,445		$2,445	$2,445	$2,445	$2,445	$6,113	$3,668	
Facilities	$3,877	$1,939	$1,939		$5,816	$5,816	$5,816	$7,754	$5,816	
First step-down	$6,322	$4,384	$1,939	$0	$14,108	$14,108	$14,108	$50,834	$23,998	$129,800

Second Step-Down	Admin	HIM	Housekeeping	Facilities	Pharmacy	Lab	Radiology	Inpatient	Outpatient	
Residual overhead	$6,322	$4,384	$1,939	$0	$14,108	$14,108	$14,108	$50,834	$23,998	$129,800
Admin		$632	$632	$948	$632	$632	$632	$1,264	$948	
HIM			$0	$0	$251	$251	$251	$3,260	$1,003	
Housekeeping				$321	$321	$321	$321	$803	$482	
Facilities					$238	$238	$238	$317	$238	
Second step-down					$15,550	$15,550	$15,550	$56,479	$26,670	$129,800

Column totals may reflect rounding of decimal places.

Labor Costs

On its financial statements, a hospital's largest single expense is human resources. Some labor costs are fixed, such as accounting and information technology. Management costs are also fixed. These fixed costs are controllable by wage levels and total staffing, but there are levels of expertise required for these positions that support the price paid for the services. Some departments have both fixed and variable labor costs. For example, in a full-service hospital, laboratory and pharmacy likely require 24-hour staffing in order to support the needs of the emergency department and unexpected inpatient demand. However, the daily staffing of the departments varies by volume. If census is low, there is no value in maintaining a staff complement on site that has no work to do.

Department managers are expected to control labor costs. One way to do that is to use a mix of labor that enables the department to flex up in times of high volume and down with low volume. Department-level evaluation of staffing needs can be accomplished through time-and-motion analysis of tasks and by **benchmarking.** Benchmarking is the comparison of the department with peer facilities and professional best practices.

Since the actual number of employees varies between facilities, one way to compare is by using the number of full-time equivalents (FTEs). Full-time employees are expected to work a set number of hours in a period. The organization decides the specific number of hours, generally ranging from 35 hours per week (7 hours per day) to 40 hours per week (8 hours per day). The total number of hours worked by all employees, divided by the normal hours in a workweek, yields the number of FTEs. Table 4.7 illustrates the comparison between two facilities. Note that City Hospital has more employees but fewer FTEs than Community Hospital.

Full-Time Employees

Full-time employees may be **exempt** or **nonexempt.** Exempt employees are paid a set salary. They are expected to work the set hours but are not paid for additional hours worked—nor are they paid less if they work fewer hours in a particular pay period. The advantage to the employer of exempt employees is that there is no additional salary expense if the employee works extra hours to complete a project. The advantage to the employee is that time-shifting and working at home are often allowed. Exempt employees are typically managerial or supervisory personnel and some professional personnel.

Table 4.7 Total number of employees and FTEs

Community Hospital HIM Department Staffing Standard Week = 40 hours		City Hospital HIM Department Staffing Standard Week = 35 hours	
	Hours per Week		Hours per Week
Director	40	Director	35
Coding Manager	40	Coding Manager	35
Coder 1	40	Coder 1	35
Coder 2	40	Coder 2	35
Coder 3	40	Coder 3	35
Coder 4	40	Coder 4	20
Coder 5	40	Coder 5	20
Coder 6	7	Coder 6	10
Coder 7	5	Coder 7	5
Coder 8	8	Coder 8	10
Data Quality Analyst	40	Data Quality Analyst	35
Release of Information Supervisor	40	Release of Information Supervisor	35
ROI Clerk 1	40	ROI Clerk 1	35
ROI Clerk 2	40	ROI Clerk 2	20
Analyst 1	40	Analyst 1	35
Analyst 2	40	Analyst 2	35
Analyst 3	40	Analyst 3	20
Analyst 4	20	Analyst 4	20
File Clerk 1	40	File Clerk 1	20
File Clerk 2	20	File Clerk 2	20
File Clerk 3	20	File Clerk 3	20
Evening Supervisor	40	File Clerk 4	20
		File Clerk 5	10
		File Clerk 6	10
		Evening Supervisor	35
Number of employees	22	Number of employees	25
Number of full-time equivalents	18.00	Number of full-time equivalents	17.43

Nonexempt employees are paid at a specified rate for work performed, generally hourly. Hours worked are paid at that rate. Hours not worked are either not reimbursed or count toward paid time off. Nonexempt employees who work in excess of the set number of full-time hours are compensated in excess of their specified rate: typically, time and a half for overtime and holidays. Some organizations may pay double or triple time in certain circumstances.

When budgeting for full-time employees, both salaries and benefits must be taken into consideration. Further, historical use of overtime should be included in the subsequent operating budget. Excessive use of overtime is one way that additional staff can be justified. For example, it may be less expensive to hire an additional employee if the current staff is routinely working overtime. Table 4.8 illustrates this calculation.

Part-Time Employees

Part-time employees work less than the set number of full-time hours. They may be eligible to participate in benefits programs, including health insurance

Table 4.8   Justifying an additional employee based on historical use of overtime

	Normal Hours	Average Overtime per Week	Gross Paid Hours
Full-time staff			
Coder 1	40	4	46
Coder 2	40	3	44.5
Coder 3	40	1.5	42.25
Coder 4	40	6	49
Coder 5	40	0	40
	200		
Per diem staff			
Coder 6	7		7
Coder 7	5		5
Coder 8	8		8
	20		
Total paid hours			241.75
Coding FTEs	5.5		6.04

In this example, the number of FTEs based on normal hours is 5.5, not enough to justify hiring another full-time coder. However, when taking the overtime hours into consideration, it may be cost-effective to hire an additional full-time coder and save the per diems for vacation coverage. The actual cost of the per diem coders should also be taken into consideration.

and paid time off. Their eligibility to participate in benefits programs is typically pro-rated—at some percentage of the full-time employee rate. Part-time employees may occasionally work a full-time schedule and may occasionally earn overtime; however, such instances should be rare.

Since part-time employees are paid for all hours worked and should not work beyond that on a regular basis, budgeting for them is based on their guaranteed hours.

Per Diem Employees

Per diem employees work on demand. They are paid at a specified rate for the number of hours worked. They may work overtime. Per diem employees may be hired on a temporary or permanent basis. However, they should not be used for long periods of time at full-time hours as their per diem status is questionable in that circumstance.

The advantage of per diem employees is that they are used only when the volume of work requires. Thus, they are brought in and dismissed to match the needs of the organization. The disadvantage of per diem employees is that they are not always available on demand or on short notice, particularly if they have other employers.

Since per diem hours are by definition uncertain, historical usage is one way to budget for these employees. Examination of historical usage may reveal that per diems are used only for vacation coverage or for projects. So, calculation of estimated vacation coverage and upcoming project needs would assist in the budget process.

Contracted Workers

Contracted workers are not employees of the organization. They are independent workers who offer their services to many organizations. They may be self-employed or they may work for an agency. In the latter case, the organization contracts with the agency, not with the individual worker.

Budgeting for contracted workers depends on how they are used. They may work full-time, part-time, or per diem. So, the budget for these workers is based on historical usage. Again, excessive use of contracted workers could help to justify additional employee staff.

The main advantage of contracted workers is that they are easily terminated. There is generally no guarantee of hours. If working with an agency, an unsatisfactory worker could be replaced upon request. The disadvantage is that they tend to be relatively expensive, because their rates include the contractor's overhead, transportation, and supplies. Care must be taken to ensure that individually contracted workers are, in fact, independent. The IRS has specific guidelines to test the employment status of independent contractors (see figure 4.4).

Needs Assessment

Benchmarking yields the standard or best practices labor levels. However, there are other factors to consider in the evaluation of workforce needs. Variations in volume, service standards, environment, and labor pool are some of the considerations.

Figure 4.4   IRS guidelines for independent contractor status

Behavioral Control   Behavioral control refers to facts that show whether there is a right to direct or control how the worker does the work. A worker is an employee when the business has the right to direct and control the worker. The business does not have to actually direct or control the way the work is done—as long as the employer has the right to direct and control the work.   The behavioral control factors fall into the categories of: • Type of instructions given   • Degree of instruction   • Evaluation systems   • Training
Financial Control   Financial control refers to facts that show whether or not the business has the right to control the economic aspects of the worker's job.   The financial control factors fall into the categories of: • Significant investment   • Unreimbursed expenses   • Opportunity for profit or loss   • Services available to the market   • Method of payment
Type of Relationship   Type of relationship refers to facts that show how the worker and business perceive their relationship to each other.   The factors, for the type of relationship between two parties, generally fall into the categories of: • Written contracts   • Employee benefits   • Permanency of the relationship   • Services provided as key activity of the business

Source: Independent Contractor (Self-Employed) or Employee? Internal Revenue Service. http://www.irs.gov/businesses/small/article/0,,id=99921,00.html.

Volume

The first issue in determining the labor levels is the volume of work. Volume in a patient service area might be visits or census. To the laboratory, volume is the number of specific tests performed. To the HIM department, it is the number of discharges from specific service areas. Based on productivity standards for specific work, the number of FTEs can be calculated.

Service Standards

The service standards—quality and volume—make up the productivity requirements for the work. Factors that affect productivity include the type of equipment used as well as the computerization of the function. What are the productivity requirements? Equipment availability? Computerization of the function?

The qualifications and requirements for different categories of the same work may be different. In the radiology department, a CT scan requires different technical skills than a simple X-ray. The length of time it takes to perform a CT scan is also different. Further, the workforce used to perform the exams may not be interchangeable. Similarly, an outpatient coder cannot necessarily be used to code inpatient records and vice versa.

Thus, budget must be calculated based on productivity standards for the specific workforce and activity. The inpatient needs will be calculated differently from the outpatient needs. Table 4.9 illustrates the application of productivity requirements to the required FTE calculation.

Environment

Although volume and productivity are the key drivers of the FTE budget, there are additional considerations that have budget implications. Education of coders is easily accomplished if they all commute to the facility. However, what are the organizational requirements if there are multiple locations? If travel is to be reimbursed, then that must be included in the budget. If telecommuters are in remote locations, teleconferencing costs must be included. Further, the costs of computer maintenance and telecommunications must be included in the budget.

Labor Pool

Another factor that impacts budget is the **labor pool** itself. Are workers scarce or plentiful? Is the organization willing to share labor with other facilities in the area? Workforce shortages can drive up salaries and make filling vacancies

Table 4.9   Impact of productivity on budgeted workforce

	Gross Paid Hours	Charts Coded per Week	Type of Charts	Average Charts per Hour
Full-time staff				
Coder 1	46	125	IP	2.7
Coder 2	44.5	200	Amb Surgery	4.5
Coder 3	27.25	375	ED	13.8
	15	25	IP	1.7
Coder 4	32	325	ED	10.2
	17	20	IP	1.2
Coder 5	40	425	Outpatient	10.6
Per diem staff				
Coder 6	7	150	ED	21.4
Coder 7	5	15	Amb Surgery	3.0
Coder 8	8	60	IP	7.5

In this view of the coding staff, the case for hiring an additional full-time coder is not as clear. Over 30% of the inpatient cases are coded by a per diem. Further, the full-time ED coders work at half the pace of the per diem. Factoring in volume productivity, therefore, is important when attempting to justify an increase in budget for human resources.

difficult. Similarly, replacement workers in a plentiful workforce may be comparatively inexpensive.

Labor Mix Issues

The determination of what mix of full-time, part-time, per diem, and contract workers is needed in a particular area is generally the responsibility of the department manager. Based solely on cost, per diem workers may be the least expensive alternative. However, most departments cannot run effectively or efficiently with solely per diem workers. Other factors to consider are consistency, reliability, training, and data quality.

Consistency

All departments provide service in one way or another: to patients, to other departments, or both. In order to provide service at expected levels of quality—consistent performance—the labor pool must be stable. Policies and procedures regarding the provision of services must be followed accurately in order to maintain compliance with organizational rules as well as regulatory and accreditation rules, guidelines, and standards.

While per diem staff may be inexpensive, they cannot be used routinely for long periods of time. Many organizations use per diems for high-volume coverage times and coverage of vacation or periodic staffing situations. For example, the HIM department may use per diems for vacation coverage or periodically for purging of paper records. Cardiology may use per diems for weekend coverage of unscheduled procedures.

Reliability

To ensure the smooth operation of a department, staffing at expected levels must be maintained. Depending on the needs of the department, the ability to flex up or down in staffing will vary. Nursing may contract with an agency that can provide coverage immediately in the event of unexpected staffing shortages and surges in census. On the other hand, the HIM department may not be able to flex quickly in the face of unexpectedly high volumes of discharges. While nursing needs staff immediately for patient care, HIM can use overtime or staff reallocation to cover unexpected volumes.

Training

Some technical aspects of departmental operations may require special training. For example, answering the telephone and taking a message are tasks that can be performed by most workers. However, release of information is not a task to be entrusted to an untrained worker. The more technical the task, the less flexibility the department will have in covering the activity. Further, upgrades in systems capabilities and changes in equipment require in-service education that must be completed prior to operation of the system or equipment. Therefore, departments that use per diems routinely for coverage must ensure that those workers are competent at the task.

In some areas, such as IT and HIM, the use of per diems to cover certain tasks is not feasible. Based on the needs of the organization, part-time or full-time workers would be needed for these activities.

Data Quality

One of the best reasons to maintain full-time employees in certain areas is data quality. To ensure that tasks are performed accurately, the department may need individuals with extensive training and deep knowledge of both the organization and its processes. Coding is a good example of a task for which this training and knowledge acquisition are facilitated by full-time employment.

Nonlabor Costs

Other costs involved in the production of revenue include supplies, education and training, rents and leases, and utilities. Generally, the budget for utilities is not the responsibility of department management because it is a global cost of operations that is allocated to the departments as described earlier in this chapter. Similarly, rents and leases are typically contractual and would be fixed elements of the budget.

All departments will contain salary and benefits lines; however, the specific costs incurred by departments vary widely, depending on the services performed. Some costs are highly specific to the service line. Surgical services will have many different types of items that are purchased, such as gowns, operating room supplies, and devices that are unique to that service line. Some costs are unique to certain departments. For example, only the HIM department would have a contract for encoding and grouping.

Cost Justification

All labor costs should be justified based on their contribution to the mission, vision, and values of the organization. To obtain approval for budget estimates that exceed historical levels, some analysis will need to be provided that helps leadership understand the potential impact of the cost. Some cost increases are easier to justify than others. For example, the development of a clinical documentation improvement program may be expensive; however, it can be justified by the increased accuracy of coding. The need for increased accuracy might be revealed by audit findings that have identified patterns of insufficient documentation.

Quality of some output is quantifiable by audit. Coding, documentation, filing, and adherence to protocols are examples of activities whose output can be audited. Therefore, desired improvements can be measured in the same way. The expense of coder education might be justified by a target improvement in coding accuracy from 95 percent to 96 percent. Since coding accuracy impacts revenue as well, there are also supporting financial justifications.

Adherence to protocols can also be measured by audit. Deep vein thrombosis prophylaxis protocols affect patient outcomes. An increase of 10 percent in compliance may be projected to result in a 15 percent reduction in length of stay for certain patient populations, defined by diagnosis. Therefore, the cost of educating for compliance is justified by the improvement in quality of care. For diagnoses that are a target of Core Measures, high levels of compliance with certain protocols must be achieved. As such, the expense of documentation tools and education help to maintain accreditation.

With the increase in audit activity by payers, notably CMS's Recovery Audit Contractor (RAC) program and the Medicaid Integrity Contractor (MIC) program, the volume of record and billing requests has increased significantly. A request for resources to handle this volume may be justified in terms of compliance with the requests themselves and also with the analysis of resultant denials. Such resources may include contracted services as well as personnel. While it is difficult to estimate what the impact would be on revenue without historical data, the immediate impact on productivity in the department can be identified by the number of hours spent on audit-related tasks as well as any backlog created by the diversion of personnel to handle the audits.

Budget Estimations

All budgets are estimates. Some contractual elements of the budget, such as fixed-price service contracts, do not vary until the contract is renewed or renegotiated. For example, the cost of encoder and grouper software is fixed during the contract period. Transcription costs, on the other hand, vary by volume. It is important that the manager identify any contracts that may expire during the new budget period in order to provide adequate information to leadership about the potential increase in costs. While it is neither necessary nor even desirable to enter into early negotiations for budget purposes, it is certainly prudent to obtain some understanding of the possibilities during the budget process. For example, if the transcription contract will expire at the end of the new budget period, this should be noted in the budget worksheet and the plan for renewal stated. If a competitive bidding process is to be initiated, that will be important information for leadership.

Estimation of salary and benefits is often the responsibility of human resources. In organizations that have a fixed-date review system, the organization may have an overall dollar amount allocated to salary and benefits that is distributed to the departments during the budget period. In this case, the department would not necessarily budget dollars but would more likely budget for FTEs.

Estimation of other line items, such as supplies, will come from the department manager. Therefore, it is important that the manager understand the drivers of each line item so that the estimate is as accurate as possible. Coding is an example of a function that is driven by volume. The HIM manager can use volume estimates to determine the budget for overload coding services.

Similarly, a projected increase in certain service lines will drive an increase in the volume, and therefore costs, of transcription services. Table 4.10 illustrates these calculations.

Because the current fiscal year has not ended at the time the budget for the subsequent year is being developed, some additional calculations may be necessary. For example, a position may be unexpectedly vacant and contract staffing is being used for the foreseeable future. Since this contracted services line item differs from the current budget, the estimates for the following year may be different from the current year's budget. Another issue that might arise is the negotiation of a contract for a service to be provided in the next budget year. The manager needs to project when those services will begin so that the budget will reflect the expense and the related cash.

An important internal control that facilitates preparation of the periodic financial statements and annual budgets as well as cash management is a system of purchase orders. Purchase orders are internal documents that define the organization's approval of purchases. Purchase orders may cover contracts for ongoing services, such as contract coding, as well as individual acquisitions such as medical devices and office supplies. Purchase orders frequently contain specific items with associated fixed prices, such as for supplies. Other purchase orders are estimates with ranges of total costs, such as consulting projects with estimated durations. Open purchase orders are useful for budget estimation, particularly when the purchase order is for a new, ongoing service that is not included in the current year's budget.

Table 4.10   Estimation of budget lines driven by volume

Current inpatient volume	12,000 per year
Projected growth	5%
Projected volume	12,600
Current coding productivity	230 charts per week
Productivity annualized	11,960
Projected shortfall	640
Shortfall per week	12.3 charts
Shortfall in overtime hours	4.6 if completed by Coder 1 7.2 if completed by Coder 3

In this example, a 5% projected growth in volume of inpatients will require, on average, completion of 12 additional charts per week. Allocation of this shortfall to a specific coder is a budget maintenance issue and will likely result in a permanent, unfavorable variance if not identified and quantified during the budget process.

Purchase orders are also important cash management tools. A purchase order signals to the accounting department that there is a potential expense that must be accrued for the period. It also provides the controller with some guidance as to the upcoming cash requirements to satisfy the resultant accounts payable. Those cumulative cash requirements are summarized in the cash budget.

Cash Budget

The **cash budget** rolls up the approved operating and capital budgets into net projected inflows and outflows of cash. This enables the organization to estimate, monitor, and control the need for funds throughout the budget year. Table 4.11 illustrates the concept of a cash budget.

For individuals, projected cash inflow is the paycheck or other income. Contractual cash outflows are the monthly payments, such as mortgage or car loan, or other period payments such as child care and tuition. An example of a project-based cash outflow is replacement of a furnace or kitchen appliance. Other cash outflows include groceries, clothing, gas, and entertainment. If an outflow is needed and cash is not available, the individual might be able to forgo the expenditure. If the expenditure is desired or necessary despite the shortfall in funds, then credit may be available. In the extreme, if payments on credit obligations exceed the inflows needed to satisfy the obligations, then refinancing or bankruptcy may ensue. Conversely, if there are excess inflows over outflows, investment is possible.

A hospital is no different—revenue is earned and bills must be paid. There are two significant differences: The dollar amounts are higher and the cash inflows are not certain. Chapter 7 addresses the cost of capital, financing, and investment issues that arise when inflows and outflows don't match. As described earlier in the revenue cycle discussion, the cash inflows in any month are not necessarily related to the revenue from that month. While expenses are matched as much as possible to revenue, the cash associated with the collection of the revenue is routinely out of sync, due to accounting on an accrual basis. Similarly, the cash outflows related to accounts payable may also take place in different accounting periods than the underlying expense.

The cash flow related to capital projects is equally complex. An additional layer of complexity is the potential source of funds. The restricted funding of particular capital projects may affect the overall cash budget, particularly if the project funding must be processed through a grant office.

Table 4.11   Cash budget

	January	February	March	April	May	June	July	August	September	October	November	December
Cash in from patient services												
Prior months	$4,000	$4,000	$4,000	$4,000	$4,000	$3,000	$3,000	$4,000	$3,000	$3,000	$4,000	$4,000
Current month	$9,000	$9,000	$8,000	$7,000	$7,000	$8,000	$8,000	$6,000	$7,000	$8,000	$8,000	$8,000
Cash in from other sources	$500	$500	$500	$500	$500	$500	$500	$500	$500	$500	$500	$500
Total cash inflows	$13,500	$13,500	$12,500	$11,500	$11,500	$11,500	$11,500	$10,500	$10,500	$11,500	$12,500	$12,500
Cash outflows from operations												
Salaries & benefits	$6,000	$6,000	$6,000	$6,000	$6,000	$6,000	$6,000	$6,000	$6,000	$6,000	$6,000	$6,000
Contracted services	$300	$300	$300	$300	$350	$350	$350	$350	$350	$350	$350	$350
Projects				$750			$750			$750		
Supplies	$5,400	$5,400	$5,000	$4,600	$4,600	$4,600	$4,600	$4,200	$4,200	$4,600	$5,000	$5,000
Other cash outflows	$600	$600	$600	$600	$600	$600	$600	$600	$600	$600	$600	$600
Total cash outflows	$12,300	$12,300	$11,900	$12,250	$11,550	$11,550	$12,300	$11,150	$11,150	$12,300	$11,950	$11,950
Net infows (outflows)	$1,200	$1,200	$600	($750)	($50)	($50)	($800)	($650)	($650)	($800)	$550	$550
Cumulative inflows (outflows)	$1,200	$2,400	$3,000	$2,250	$2,200	$2,150	$1,350	$700	$50	($750)	($200)	$350

This example illustrates how a hospital can be cumulatively profitable yet need funding for net cash outflows. This example does not take into consideration any required minimum balances.

Working Capital

In order to pay the bills, the organization must have enough resources to satisfy its obligations. This ability to satisfy obligations is measured as the net of short-term assets and short-term liabilities, or **working capital.** Effectively, though, the most important short-term asset for paying the bills is cash. Revenue from services provided is not cash; it is merely a reflection of the amount of services provided. Revenue, when booked, is balanced by accounts receivable. It is the collection of accounts receivable that provides the cash with which organizations in turn pay their bills, thereby reducing accounts payable. See figure 4.5 for a review of this concept.

The ability of an organization to satisfy its debts (pay its bills) ongoing is critical to the organization's financial health. Two concepts that are relevant to that issue are cash flow and creditworthiness.

Key Cash Budget Considerations

Cash flow is the outgoing cash and the incoming cash. The Statement of Sources and Uses of Cash summarizes how the organization used its cash in a prior fiscal period. For budget purposes, cash flow is an estimate of the levels of cash available during the year. Since it is nearly impossible to exactly predict the cash received and the cash needed to pay bills, cash budgets are always estimates, derived from the operational and capital budgets submitted for the coming period.

Figure 4.5   How revenue becomes cash

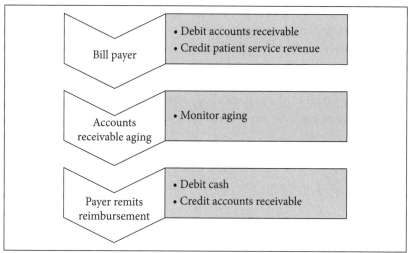

Creditworthiness is the ability of the organization to satisfy its debts. If there is a cash shortfall at any time and bills need to be paid, the organization must be able to borrow to stay in business. The cost of raising cash and the impact of credit on interest rates are discussed in chapter 7.

The organization's need for cash is driven by the timeliness of turning revenue into cash and the resolution of obligations arising from the generation of revenue. Although revenue and expenses are defined when earned or incurred, the resultant cash flow is less predictable.

Revenue/Accounts Receivable

As departments develop their operating budgets, they project revenue. That revenue is not realized unless and until services are actually performed. Small amounts of cash may be collected at point of care in the form of copays and deposits. However, the bulk of revenue is booked as a receivable, at which point the organization must wait for the payer to clear and pay the claim. Some payers, such as Medicare, pay in predictable patterns. So, presuming the bill is dropped and submitted on a timely basis, the organization can expect payment from Medicare within two to three weeks of discharge. To a hospital, all of the activities that identify, record, and collect payments (from preregistration through bill collection and cash posting) are collectively referred to as the **revenue cycle.**

The key variables on the hospital's side of the revenue cycle are **bill hold** and **claims correction.** Bill hold is the number of days, determined by the hospital, that a claim will remain on the list of **discharged and not final billed** (DNFB) accounts waiting for late charges, coding, error correction, and final documentation. The hospital does not have to hold bills at all and could theoretically declare a zero bill hold. However, the coding process will delay the claims anyway, and a standard bill hold gives staff a grace period in which to review the claims and make any necessary corrections. A clean claim is one that flows through to the payer without error. With a three-day bill hold, a clean claim can reach the payer by day four after discharge and cash may be received within two weeks. Technical coding and charging errors are caught by edits, the correction of which delays the claim from reaching the payer. An example of a bill error is a claim that is missing a charge. The claims correction process can delay billing for days or even weeks.

There are many reasons why a claim can be delayed. The record might not be coded because there is missing documentation. Even if coded, the bill might not drop because there is a technical error such as missing or duplicate charges. Even if the bill drops, it might be held up at the clearinghouse for a different technical error. Part of managing cash flow is understanding this revenue cycle process, setting clear thresholds and expectations, and acting quickly when expectations are not met. The DNFB report is one measure of expectation. If total DNFB exceeds 7 percent of total accounts receivable, then an investigation into the root cause ensues and corrective action is taken.

Organizations will set monthly goals for cash receipts as a part of the cash budget process, based on projected revenue. However, there are cash outflows that must happen more frequently, such as payroll.

Payroll and Benefits

Human resources is the largest expense for hospitals. Salaries and benefits can easily exceed 50 percent of total expenses. Payroll distributions occur on a regular, predetermined schedule—usually twice a month or every other week. In addition, payroll taxes as well as contributions to pension accounts and payment of health insurance premiums must be remitted.

These cash outflows cannot be avoided. However, the amounts are relatively stable in comparison with other outflows, such as vendor payments. Therefore, while large dollar amounts, they provide a baseline of sorts in the cash budget.

Self-Funded Accounts

Some organizations fund their own health insurance plans. They do not pay premiums to an insurance company; rather, they set aside funds from operations to pay any costs of care for covered lives. Depending on how the plan is set up, there may be an actual escrow account that requires funding at predetermined levels. Alternatively, there may be only an accrued liability or restricted fund balance. If cash funding is required, then the amounts must be included in the cash budget.

Expenses/Accounts Payable

Payments not tied to payroll are often distributed in nonpayroll weeks. Biweekly, rather than bimonthly, payroll facilitates this process. Many organizations also distribute payments only once a week, which facilitates cash budgeting.

Invoices from vendors are received monthly for ongoing services or periodically when services are rendered. Office supply vendors may deliver goods all month long but render an invoice at the end of the month. Surgical devices that are specific to the patient may be invoiced upon delivery.

Some payments are the result of contractual obligations. Contracted services may be fixed price, which puts the risk of loss on the contractor; variable price, which is tied to volume and puts the risk on the hospital; or a mixture of the two. Some contracts may be written with a fixed payment that is reconciled to volume at the end of the year. When planning the cash budget, it is important to understand the terms of the contracts: not only how the contractor is paid, but also when payment is due. Mortgage payment is an example of a fixed contractual obligation.

Invoices received from vendors have specific terms of payment, which are typically defined in the contract or the price quotations. Commonly, payment is due in a specified number of days, such as 30 days or 60 days. Some vendors offer a discount for early payment. Payments not made within the vendor's specified period may be subject to penalties, such as interest on the balance due. Organizations establish policies and procedures to determine how to prioritize the payment of invoices. Part of the decision is the vendor's terms. The other major consideration is the cash available. One way that organizations manage shortfalls in cash available is to delay payment on some invoices.

It is important to remember that payment of invoices, which relates to the cash budget, is not the same as expenses, which relate to the operating budget. The invoice for transcription services rendered in March will be recorded as a March expense for financial accounting and budget analysis purposes. However, the cash payment to the transcription vendor will not be distributed until April or even May, depending on when the invoice is received. So, even though cash is related to expenses, just as cash is related to revenue, the timing of the cash flow is different from the financial accounting for same.

Cash Shortfall and Surplus

Cash shortfall and cash surplus must be addressed in a timely fashion. A key purpose of the cash budget is to determine when those projected shortfalls might be and to obtain the appropriate financing. The negotiation of financing to cover shortfalls is done in advance of the actual needs of the organization. The most favorable terms will be realized if the organization plans in advance and establishes a working relationship with the lender. Similarly, short-term investment of a cash surplus is best accomplished through an existing account with a financial institution. Financing and investment issues are discussed in detail in chapter 7.

Summary

Financial statements are useful to external users; however, internal users need a different approach in order to control financial performance. Budgets are developed for the coming year; management reporting during the year compares the budgeted amounts with the actual financial performance. The budget process starts with the development of the statistical budget, then the operating budget and capital budgets are developed, approved, and implemented. Actual financial results are compared to budgeted results during the year, usually monthly. Variances between budget and actual performance are identified and analyzed in order to improve performance. To develop a budget, revenue and expenses must be projected. Revenue projections are based on volume, using historical experience, market analysis, and knowledge of service line development. Expenses are projected using revenue estimates and consideration of labor and nonlabor costs. Departmental or functional costs consist not only of department-specific expenditures, but also of overhead costs. Costs associated with overhead services provided to revenue-producing areas are allocated using one of four methods: direct, step-down, double step-down, or simultaneous equations. Using the projected revenue and expense budgets, the organization projects a cash budget, which is used to control cash flow and to determine financing needs.

CHECK YOUR UNDERSTANDING

1. A hospital's operating budget addresses what period of time?
   a. A quarter
   b. A calendar year
   c. A fiscal year
   d. A project
2. Which of the following is a component of an organization's statistical budget?
   a. Desired rate of growth
   b. Estimated revenue by service line
   c. Quarterly cash projections
   d. Capital budget
3. The budgeted salary expense for May in the HIM department is $150,000. The actual expense is $145,000, due to the departure in April of the lead coder. Which of the following best describes this variance?
   a. Permanent, favorable
   b. Permanent, unfavorable
   c. Temporary, favorable
   d. Temporary, unfavorable

4. The budgeted salary expense for May in the HIM department is $150,000. The actual expense is $145,000, due to the departure in April of the lead coder. Which of the following expense line items is most likely to reflect a permanent, unfavorable variance as a result of this coder's departure?
   a. Salary
   b. Supplies
   c. Consulting fees
   d. Benefits

5. The HIM department budget for contracted services is $4,500 per month, based on a 300-chart backlog generated from 1,200 discharges. The actual discharges in May were 900 and the contracted services were zero for May. If the hospital uses a traditional budget, which of the following best describes the budget variance?
   a. Permanent, favorable
   b. Permanent, unfavorable
   c. Temporary, favorable
   d. None of the above—there is no variance

6. The HIM department budget for contracted services is $4,500 per month, based on a 300-chart backlog generated from 1,200 discharges. The actual discharges in May were 900 and the contracted services were zero for May. If the hospital uses a flexible budget, which of the following best describes the budget variance?
   a. Permanent, favorable
   b. Permanent, unfavorable
   c. Temporary, favorable
   d. None of the above—there is no variance

7. The hospital's target Medicare case-mix index is 1.35; its blended rate is $6,800. What is the expected revenue from 4,300 Medicare cases?
   a. $5,805
   b. $9,180
   c. $21,659,259
   d. $39,474,000

8. To the Surgical Services department, which of the following best describes the cost of surgical supplies (gown, gloves, and suture kit, for example) as it relates to an individual patient's surgery?
   a. direct, fixed, controllable
   b. direct, variable, controllable
   c. direct, fixed, uncontrollable
   d. direct, variable, uncontrollable

9. Which of the following cost allocation methods is required for Medicare cost reporting?
   a. Direct allocation
   b. Step-down allocation
   c. Double step-down allocation
   d. Simultaneous equations

10. The need for short-term borrowing to meet vendor payment obligations in the month of June will be determined by reviewing the:
   a. Operating budget
   b. Capital budget
   c. Working capital
   d. Cash budget

Variance Analysis

Learning Objectives

- Define budget variances
- Define various approaches to objectively defining significant budget variances
- Analyze budget variances to understand the root cause

Key Terms

Average	Root cause
Bell-shaped curve	Sensitivity
Budget variance	Specificity
Controllable costs	Standard deviation
Cost center	Statistical process control
Decision theory	Threshold
Decision tree	Unfavorable variance
Favorable variance	Unit price
Intensity of service	Variance
Normal distribution	Variance analysis

Budget Control

Budgets are managed by performing a **variance analysis** to determine if actual revenue and expenses are deviating from the budgeted amounts. The difference between the actual and budgeted figures is called a **variance.** If the actual expenses are lower than budget or the actual revenue is higher than budget, then the variance is referred to as a **favorable variance.** Conversely, if the actual expenses are higher than budget or the actual revenue is lower than budget, then the variance is an **unfavorable variance.** A variance analysis often includes looking back at a previous period's performance to determine the **root cause** of the difference between budget and actual performance.

Budgets are built based on an organization's financial history and assumptions about future activity. When the actual performance is different from the budget, action may be required to either change the operational activity to conform to budget or adjust the budget to reflect new information about the financial position of the organization. If budget variances are addressed quickly, it is typically less expensive and less time-consuming to correct the operational issue. If the budget variance is due to an environmental change outside the control of the organization, an early revision to the budget will assure that budget and reality are closely aligned. Figure 5.1 displays the budget review and control cycle. The manager or person responsible for the performance of the department drives the budget control cycle.

The budget report in figure 5.2 shows an example of actual and budgeted expenses and revenues. The **budget variance** for each line is also calculated along with an indicator of whether the budget variances are favorable or unfavorable. This presentation allows the user to quickly identify which budget items are higher or lower than expected. Notice that the only line in the budget without a variance is the rent expense. Since the rent expense is likely fixed by a long-term lease arrangement, the value will not vary. All of the other expenses and revenue are based on assumptions regarding staffing, volume, payer mix, and type of procedure performed, as discussed in chapter 4. Since some level of budget variances is the norm, the organization must have a method for identifying variances that require further analysis.

Figure 5.1   Budget control cycle

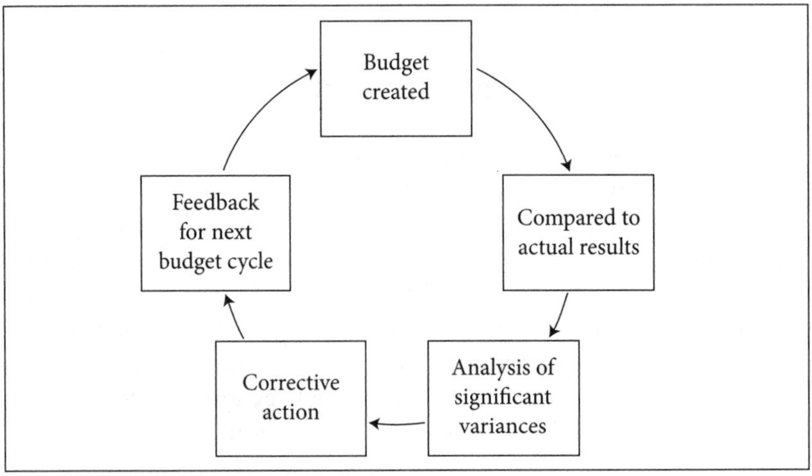

Figure 5.2   Example of a budget variance report

January Budget Comparison **XR Radiology**				
Category	**Actual**	**Budget**	**Variance**	**Favorable (F) or Unfavorable (U)**
Expense				
Administration	$9,354	$10,000	($646)	F
Salary and benefits	$23,980	$20,000	$3,980	U
Rent	$7,500	$7,500	$0	
Supplies	$6,730	$5,000	$1,730	U
Maintenance	$239	$500	($261)	F
Total expenses	$47,803	$43,000	$4,803	U
Revenue				
Third-party payments	$45,670	$40,000	$5,670	F
Patient payments	$1,540	$1,000	$540	F
Total revenue	$47,210	$41,000	$6,210	F
Net income	($593)	($2,000)	$1,407	F

Identifying Significant Budget Variances

Identifying when a budget variance is worthy of investigation should be accomplished using objective criteria. The criteria should be sensitive enough so that significant variances are identified quickly but specific enough that small natural fluctuations in the budget lines do not cause undue investigation and additional cost. In data analytics, **sensitivity** refers to the ability of a decision rule to detect a true difference. **Specificity** refers to the ability of the decision rule not to falsely identify a variance as significant or a false positive.

Thresholds

One strategy that was presented in chapter 4 is to set budget variance **thresholds** based on fixed dollar amounts or percent variance from budget for a single time period or multiple time periods. Some example thresholds are set to investigate all budget variances that are more than:

- $10,000
- 10 percent
- $5,000 for two successive periods

The threshold should be selected so that variances that represent systemic issues in a department are identified and addressed as quickly as possible. A threshold that is set too low may be too conservative and may cause unneeded expense to investigate small issues that may self-correct without intervention. Conversely, a threshold that is too high will result in missed opportunities to improve performance and track closer to budget. In healthcare, the business environment can change very quickly. Variance thresholds may require adjustment over time.

For example, suppose a radiology manager is presented with the monthly budget results displayed in figure 5.2. Note the supply cost for the department is $1,730 above budget. The practice has a policy of investigating budget variances larger than $1,500. The manager embarks on an investigation to determine the root cause of the variance. She knows the supply cost in the department is a function of the amount paid for individual supplies, the number of procedures performed, and the type of procedures performed. Each of these cost drivers is investigated, and she determines the cost increase is due to an unexpected volume increase. The manager further notes that volume has been increasing gradually over the last three months. It is likely that the following months will follow this growth trend and continue to trigger the budget variance threshold. The action taken in this case is to formulate a flexible budget based on the growing volume. Instead of using a threshold based on total cost, a new threshold based on cost per unit is developed so that variances attributable to factors other than volume may be identified.

Statistical Process Control Charts

Many departments in a healthcare entity will experience a certain amount of random variation in their expense and revenue amounts. This may be due to seasonality, changes in contract terms, or even shifts in the underlying population. Statistical process control is a tool that may be used to identify budget variances that go beyond random occurrences. **Statistical process control** may be applied to the monthly budget variances by creating a control chart to examine monthly figures and determine if the values stray beyond probable limits.

The **normal distribution** or **bell-shaped curve** may be used to set up data-driven thresholds for determining which budget variances are unusual enough to be investigated. Recall from elementary statistics that a normal distribution is centered at its mean. The **standard deviation** of the normal distribution describes how steep the sides of the bell-shaped curve descend. The standard deviation is a common statistic that is used to describe the spread or consistency of a distribution. If we can assume that the budget items are varying randomly around the budgeted amount and there are no significant nonrandom factors causing the budget variances, then it is reasonable to use a normal distribution to approximate the difference between the budget and actual amounts for the various budget lines. If these assumptions are reasonable and there is no significant bias in our budget process, then the distribution of the budget variances may be approximated by a normal distribution.

In a normal distribution, the chance of a value being within one standard deviation of the mean is approximately 68 percent, the chance of a value being within two standard deviations of the mean is approximately 95 percent, and the chance of a value being within three standard deviations is approximately 99.7 percent. These relationships are depicted in figure 5.3.

From these properties of the normal distribution we can infer that if a particular value is outside two or three standard deviations from the **average,** then it is unlikely to be a random occurrence and therefore may require investigation. Although a series of values encountered in practice will not follow a bell-shaped curve exactly, the number of standard deviations a value is from the series mean still offers excellent criteria for identifying unusual values. This approach may be applied to monthly volume, cost, or any other values that are

Figure 5.3 Normal distribution or bell curve

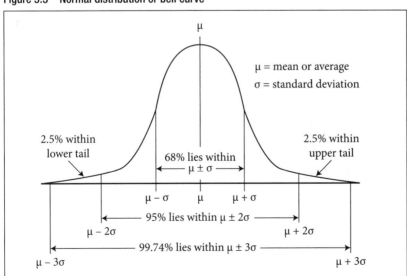

tracked on a periodic basis by setting an upper control limit (UCL) and lower control limit (LCL) based on a set number of standard deviations from the mean value.

For example, suppose the cost per month at Exact Laboratory is directly related to the number of tests performed. The director tracks the number of tests performed each month as an indicator of performance. In studying the volume over the last 12 months, he calculates that the average number of tests per month is 1,000. The standard deviation of the number of tests is 150. The director opts to set the threshold for investigating budget variances two standard deviations higher or lower than the average. Thus, any months with volume greater than 1,300 or less than 700 should be investigated. The probability of observing monthly volume outside of those limits is approximately 5 percent. Further, since the normal distribution is symmetric, we can infer that there is a 2.5 percent chance of observing a monthly volume greater than 1,300 and a 2.5 percent chance of observing a monthly volume lower than 700 due to random chance. Certainly, volumes with such a small chance of occurring randomly should be investigated. Figure 5.4 shows a statistical process control chart with two standard deviation limits around the average number of tests per month. The volume for the month of August exceeds the UCL of 1,300 tests. The manager should investigate that month to determine the cause of the shift in volume.

Figure 5.4   Exact Laboratory monthly test volume control chart

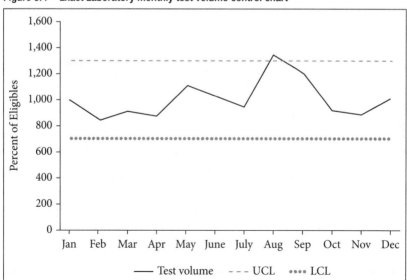

Decision Theory

Decision theory may also be used to identify budget variances that require further investigation. In decision theory, the expected cost of investigating and not investigating a budget variance are calculated and compared to determine the most cost-effective alternative. The end result will be the expected payoff or cost of investigating and correcting a budget variance. There are essentially four potential endpoints in determining if a budget variance is worth investigating. Table 5.1 shows the various decision endpoints and the cost of each.

Each of the costs represented in figure 5.5 has a probability of occurring. The expected cost of each alternative may be calculated by summing the cost of each alternative multiplied by the probability of each alternative occurring. A **decision tree** is an effective presentation of the various decisions and their associated probabilities. Figure 5.5 displays a decision tree that may be used to determine if investigation of a budget variance is cost-effective. To calculate the expected value or expected utility of the alternatives, a probability of each of the outcomes must be assumed. The probability may be derived from prior experience or may be approximated by assuming that the actual values are approximately normally distributed. For instance, in applying decision theory to the previous laboratory example, suppose we observed a test volume of 700 in January. Because the monthly test volume is approximately normally distributed, we know from the previous example that the probability of this occurring by chance if the process is in control is 2.5 percent. The probability of the presence of some other event causing the low volume is 97.5 percent. This probability along with the cost to investigate the issue may be combined to formulate the decision tree in figure 5.5.

Table 5.1   Decision theory method costs

Decision	Cost of Decision	**Actual State**	
		Variance represents a true performance issue	Variance does not represent a true performance issue
	Investigate	Cost of investigation and corrective action minus any benefit for corrective action	Cost of investigation
	Do not investigate	Cost is loss of benefit from corrective action	No cost

Figure 5.5   Budget variance decision tree

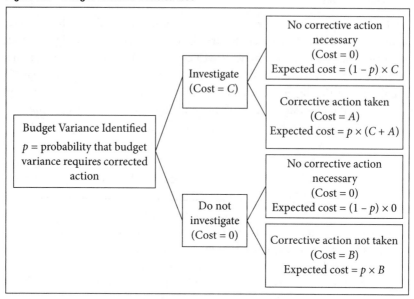

The expected cost of investigation versus no investigation may be calculated by summing up the expected costs of each branch of the decision tree:

$$\text{Expected Cost of Investigation} = (1-p) \times C + p \times (C + A)$$
$$\text{Expected Cost of No Investigation} = (1-p) \times 0 + (p \times B) = (p \times B)$$

For example, suppose an HIM director tracks coding backlog as an indicator of departmental budget performance. He knows that the coding backlog exceeded 100 charts on seven days last year and that the staffing level and patient volume have remained relatively stable since that time. The coding backlog is now 110 charts, and he is considering bringing in a consulting firm to investigate the reason for the increased backlog. The cost of the investigation is estimated to be $5,000 and the expected cost to the facility in terms of cash flow is estimated to be $7,500. The manager estimates that the cost of corrective action will be $2,000 due to hiring contract coders or paying overtime to internal staff. Should the variance be investigated?

From historical information, we know that the probability of observing more than 100 charts in the backlog is 7/365 or 1.9 percent. Therefore, the probability that a backlog of 110 charts is not due to random variation alone is 1 − 0.019 or 98.1 percent.

Relevant information for expected cost calculation:

$$p = 1 - 7 / 365 = 98.1 \text{ percent}$$
$$A = \$2,000 \text{ (cost of corrective action)}$$
$$B = 7,500 \text{ (loss due to not fixing issue)}$$
$$C = \$5,000 \text{ (cost of investigation)}$$

$$\text{Expected Cost of Investigation} = (1-p) \times C + p \times (C + A)$$
$$\text{Expected Cost of Investigation} = (1-0.981) \times 5,000 + 0.981 \times (5,000 + 2,000)$$
$$\text{Expected Cost of Investigation} = 95 + 6,867 = 6,962$$

$$\text{Expected Cost of No Investigation} = (1-p) \times 0 + (p \times B)$$
$$\text{Expected Cost of No Investigation} = (1-0.981) \times 0 + (0.981 \times 7,500)$$
$$\text{Expected Cost of No Investigation} = 0.981 \times 7,500 = 7,358$$

Because the expected cost of investigating is lower than the cost of not investigating, the variance should be investigated.

The strength of this approach is that the cost of taking no action or not investigating the variance is quantified and compared to the cost of investigating and correcting a potential issue. In practice, there are situations where the most cost-effective solution is watchful waiting. For instance, in the coding backlog example, if the cost to the facility were less than $7,097 ($6,962/0.981) then the most cost-effective decision would be not to investigate the variance.

Identifying the Source of Budget Variance

The root cause of a budget variance should be investigated in a methodical manner. Once the root cause is identified, a strategy to correct the variance must be developed for **controllable costs** or revenue drivers. If the issue is noncontrollable, then budget adjustments or other strategic changes may be necessary to improve performance.

The strategies used to investigate cost and revenue variances are similar. The source of a budget variance typically falls into one of the following three categories:

1. Volume
2. Unit price
3. Intensity

The metrics used to measure each of these variance components is dependent on the context of the analysis. Volume refers to the quantity of items produced or purchased to derive the budget line. Common measures of volume include laboratory tests, discharges, charts, employees, or clinic visits. **Unit price** is the cost to produce the unit of volume or the revenue per unit volume. The term price is used here to represent the monetary value per unit in either the revenue or cost variance setting. The unit used to determine the unit price must be the same as the units measured for the volume component. For instance, if volume is defined to be discharges, then the unit price must be cost or revenue per discharge.

Intensity of service is often the most difficult component to measure. The intensity metric should be relevant to the department or **cost center** studied. There is no one-size-fits-all intensity measure in healthcare. Table 5.2 lists some example intensity measures.

The first step in investigating a significant budget variance is to divide the variance into the volume and unit price components. The volume component is estimated by multiplying budgeted unit price by the difference between the actual and budgeted volume. Next, the unit price portion is estimated by taking a flex-budget approach. In other words, estimate the budgeted amount based on the actual volume and compare that figure to the actual. The unit price component is the difference between the actual and budgeted unit price multiplied by the actual volume. The notation and formulas for these calculations are presented in figure 5.6.

The portion of the variance attributed to unit price may be due to **intensity of service** or the price of inputs into the production of the budget units. For instance, if the salary cost for a radiology department is above budget and the majority of the budget variance is due to unit price, the root cause may be the mix of CT versus MRI scans (intensity) or the hourly rate for the staff (price).

Table 5.2   Example intensity measure for services

Context	Intensity Measure
Hospital inpatient services	Case-mix index
Physician clinic	Resource-based relative value scale (RBRVS)
HIM department	Inpatient versus outpatient claims
Radiology	Average APC weight of tests performed
Nurse staffing	RN to LPN ratio

Figure 5.6   Budget variance components

Variance Component	Actual Value	Budget Value
Volume (V)	V_A	V_B
Unit price (P)	P_A	P_B
Total (T)	T_A	T_B
Volume Variance Component $(VVC) = (V_A - V_B) \times P_B$		
Price Variance Component $(PVC) = (P_A - P_B) \times V_A$		
Total Variance $(TV) = T_A - T_B = VVC + PVC$		

In studying the impact of intensity on the unit price, measurement of intensity and input price must be matched much like the volume and the unit price are in the previous discussion. In the radiology example, if the intensity is to be measured as the time to perform each test in hours, then the input price should be measured as salary per hour.

The basic steps for investigating a budget variance are as follows:

1. Determine if the budget variance is significant
2. Identify the key drivers of the cost or payment
3. Identify the data elements needed to measure volume, unit price, and intensity
4. Break the budget variance into volume and unit price components
5. If necessary, further break the unit price component into input price and intensity

This hierarchical approach to identifying sources of variance is best demonstrated through example. The following examples include investigations of both cost and revenue budget variances.

Cost Variance Examples

Case Study 5.1: Labor Cost

The HIM director at University Medical Center (UMC) notices that the cost for contracted coding services was significantly over budget last month. The actual cost was $7,875 compared to the budget of $6,250. UMC uses Quick Coders with an hourly rate of $50 for outpatient claims. The annual budget for contract coding was constructed based on an assumption of outsourcing the coding of 500 claims per month and a production rate of four outpatient claims per hour. The actual number of claims sent to Quick Coders was 525. What is the likely cause of the budget variance?

The director knows that the source of the budget variance must be one of three factors:

Volume: Total number of claims
Cost per unit: Cost per claim for review
Intensity: Type of claim

Because this example includes only outpatient claims, we will assume that the intensity or time to code is similar for all claims. Therefore, the intensity is likely not a source of budget variance in this case. The volume of cases is higher than budgeted. The amount of budget variance attributed to volume may be calculated by comparing the total projected cost based on budgeted and actual volumes using the budgeted cost of $12.50 per claim:

Amount of budget variance due to volume:

$$(\text{Actual Volume} - \text{Budget Volume}) \times [\text{Budget Cost per Unit}] =$$
$$(525 - 500) \times 12.50 = \$312.50$$

The amount of budget variance attributed to cost per unit may be calculated by comparing the projected total cost based on budgeted and actual cost per unit using the actual volume of 525 claims. The actual cost per claim is $7,875/525 = $15.

Amount of budget variance due to cost per unit:

$$(\text{Actual Cost per Unit} - \text{Budget Cost per Unit}) \times [\text{Actual Volume}]$$
$$= (15.00 - 12.50) \times 525 = \$1,312.50$$

The majority of the budget variance is driven by the cost per unit.

The HIM director questions the Quick Coders representative about the cost per coded claim. The contract estimate was based on an average of four outpatient claims coded per hour at an hourly rate of $50. The invoice received for last month stated 170 hours ($8,500/$50 per hour). If 525 claims were coded during the month, then the average time per claim is 0.324 hours per claim or approximately 19 minutes per claim. The Quick Coders representative explains that the estimates were based on the historical mix of surgical and ancillary cases at the client's facility and it appeared that mix has changed. The previous fiscal year mix was 50 percent ancillary cases and 50 percent surgical cases. Ancillary cases take approximately 10 minutes to code, while surgical cases take 20 minutes on average. The actual mix of ancillary and surgical cases was 30 percent/70 percent.

The director wishes to test the Quick Coders rep's claim and determine if the intensity shift explains the variance in cost per claim. The claims coded per hour can be interpreted as an intensity measure. The budgeted intensity is 15 minutes or 0.25 hours per claim. The actual intensity may be calculated using the following steps:

1. Convert minutes to fractions of hours:
   Ancillary: 10 minutes = 10/60 = 0.17
   Surgical: 20 minutes = 20/60 = 0.33
2. Calculate the weighted average of the hours per claim using the actual percentage of each category as the weight:
   Intensity = $0.30 \times 0.17 + 0.70 \times 0.33 = 0.282$

Amount of budget variance due to intensity:

(Actual intensity – budget intensity) × actual cost per claim × actual volume =
$(0.282 - 0.25) \times 50 \times 525 = \$840$

Amount of budget variance due to cost that is not explained by intensity shift:

$\$1,312.50 - \$840 = \$472.50$

Conclusion: Intensity or claim type mix explains a portion of the variance in cost per unit. The HIM director should consider renegotiating the contract with Quick Coders to be based on per-claim terms to allow more budgetary control.

Case Study 5.2: Treatment Pathways

The medical director at North Hospital notices that the cost for antibiotics dispensed during January was significantly above the budgeted amount. By analyzing the antibiotic cost per case by MS-DRG, he is able to isolate the cost variance to pneumonia cases. The total cost of antibiotics dispensed for pneumonia cases during January was $312,400 versus the budgeted amount of $250,000. The budget was constructed using an assumption of 1,000 cases per month and a typical antibiotic cost of $250 per discharge. The relevant statistics are presented in figure 5.7.

Figure 5.7   Treatment pathway data: Variance analysis for pneumonia cases

	Actual	Budget	Variance
Total cost	$312,400	$250,000	$62,400
Volume: Pneumonia cases	1,100	1,000	100
Unit price: Antibiotic cost per case	$284	$250	$34

Volume Variance Component (VVC) = (1,100 − 1,000) × 250 = $25,000
Price Variance Component (PVC)   = (284 − 250) × 1,100   = $37,400
Total Cost Variance   = $62,400

Source: Adapted from QualityNet 2010.

The volume and unit price are both higher than budgeted, but the PVC makes up 60 percent of the cost variance. The medical director would like to understand whether the unit price variance is due to intensity or input price. He knows that the unit price is driven by two primary factors: length of stay (intensity) and the antibiotic prescribed (input price). The budget was created using the historical length of stay and antibiotics cost for the previous year. The average length of stay was 5.7 days and the average cost per day for antibiotics was $43.86. The medical director requests a report of the average length of stay and cost per unit for antibiotics prescribed to pneumonia patients treated during January. The results of that report and the calculation of the variance components appear in figure 5.8.

The intensity or length of stay variance component makes up 75 percent (25/34) of the unit price variance. The medical director may decide to monitor the length of stay in subsequent months or investigate long-stay cases to determine if case management guidelines require revision. The decision theory methods described earlier in this chapter may be used to determine if it is more cost-effective to monitor or actively investigate the length of stay variance.

Figure 5.8   Treatment pathway data: Variance analysis for cost of antibiotics, January

	Actual	Budget	Variance
Unit price: Antibiotic cost per case	$284	$250	$34
Intensity: Length of stay	5.8	5.7	0.1
Input price: Antibiotic cost per day	$45.41	$43.86	$1.55

Intensity Variance Component (IVC)   = (5.8 − 5.7) × 250   = $25.00
Input Price Variance Component (IPVC) = (45.41 − 43.86) × 5.8 = $9.00
Total Unit Price Variance   = $34.00

Source: Adapted from QualityNet 2010.

Case Study 5.3: Productivity

After receiving a monthly management report, the HIM director at Memorial Hospital discovers that the level of revenue in the discharged and not final billed (DNFB) category is significantly above budget. Since the director knows that a high level of DNFB is one of the contributing factors to a cash flow issue currently under investigation at Memorial Hospital, she returns from her meeting ready to investigate the root cause of the DNFB variance.

The most recent productivity reports for the HIM department show that the average number of records coded per eight-hour shift is 730 for the most recent quarter. The budget calls for an average of 760 records per shift. Based on productivity standards found in the literature (Hughes 2003) and the historical mix of services provided at Memorial, the director calculates that the average coder should complete 152 records per shift. The productivity standards are 4 inpatient records per hour, 9 observation/outpatient surgery records per hour, and 30 other outpatient records per hour. The historical mix of services is 10 percent inpatient, 40 percent outpatient surgery, and 60 percent other outpatient records. The budgeted staffing level required to code 760 records per shift is five coder FTEs.

The budget variance analysis for records per shift appears in figure 5.9. No calculation is necessary here. All of the variance is due to coder productivity, since there is no variance between actual and budget in staffing level. The unfavorable variance of 29.2 records per shift represents more than 2,500 records over the course of the quarter. The reduction in coding throughput will cause a significant delay in cash flow.

The director must determine if the variance in the number of records coded is due to coder productivity or the mix of services provided by Memorial Hospital. In this example, coder productivity is a measure of input unit price, and it will be measured as the number of records coded per hour for each of the three types used to calculate the budget (inpatient, observation/outpatient surgery, and other outpatient). The measure of intensity will be the actual percentage of cases in each category experienced during the most recent quarter. The actual and budget values for each of these statistics are listed in figure 5.10.

Figure 5.9 Productivity data: First quarter averages of records coded

First Quarter Averages	Actual	Budget	Variance
Total records coded per shift	730.8	760	(29.2)
Volume: Coder FTEs	5	5	—
Price: Number of records coded	146.2	152	(5.8)

Figure 5.10   Productivity data: Coding by record type

Record Type	Budget Records Coded	Actual Records Coded	Budget Percentage of Records	Actual Percentage of Records
Inpatient	4.0/hour 32.0/shift	4.0/hour 32.0/shift	10	15
Observation/ Outpatient surgery	9.0/hour 72.0/shift	9.2/hour 73.6/shift	40	35
Other outpatient	30.0/hour 240.0/shift	28.9/hour 231.2/shift	50	50

Prior to any calculations, it appears that the variance is due to a combination of the percentage of records in each category and the number of records per shift per FTE coded. A variance analysis will help the director understand which of these factors is causing more of the variance in the number of records coded per shift. The variance in the number of records coded per shift may be divided into intensity (record mix) and input price (records of each type coded per shift) components:

$$\text{Intensity Variance Component (IVC)}$$
$$= (0.15 - 0.10) \times 32.0 + (0.35 - 0.40) \times 73.6 + (0.50 - 0.50) \times 231.2 = (2.1)$$

$$\text{Input Price Variance Component (IPVC)}$$
$$= (32.0 - 32.0) \times 0.10 + (73.6 - 72.0) \times 0.40 + (231.2 - 240.0) \times 0.50 = (3.8)$$

The director can now see that 66 percent (−3.8/−5.8) of the variance in coded records per shift is due to coder productivity. The record mix is more intense than assumed in the budget process with a percentage of inpatient cases of 15 percent versus 10 percent, but the impact of the lower-than-expected productivity in the "other outpatient" category is the primary source of the budget variance. The director may now decide if the productivity expectation of 30.0 per hour is reasonable or if the coders need incentives or educational programs to improve their productivity in coding the other outpatient records.

Revenue Variance Examples

Case Study 5.4: Inpatient Hospital

The CFO at Critical Medical Center (CMC) noted a trend down in the Medicare inpatient service revenue. Since Medicare inpatient payments are driven primarily by volume and case mix, he decided to perform a variance analysis

Figure 5.11   Inpatient hospital data

	Actual	Budget	Variance
Medicare inpatient revenue	$48,267,656	$54,164,138	($5,896,482)
Medicare inpatient volume	4,625	4,950	(325)
Medicare case mix	1.65	1.73	(0.08)
Medicare base rate	$6,325	$6,325	—
VVC (Discharge Volume) $= (4,625 - 4,950) \times 1.73 \times 6,325 = (\$3,556,231)$			
IVC (Case Mix) $ = (1.65 - 1.73) \times 4,625 \times 6,325 = (\$2,340,250)$			

to determine if CMC is losing volume to competitors or if the case mix is the cause of the revenue shift. The Medicare inpatient revenue budget was constructed assuming a 10 percent increase over the previous year's volume of 4,500 discharges and rolling the previous year's case mix of 1.73 forward. The CFO also assumed that outlier payments would have a minimal impact on the overall revenue. Based on CMC's Medicare base rate of $6,325, the budgeted annual inpatient service revenue was $54.2 million. The relevant budget versus actual data appears in figure 5.11. Prior to calculating the variance components, it is clear that both volume and intensity are an issue in this case. The variance in case mix results in a reduction in net revenue of $500 per case. This figure is derived from multiplying the difference between the actual and budgeted case mix times the Medicare base rate of $6,325.

After calculating the two components of variance, it is clear that the volume of cases is the stronger component, accounting for 60 percent of the variance in Medicare inpatient revenue. The CFO schedules a meeting with the director of marketing to discuss the results of his analysis.

Case Study 5.5: Physician Clinic

Good Care is a physician practice with three physician owners: Dr. Onesy, Dr. Shelly, and Dr. Wiley. The total revenue for Good Care was 10 percent lower than budget last year. Dr. Onesy has noticed that Dr. Shelly comes to the office only four days a week and therefore sees significantly fewer patients than the other two partners. The practice divides the revenue and expenses for the year three ways. Dr. Onesy believes that Dr. Shelly should not receive a full third of the revenue because of his work habits. Dr. Onesy and Dr. Wiley both billed the approximately 3,000 visits per year used to determine the revenue budget. Dr. Shelly billed only 2,450. Dr. Shelly argues that his visits are at a higher intensity level and therefore bring in more revenue per visit.

The three partners hire a consulting firm to determine if Dr. Shelly's assertion is correct. The majority of the contracts between Good Care and third-party

Figure 5.12   Physician clinic data

	Actual	Budget	Variance
Practice gross revenue	$324,625	$300,000	$5,025
Volume: Visits	2,450	3,000	(550)
Intensity: RVU per visit	2.49	2.00	0.49
Average conversion factor	$50	$50	—

VVC (Discharge Volume) $= (2,450 - 3,000) \times 2.00 \times 50 = (\$55,000)$

IVC (Case Mix) $\qquad = (2.49 - 2.00) \times 2,450 \times 50 = (\$60,025)$

payers are based on relative value units (RVUs) and pay an average of $50 per RVU. The consulting firm recommends using variance analysis techniques to break the revenue into an intensity component measured by the RVU per visit and a volume component measured by the number of visits per physician. The practice based their revenue budget on an average of 15 visits per day for 200 worked days or a total of 3,000 visits per physician. The revenue per visit was assumed to be $100. Therefore the budgeted revenue per physician was $300,000. The budget and actual number of visits and average RVU per visit for Dr. Shelly are presented in figure 5.12.

The variance analysis shows that although Dr. Shelly does see significantly fewer patients than projected, his gross revenue is slightly better than budget due to the increased intensity for his cases. The next step in this analysis may be to determine the reason for the different average RVU per visit among the physicians.

Case Study 5.6: Capitated Contract

Capitated contracts are difficult to manage and negotiate for both providers and third-party payers. The payer agrees to a fixed payment per member. This is typically called a per-member-per-month or PMPM rate. The provider must provide all necessary healthcare services to the members while receiving the flat PMPM rate per member. Capitated contracts are considered to be risky for providers for a number of reasons. The amount of care required by a group of subscribers is a function of their underlying health condition and their need for services. Calculating that expected cost per member is a complex actuarial calculation that most providers are not equipped to make without outside guidance. The cost of the care provided to members is difficult to track also. Electronic health records will allow a more rigorous analysis of the actual services provided to members, but estimating the cost of each service is often a difficult task for providers.

Suppose that United Hospital agreed to a capitated contract with Cap Health Plan. Cap agreed to pay United $55 PMPM for an estimated 5,000 members. Cap provided United with a utilization history for the membership to be covered under the agreement. The reports showed that the average cost for care was $50; thus, United would yield 10 percent profit on the book of business. United agreed to the contract, but after the first year they found that the actual net revenue from the contract was $258,264 versus the budgeted $300,000. The budgeted net revenue was based on the $5 PMPM or $60 per member per year multiplied by 5,000 members.

The net revenue per member was actually 20 percent higher than the budgeted amount at $6 PMPM or $72 per member per year. The executives at United were aware that the membership was lower than budgeted but thought that the improved net revenue per member would offset the lower membership figures. They performed a variance analysis to determine the relative impact of volume (number of members) and price (net revenue per member). The relevant data are found in figure 5.13.

The VVC is nearly twice the PVC in this case. An interesting follow-up question might be to determine the number of members required to break even under the current net revenue per member. Setting up a spreadsheet to represent this situation allows a series of "what-if" analyses to be completed.

Entering the relevant data into Excel or another similar spreadsheet software package will allow the calculation of the number of members required for the PVC to offset the VVC. Because changing the number of members in the scenario impacts both the PVC and VVC, an iterative search method may be used to explore the relationship between members, PVC, and VVC. Figure 5.14 displays the formulas required to perform the analysis.

Figure 5.13 Capitated contract data

	Actual	Budget	Variance
Net revenue	$258,264	$300,000	($41,736)
Volume: Members	3,587	5,000	(1,413)
Price: Net revenue per member	$72	$60	12
Volume Variance Component (VVC) = (3,587 − 5,000) × 60 = ($84,780)			
Price Variance Component (PVC) = (72 − 60) × 3,587 = $43,044			

Figure 5.14   Spreadsheet formulas for capitation case

	A	B	C	D
1		Actual	Budget	Variance
2	Net Revenue	=B3*B4	=C3*C4	=B2-C2
3	Volume: Members	3,587	5,000	=B3-C3
4	Price: Net Revenue per Member	$ 72.00	$ 60.00	=B4-C4
5				
6	VVC			=(B3-C3)*C4
7	PVC			=(B4-C4)*B3

The VVC is currently $41,736 more in loss than the PVC is in gain. The impact of an increase in members may be calculated by changing the 3,587 to 4,000 in the formula. Making this change in the spreadsheet should result in a value of VVC of –$60,000 and PVC of $48,000. This leaves the facility $12,000 from breaking even or having the loss from VVC offset the gain from PVC. Moving to a volume of 4,500 leaves a VVC of –$30,000 and a PVC of $54,000. Using an iterative "guess and check" approach results in a volume of 4,167, resulting in both a VVC and PVC of approximately $50,000. Therefore, if United Hospital can maintain its actual net revenue per member of $72 and recruit 580 (4,167 – 3,587) members, it will meet its net revenue budget because the VVC will offset the PVC.

Summary

To successfully manage the financial performance of a healthcare organization, the budget must be monitored and controlled. A critical component of budget control is the identification of significant budget variances. Selection of a consistent data-based method to identify budget variances that require further investigation will save the organization the time and money required to investigate small insignificant variances that may represent normal business fluctuations.

Once significant budget variances are identified, a number of steps should be followed to investigate the root cause of the budget variance. A correction to a process or to the budget cannot be made until there is a full understanding of which of the key cost or payment drivers are behind the variance. This chapter outlined an approach that uses operating data to narrow down the likely cause of the budget variance so that corrections may be implemented quickly.

CHECK YOUR UNDERSTANDING

1. Positive variances are always favorable. (True/False)
2. All budget variances should be fully investigated. (True/False)
3. In decision theory, a fixed threshold is set for budget variance materiality. (True/False)
4. In calculating the volume variance component, the difference between the actual and budget volume is multiplied by budget price per unit. (True/False)
5. The total variance can be divided into a volume variance component and a price variance component. (True/False)
6. In statistical process control, the probability of observing a value within two standard deviations from the mean of the process is:
   a. 68 percent
   b. 99.7 percent
   c. 95 percent
   d. 50 percent
7. Which of the following is typically not selected as a budget variance threshold?
   a. More than $10,000
   b. More than 20 percent variance
   c. Probability of an error greater than 10 percent
   d. Less than 20 percent decrease in volume
8. A variance analysis is performed to:
   a. Investigate favorable variances
   b. Formulate next year's budget
   c. Determine a manager's salary for the next year
   d. Determine if actual revenue differs from budgeted levels
9. Which of the following is a measure of intensity of service?
   a. Number of MRI procedures
   b. Cost per lab test
   c. Case-mix index
   d. Price of surgical supplies
10. The expected cost of an investigation is a function of:
    a. The probability that budget variance requires action, the cost of an investigation, and the cost of taking corrective action
    b. The cost of investigation and the cost of taking corrective action
    c. The probability that a corrective action is successful, the cost of taking the corrective action, and the cost of investigation
    d. The cost of not taking corrective action and the cost of investigation

References

Hughes, G. 2003. Practice brief: Using benchmarking for performance improvement. *Journal of AHIMA* 74(2):64A–64D.

QualityNet. 2010. MedQIC Pneumonia Antibiotic Consensus Recommendation Hot Card. http://www.qualitynet.org/dcs/BlobServer?blobkey=id&blobwhere=1228885435714&blobheader=application%2Fpdf&blobheadername1=Content-Disposition&blobheadervalue1=attachment%3Bfilename%3D968%2F533%2FPNE_ABX_Consensus_Recommendations_4Q10-1Q11.pdf.

Third-Party Contract Analysis

Learning Objectives

➤ Explain Medicare payment methodologies
➤ Analyze the risk level of various contract models
➤ Describe contract negotiation strategies

Key Terms

Accountable care organization (ACO)
Ambulatory payment classification (APC)
Balanced Budget Act (BBA)
Capitated rate
Carve-out
Commercial payer
Contractual allowance
Disproportionate share payment
Fee-for-service
Formulary
Geometric mean length of stay
Grouper
Health maintenance organization (HMO)
Indemnity plan
Indirect medical education payment
IPPS PC Pricer
Managed care

Medicare severity diagnosis-related group (MS-DRG)
MedPAC
Outlier
Per-diem rate
Per member per month (PMPM)
Physician–hospital organization (PHO)
Preferred provider organization (PPO)
Private fee-for-service (PFFS)
Prospective payment system (PPS)
Retrospective payment system
Revenue code
Risk
Social Security Act
Stop-loss
Third-party contract
Third-party payer
Value-based purchasing (VBP)
Wage index

The financial analysis of **third-party contracts** is an important aspect of healthcare financial management. Healthcare entities provide services to patients, but the majority of payments are received from **third-party payers.** The level of profit or loss from a population of patients depends on the cost of care provided to those patients and the payment terms that determine the level of reimbursement. Some contracts, such as Medicare and Medicaid, are non-negotiable. The provider either participates in the program and accepts the payment as defined in federal or state regulations or opts not to accept patients that are covered by those programs. Table 1.1 in chapter 1 lists a number of health insurance terms that may be helpful in understanding this discussion about payment methodologies.

The amounts due from third-party payers are recorded in the balance sheet as accounts receivable. Accounts receivable may be reported internally as either gross or net values. Gross accounts receivable reports the total charges for all services posted during the reporting period. The value of the net accounts receivable represents the actual amount expected to be paid by the payer and not the charge for the services provided to the patient. The difference between the amount paid for services by either a third-party payer or the patient and the charge amount is recorded as a **contractual allowance** or contractual adjustment in the financial records of the provider. The net patient accounts receivable recorded on the income statement is the amount charged for services provided to patients net of any contractual adjustments. In any discussion of accounts receivable, it is important to clarify whether the figures are gross or net of contractual allowances.

Net Accounts Receivable = Gross Accounts Receivable − Contractual Allowance

The level of contractual adjustments for government payers is reported on IRS 990 Schedule H as a measurement of community benefit. Accurate projection of contractual adjustments for future services is an important component of budgeting and strategic planning. The accurate estimation of present and future contractual adjustments depends on the calculation of expected payment amounts for the payers with significant volume at a provider.

As discussed in chapter 1, the healthcare delivery business model is relatively complex. Figure 1.3 shows the interaction between the third-party payer and the provider as a two-way relationship. The provider submits a claim to the third-party payer for reimbursement. The third-party payer then remits a payment to the provider based on the terms of a negotiated contract. Providers may provide services to patients who are enrolled in health plans without a contract with the provider. The noncontracted third-party payer is expected to pay full charges for the services provided to its enrollees. To avoid this situation, third-party payers may only allow their enrollees to receive services from a limited roster of providers.

Third-party payers reimburse providers based on either a **prospective payment system** (PPS) or a **retrospective payment system.** In a PPS, the payment for the services provided to an enrollee is determined prior to the delivery of those services. Examples of prospective payment systems are case rates, diagnosis-related group (DRG)-based payment per diem rates, and fee schedules. The payment for these services is known by both the provider and the payer at the beginning of a contract term. A PPS payment typically includes an **outlier** threshold to limit the **risk** of the provider agreeing to the payment rate without knowing if an unusually costly patient may present to the provider for treatment. An outlier threshold is typically based on the length of stay or charges incurred by a patient. The payment for an unusually long or expensive encounter may include extra payment to the provider. This extra payment is referred to as an outlier payment.

One of the justifications for PPS payments is that they provide an incentive for providers to use their resources carefully. The Medicare IPPS system, for example, pays the same amount if a provider uses $10,000 or $15,000 in resources to treat a patient assigned to a particular **Medicare severity diagnosis-related group** (MS-DRG). To be financially successful under PPSs, providers must have a good mechanism for measuring and controlling the resources expended in treating patients. This is a best practice in treating any patient but has more dire financial consequences for patients who are enrolled in government health plans that pay via PPSs and are non-negotiable.

In retrospective payment systems, the payment for services is determined after care is delivered. Examples of retrospective payment systems include contracts that pay providers based on a percentage of the charged amount or cost-based payments. The majority of recent third-party contracts are based on PPS terms. In a PPS situation, a limited number of services may be carved out of the contract for retrospective payment. Those services may include high-cost drugs and devices. The purpose of a **carve-out** term in a third-party contract is to ensure that the provider is fairly compensated for unusual circumstances. This is different from an outlier threshold in that the third-party payer is carving out particular items and services. An outlier threshold is used to pay an additional amount if the entire encounter is more resource-intense than was expected when the payment terms were negotiated.

Types of Insurance Plans

There are three primary types of insurance plan designs that are used by private insurance companies:

1. **Preferred provider organization** (PPO)
2. **Health maintenance organization** (HMO)
3. **Indemnity plan**

New health plan designs are released into the marketplace on a regular basis, but they typically are a variation on one of these three plan types. Each of these types of plans offers different levels of freedom of provider choice for the member or enrollee and different levels of cost control for the payer or insurance company.

HMO plans are the most restrictive in terms of flexibility for the patient. The HMO has a list of member providers, and to receive coverage the patient must go to one of the member providers to receive care. An HMO will also typically have a policy that requires the patient to obtain a referral from the primary care provider (PCP) prior to any visits to specialists and preapproval for most diagnostic tests. In exchange for following the restrictions in coverage found in HMO plans, enrollees are rewarded with lower or no copayments and/or deductibles. The HMO is able to contain costs by predicting the payments it will be required to make to a limited set of providers that have agreed to lower payment rates in exchange for a potential increase in market share by attracting the HMO's enrollees.

PPO plans are less restrictive to the enrollee than HMO plans but still encourage the enrollee to use providers in the PPO's network. An enrollee is subject to lower copayment and deductible amounts when receiving care at a network provider than if they used a non-network provider. The PPO relies on financial incentives to direct enrollees to the providers that have a contractual relationship with the PPO.

Indemnity plans offer the most flexibility to the enrollee and typically have the highest premium cost. The enrollee pays a higher premium in exchange for not having to stay with an in-network provider. That flexibility hinders the ability of the plan administrators to accurately estimate the cost of care for the enrollees. Therefore, they must charge a higher premium to ensure that the costs are covered during the plan year. Indemnity plans are also sometimes referred to as **fee-for-service** plans.

Medicare Payment

Medicare and Medicaid account for 56 percent of the typical hospital's business (American Hospital Association 2010). Providers cannot negotiate payment rates for traditional Medicare and Medicaid but have some negotiating ability in the **managed care** plans associated with these programs. Since these plans make up such a significant proportion of a provider's book of business, it is important to have a solid knowledge of the payment methodologies they utilize. In this section we will study Medicare payment methodologies at a high level. More in-depth information may be found in reimbursement texts on the CMS website (www.cms.hhs.gov).

The Medicare program provides coverage for individuals 65 years and older, those with end-stage renal disease (ESRD), and those who are permanently disabled in the United States. The Medicare program was formed under Title XIX of the **Social Security Act** in 1965. Medicare coverage is segmented into four parts (CMS 2011d):

1. Part A—Inpatient hospital and rehabilitation, skilled nursing facility, and home health and hospice coverage
2. Part B—Outpatient hospital facility, freestanding ambulatory surgery center, and physician office coverage
3. Part C—Managed Advantage
4. Part D—Prescription drug coverage

Providers that accept Medicare patients must accept the government-defined payment as payment in full for services provided to beneficiaries. Providers may not balance bill the patient. In other words, if the charge for a service is $100 and the total Medicare payment is $40, then the provider must accept the $40 as payment in full and take the unpaid $60 as a contractual adjustment. Providers may charge Medicare enrollees directly for noncovered services if they inform the patient that the service will not be paid by Medicare prior to delivery of the service. The patient must sign an advanced beneficiary notice (ABN) to acknowledge that they are financially obligated to pay for the services directly.

Medicare Part A—Inpatient

Medicare Part A includes services provided to Medicare enrollees in the hospital inpatient setting, skilled nursing facilities, and home health and hospice care. Hospitals are reimbursed for inpatient services provided to Medicare beneficiaries via a PPS. Table 6.1 presents the various care settings covered under Medicare Part A and a general description of the payment methodology for each.

The payment for hospital inpatient services under Medicare Part A is based on MS-DRGs. The diagnoses and procedures assigned to a discharge are combined to assign an MS-DRG using a **grouper.** Each MS-DRG has a relative weight that is combined with a provider-specific base rate to determine the payment for the discharge. The general formula for the calculation of Medicare Part A reimbursement is presented in figure 6.1.

The relative weight of each MS-DRG is determined based on the cost of treating patients who are grouped or assigned to that MS-DRG. A higher weight results in a higher payment. The relative weights are recalculated by CMS on an annual basis based on Medicare claims experience. Table 6.2 shows the relative weights for sample MS-DRGs from federal fiscal year 2011. The Medicare relative weights for all MS-DRGs may be found in appendix 6.1.

Table 6.1   Medicare Part A payment settings

Provider Setting	Classification System
Inpatient acute care hospital	Medicare Severity Diagnosis Related Groups (MS-DRGs)
Inpatient rehabilitation hospital or distinct unit	Case-Mix Groups (CMGs)
Skilled nursing facility	Resource Utilization Groups, Third Version (RUG-III)
Home health agency	Home Health Resource Groups (HHRGs)
Hospice	Each day of care is classified into one of four levels of care
Long-term acute care hospital	Medicare Severity Diagnosis Related Groups—Different relative weights than acute care hospitals

Figure 6.1   Basic MS-DRG payment formula

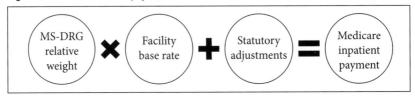

Table 6.2   MS-DRG weights—sample from FFY 2011

MS-DRG	Type	MS-DRG Title	Weight
088	MED	Concussion W MCC	1.4872
089	MED	Concussion W CC	0.9667
090	MED	Concussion W/O CC/MCC	0.6927
163	SURG	Major Chest Procedures W MCC	5.0828
164	SURG	Major Chest Procedures W CC	2.6236
165	SURG	Major Chest Procedures W/O CC/MCC	1.7758
190	MED	Chronic Obstructive Pulmonary Disease W MCC	1.1924
191	MED	Chronic Obstructive Pulmonary Disease W CC	0.9735
192	MED	Chronic Obstructive Pulmonary Disease W/O CC/MCC	0.7220
242	SURG	Permanent Cardiac Pacemaker Implant W MCC	3.7277
243	SURG	Permanent Cardiac Pacemaker Implant W CC	2.6508
244	SURG	Permanent Cardiac Pacemaker Implant W/O CC/MCC	2.0398
291	MED	Heart Failure & Shock W MCC	1.4943
292	MED	Heart Failure & Shock W CC	1.0302
293	MED	Heart Failure & Shock W/O CC/MCC	0.6853
374	MED	Digestive Malignancy W MCC	2.0674
375	MED	Digestive Malignancy W CC	1.2801
376	MED	Digestive Malignancy W/O CC/MCC	0.8478
466	SURG	Revision of Hip or Knee Replacement W MCC	4.9144
467	SURG	Revision of Hip or Knee Replacement W CC	3.2321
468	SURG	Revision of Hip or Knee Replacement W/O CC/MCC	2.5728
469	SURG	Major Joint Replacement or Reattachment of Lower Extremity W MCC	3.4724
470	SURG	Major Joint Replacement or Reattachment of Lower Extremity W/O MCC	2.1039
471	SURG	Cervical Spinal Fusion W MCC	4.7301
472	SURG	Cervical Spinal Fusion W CC	2.7722
473	SURG	Cervical Spinal Fusion W/O CC/MCC	2.0768
682	MED	Renal Failure W MCC	1.6407
683	MED	Renal Failure W CC	1.0243
684	MED	Renal Failure W/O CC/MCC	0.6587

Source: CMS 2011b.

The payment for claims that are grouped into the various MS-DRGs in table 6.2 may be calculated using the relative weight from the table and the base rate for the facility of interest. For the purpose of these examples, we will assume that no transfer reduction or outlier payments are required for the claim. Notice that the MS-DRGs appear in groups or families, each with one of the following suffixes: MCC (major complication or comorbidity), CC (complication or comorbidity), and W/O CC/MCC. The relative weights for the MS-DRGs are based on the resource intensity required to treat the typical patient whose claim groups to that MS-DRG. Notice that the weights for the MCC are the highest in the various families, CC is next, and finally W/O CC/MCC. Patients with major complications or comorbidities require more resources to treat and therefore are paid at a higher rate. If a facility's base rate is $5,000, then the payment for MS-DRG 090 (Concussion W/O CC/MCC) is $0.6927 \times 5,000 = \$3,463.50$. The payment for a claim that groups to MS-DRG 088 (Concussion W MCC) is $7,436.00. The facility's base rate is a function of a number of attributes that influence the cost of the resources required to treat patients.

The Medicare IPPS base rate is comprised of two components: operating payment and capital payment. Both components are adjusted for the cost of living based on the **wage index** assigned to the core-based statistical area (CBSA) of the facility's location. Wage indices are standardized to a value of one. CBSAs with a wage index of more than one have a higher cost of living than those with a wage index of less than one. Since only a portion of the care provided requires personnel costs, only a portion of the base rate is adjusted for wage index. In 2011, 68.8 percent of the base rate was adjusted for wage index if the facility's wage index was greater than or equal to one and 62.0 percent if the facility's wage index was less than one. For example, in 2011 the wage index for Buffalo, New York, was 0.958 and the wage index for New York City was 1.3122. The operating payment component of the base rate was $5,164.11 for federal fiscal year 2011 (CMS 2011b). The wage-adjusted operating payments or blended rates for facilities in these two locations are as follows:

Buffalo: $(0.62) \times (5,164.11) \times (0.958) + (0.38) \times (5,164.11) = \$5,029.64$
New York City: $(0.688) \times (5,164.11) \times (1.3122) + (0.312) \times (5,164.11) = \$6,273.33$

A facility in New York City would receive a 24 percent higher operating payment than a facility in Buffalo for a claim that was assigned to the same MS-DRG. Notice that the proportion of the payment that is adjusted for wage index is higher in the high wage index areas. The capital portion of the base rate is adjusted in a similar way.

The base rate may be adjusted for the proportion of uninsured treated via the disproportionate share hospital payment. The disproportionate share payment is based on the proportion of inpatient days paid via Medicaid. It is used as a proxy to measure the level of indigent care provided by the facility. Other adjustments to the base rate may be based on urban versus rural location, the existence of a teaching program, and the volume of Medicare patients treated (CMS 2011b). A facility's Medicare base rate may also be referred to as the blended rate, because a portion of the rate is based on the facility and a portion is a national rate for the MS-DRG. The details of the Medicare Part A inpatient hospital payment calculation may be found in appendix 6.2.

The statutory adjustments include a reduction in payment if the patient is transferred to another facility for a subset of MS-DRGs, an outlier payment for cases with extremely high cost, and add-on payments for the use of new technology. Outlier and new technology payments are a rare occurrence, but the reduction of payments due to transfers can have a significant impact on the payment received for Medicare inpatient cases. If the length of stay prior to transfer is below the **geometric mean length of stay** for selected MS-DRGs, then the payment will be adjusted for the number of days of treatment prior to the transfer.

CMS updates the MS-DRG weights for each federal fiscal year, which begins on October 1. Although the basic components of the calculation of Medicare IPPS payment appears in figure 6.1, the precise calculation of the statutory adjustments requires provider-specific data elements that may be updated during the fiscal year. Keeping track of the components and meshing that with the discharge date of claims can become quite involved. CMS distributes free software that may be used to calculate the payment for any MS-DRG and IPPS-paid provider on their website. The software is called the PC Pricer and as of the print date of this book may be found on this webpage: http://www.cms.gov/PCPricer.

The calculation of a small number of claims can be performed using the **IPPS PC Pricer** by professionals with no programming ability. Inputting various MS-DRG and provider scenarios is an excellent strategy to begin to understand the impact of MS-DRG weights and provider attributes on the Medicare IPPS payment that a hospital receives.

The key financial performance indicator for Medicare Part A is the case-mix index (CMI). The CMI is the average relative weight for the MS-DRGs assigned to the discharges from a provider. Since Medicare IPPS payment is a function of the MS-DRG relative weight, tracking the CMI over time allows providers to predict the revenue received for inpatient services provided to

Medicare beneficiaries. The CMI is often used to determine the net revenue budget for Medicare services with the following formula:

$$\text{Medicare Inpatient Net Revenue} = \\ [\text{Medicare discharges}] \times [\text{CMI}] \times [\text{Medicare base rate}]$$

The remaining Medicare Part A providers listed in table 6.1 are also paid via PPS. The logic used to group the cases is different, but the concept of a base rate multiplied by a relative weight is consistent in these providers. The relative weights for the case groupings are set based on the expected resource intensity derived from claims history in each of the settings. The CMI is useful for both budgeting and benchmarking in all of the Part A providers.

Medicare Part B—Outpatient

Hospitals are reimbursed by Medicare for outpatient services based on the outpatient prospective payment system (OPPS). The OPPS is comprised of three components: **ambulatory payment classifications** (APCs), fee schedules, and cost-based payments. Outpatient surgical procedures, radiology services, clinic visits, emergency department visits, and separately paid drugs and biologicals are all paid via APCs. Fee schedules are used to determine reimbursement for laboratory services, ambulance services, physical therapy, occupational therapy, and speech therapy. Cost-based payments are made for therapeutic radiopharmaceuticals and select new devices. The OPPS system is considered prospective since the payment is determined prior to the delivery of services.

Each APC is assigned a relative weight, and the payment for each service is set to the relative weight multiplied by a wage-index adjusted base rate much like the IPPS system. There is an important difference between the APC payment system and the MS-DRG payment system used in the inpatient setting. Under IPPS, each case is assigned one MS-DRG code. Under OPPS, each APC-payable service is assigned to an APC and may be assigned a payment amount. The full APC payment may be discounted for multiple procedures for some services. A number of services are not paid separately but instead are packaged or paid as a portion of the reimbursement received for the main procedure performed.

Laboratory services provided in the hospital outpatient setting are paid via a fee schedule. Therapy services such as physical therapy, occupational therapy, and speech therapy are also paid via a fee schedule. A fee schedule is a listing of the procedure codes that are payable and the payment amounts. Table 6.3 lists example Medicare fee schedule payments for selected laboratory procedures

Table 6.3   Medicare laboratory fee schedule example

HCPCS Code	Description	Ohio	Texas	Tennessee
36415	Routine venipuncture	$3.00	$3.00	$3.00
80048	Metabolic panel (calcium total)	$10.33	$11.91	$9.71
80051	Electrolyte panel	$6.37	$9.87	$8.15
80053	Comprehensive metabolic panel	$14.87	$14.87	$12.13
80061	Lipid panel	$17.89	$18.85	$18.85

Source: CMS 2011a.

and states for calendar year 2011. A facility in Ohio received a payment of $17.89 for providing a lipid panel test to a Medicare beneficiary during 2011.

The payment for a claim is the sum of the payments for the individual services. The APC and fee schedule payments are based on the Healthcare Common Procedure Coding System (HCPCS) code used to bill the service performed. Therefore, the accurate submission of HCPCS codes is critical to receiving the proper payment for services provided under the APC payment system. The average APC relative weight per claim (RWI) is analogous to the inpatient CMI. Tracking the RWI over time can help managers detect the cause of variances in net patient revenue for Medicare outpatient services.

The program logic for the OPPS pricer may be downloaded from the CMS website here: https://www.cms.gov/PCPricer/OutPPS/list.asp. The programming logic is supplied in a computer programming language called Common Business-Oriented Language (COBOL) and must be adapted for use unless the provider has the capacity to implement a COBOL program. The logic is updated each quarter and is available for no charge. Unfortunately, there is no PC program version of the OPPS pricer that will run directly on provider computers as found in the IPPS setting. This makes the calculation of expected payment more challenging for providers under OPPS than IPPS.

Freestanding ambulatory surgery centers are also paid via the APC system. The relative weight assigned to each APC is a fraction of that paid in the hospital-based outpatient service setting, but the APC groupings are the same for both provider types. Physicians are paid by a fee schedule under Medicare Part B.

Medicare Part C—Medicare Advantage

Medicare Advantage is a program that allows Medicare beneficiaries to be covered under commercial insurance companies (MedPAC 2010c). CMS reimburses the insurance companies for providing coverage to the beneficiaries.

Many Medicare Advantage plans provide a richer set of benefits than traditional fee-for-service Medicare coverage. The additional benefits may come with the requirement that the beneficiary receive care only from providers that are in the commercial health plan's network.

Medicare Advantage plans are typically HMOs, PPOs, **private fee-for-service** (PFFS), or special needs plans (SNPs) (CMS 2010b). SNPs are available for Medicare beneficiaries with a select set of chronic diseases including diabetes, congestive heart failure, a mental health condition, or HIV/AIDS, or if the beneficiary lives in a nursing home (CMS 2010b).

Providers may negotiate payment terms for services provided to beneficiaries enrolled in Medicare Advantage plans. This is the only type of Medicare coverage for which providers have control over negotiating the payment rates. Providers must be careful in determining that a patient covered under a Medicare Advantage plan is an enrollee to a plan with which they have a contractual relationship. If not, it could be difficult for the provider to collect the payment to which they are entitled without additional negotiation with the sponsor of the beneficiary's plan.

Medicare Part D—Prescription Drug Coverage

Medicare Part D provides prescription drug coverage for Medicare beneficiaries through Medicare Prescription Drug Plans (PDPs). Beneficiaries enrolled in traditional Medicare, Medicare PFFS, and some Medicare Medical Savings Accounts are eligible to enroll in Part D. Beneficiaries who are enrolled in either Medicare Advantage HMO or PPO plans receive drug coverage through those plans and are not eligible to enroll in Part D.

Part D was established by the Medicare Modernization Act of 2003 and was enacted on January 1, 2006 (CMS 2011e). Beneficiaries may select from a number of different plans. Each has its own **formulary,** benefit structure, and monthly premium to be paid by the beneficiary. CMS provides a Plan Finder (https://www.medicare.gov/find-a-plan/questions/home.aspx) that assists beneficiaries in finding the best plan for their particular prescription drug utilization and location.

There is a coverage gap in the Medicare Part D program that is sometimes referred to as the donut hole. Beneficiaries enrolling in Part D must pay a deductible ($310 for 2011). The PDP will pay for drugs according to the individual plan terms up to a limit ($2,850 for 2011). After reaching the coverage limit, beneficiaries are responsible for paying for their prescription drugs until

Figure 6.2   Medicare beneficiary prescription drug coverage as of February 2011

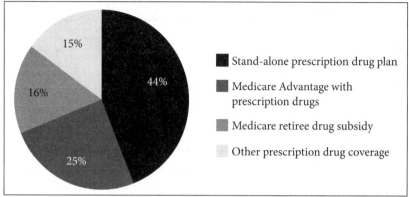

Source: CMS 2011e.

they hit a catastrophic coverage limit ($4,450 for 2011). Beneficiaries are able to take advantage of a 50 percent discount on brand-name drugs and a 7 percent discount on generic covered prescription drugs while in the coverage gap prior to reaching the catastrophic coverage limit (CMS 2011c).

As of February 2011 (CMS 2011e) 86 percent of all Medicare beneficiaries eligible for Part D received some form of prescription drug coverage. The source of that coverage was through a PDP, the Medicare Advantage plan, a retiree subsidy from a previous employer, or other state-subsidized plans. Figure 6.2 presents the distribution of the various prescription drug coverage sources utilized by Medicare beneficiaries.

Medicare Part D coverage is not available for drugs supplied to patients during an inpatient stay or during treatment in an outpatient setting.

Medicaid Coverage and Payments

The Medicaid program was created under Title XIX of the Social Security Act in 1965 (CMS 2011a). Medicaid is jointly funded by federal and state governments. Medicaid programs are actually administered at the state level. Therefore, the exact payment terms and eligibility requirements vary by state. To receive federal funds for their Medicaid programs, the states must supply the benefits listed in figure 6.3 at a minimum.

Many states offer managed care options to residents eligible for Medicaid. According to CMS figures, the enrollment in Medicaid managed care plans has

Figure 6.3   Medicaid required services

Inpatient hospital services
Outpatient hospital services
Physician services
Medical and surgical dental services
Nursing facility services for individuals aged 21 or older
Home health care for persons eligible for nursing facility services
Family planning services and supplies
Rural health clinic services
Laboratory and x-ray services
Pediatric and family nurse practitioner services
Federally qualified health center services
Nurse-midwife services
Early and periodic screening, diagnosis, and treatment services for individuals under age 21

Source: Casto and Layman 2011, 85.

grown significantly since 2000 (CMS 2010a). Figure 6.4 shows the pattern in the growth from 56 percent in 2000 to 72 percent in 2009.

As noted for the Medicare program, providers are not able to negotiate payment rates with traditional Medicaid programs. They are able to negotiate somewhat with Medicaid managed care plans. The increase in the proportion

Figure 6.4   Percentage of Medicaid eligibles enrolled in managed care plans

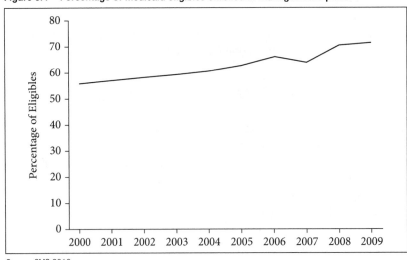

Source: CMS 2010a.

of Medicaid beneficiaries enrolling in managed care plans allows providers to have more control over the finances of providing care to this population. The federal restrictions on plan offerings and coverage limit the negotiating ability of both the plan and the provider.

Impact of Legislation on Government Payment Systems

The Medicare Modernization Act (MMA) of 2003, the Deficit Reduction Act (DRA) of 2005, the American Recovery and Reinvestment Act (ARRA) of 2009, and the 2010 Affordable Care Act (ACA) included a number of provisions that have impacted and will continue to impact the payments providers receive from government payers. In response to this and other legislation, CMS released a report titled "Roadmap for Implementing Value Driven Healthcare in the Traditional Medicare Fee-for-Service Program" (CMS 2009). This report outlines the various pilot projects and quality measurement programs that CMS sponsored. The long-term CMS goal in expanding its **value-based purchasing** (VBP) plans is summarized in this excerpt from the report:

> To help address these concerns, CMS during the current Administration and with direction from Congress (e.g., through enactment of provisions in the Medicare Modernization Act, Deficit Reduction Act, and other provisions) has begun to transform itself from a passive payer of services into an active purchaser of higher quality, affordable care. Further future efforts to link payment to the quality and efficiency of care provided, would shift Medicare away from paying providers based solely on their volume of services. The catalyst for such change would be grounded in the creation of appropriate incentives encouraging all healthcare providers to deliver higher quality care at lower total costs. This is the underlying principle of value-based purchasing (VBP). The cornerstones of VBP are the development of a broad array of consensus-based clinical measures, effective resource utilization measurement, and the payment system redesign mentioned above. The overarching goal would be to foster joint clinical and financial accountability in the healthcare system. (CMS 2009, 1)

The report also presents the concept of an **accountable care organization** (ACO). ACOs are collaborations among physicians, hospitals, and other providers that are clinically and financially accountable for the healthcare delivery in their communities (CMS 2009, 2). CMS released proposed rules regarding the structure of ACOs and the potential financial incentives available to the organizations. Although as of the printing of this text the rules have not been finalized, it is clear that some collaboration among providers is an essential component in improving both the quality and efficiency of care delivered in the United States. This is true for all patients and providers, not only those associated with the Medicare program.

CMS presents a template for VBP that may be used in all provider settings and even with ACOs (CMS 2009, 4):

- Identification and promotion of the use of quality measures through pay for reporting,
- Payment for quality performance,
- Measures of physician and provider resource use,
- Payment for value—promote efficiency in resource use while providing high-quality care,
- Alignment of financial incentives among providers, and
- Transparency and public reporting.

CMS started down this path in 2007 with the implementation of pay-for-reporting in the hospital inpatient setting. CMS required hospitals to submit data for release on their Hospital Compare site in order to receive full payment for IPPS claims. The number of reported quality indicators grew to 44 by federal fiscal year 2010. CMS is working toward implementing pay-for-reporting in both the physician and ambulatory surgery center settings. The current pay-for-reporting system will transform into a pay-for-performance system, which CMS listed as one of the essential components of a VBP.

In chapter 1 we discussed the concept of community benefit or value. Value should be a function of both quality and cost. In businesses outside of healthcare delivery, a company can demand a higher price for a higher quality product. For instance, we pay more for a new model of a car than a 10-year-old model. The perceived value of the new car is higher: more dependable, better looking, and so forth. In healthcare the value equation is more difficult to define.

Government Contract Management

As discussed in chapter 3, the ultimate measure of a provider's financial performance in treating patients is the operating margin. Recall that the formula for operating margin is as follows:

$$\text{Operating Margin} = \frac{\text{Operating Income}}{\text{Operating Revenues}}$$

An operating margin may be calculated for the entire facility, as presented in chapter 3, or for a particular set of patients or product lines. A Medicare or

Medicaid operating margin may be used as a key performance indicator for that portion of a provider's business.

MedPAC, an agency that advises Congress on Medicare payment issues, tracks a number of statistics regarding hospital financial performance and releases the results in their annual data book. Figure 6.5 shows the trend in inpatient operating margin for acute care hospitals from 1998 to 2004. The statistics are based on financial information reported in the Medicare Cost Report for hospitals that are paid via IPPS. The **Balanced Budget Act** (BBA) of 1997 is likely the cause of the dramatic decline starting in 1997. This dramatic decline in Medicare inpatient margin demonstrates the difficulty in achieving a positive margin for this portion of a hospital's business. Often, managing the financial results of a Medicare contract is focused on limiting the loss to levels that are comparable to regional or national results.

Although hospitals cannot negotiate with CMS to modify the payment rates or methodology, estimating expected payment is critical for accurate budgeting. A provider has control over three factors in determining its inpatient payment. It can control the proportion of cases that are transferred and the timing of those transfers. It can control the pricing and cost structure that may impact outlier payments. The single most important factor in the provider's control is the proper documentation and assignment of diagnosis and procedure codes to ensure an accurate MS-DRG assignment.

The CMI is used as a key performance indicator for the effectiveness of MS-DRG assignment. The CMI is the average weight of the MS-DRGs assigned during a period of time. A higher CMI value results in more revenue for

Figure 6.5   Medicare acute inpatient margin, 1994–2008

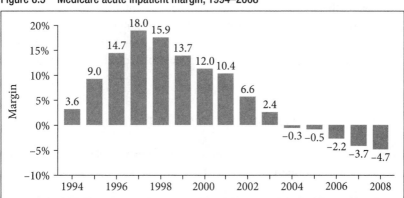

Source: MedPAC 2010a, 86.

Medicare inpatient services. A drop in CMI may be indicative of a coding and documentation issue or a change in the referral patterns in the provider's service area. The CMI is sometimes tracked excluding transfers and transplant patients. Transfers are excluded because the IPPS transfer reduction influences the direct relationship between CMI and reimbursement. Transplants are excluded because their MS-DRGs have significantly higher relative weights, and therefore a few cases can heavily influence the CMI.

The volume of cases and CMI are used to drive the budgeted amounts for Medicare patient net revenue for the inpatient setting. Small shifts in the CMI can cause significant changes in the net revenue realized for Medicare patients. For instance, a 0.5 shift in CMI reduces the average payment per claim by approximately $2,500. If this $2,500 per claim reduction is projected on an annual basis for a hospital with 1,000 Medicare inpatient admissions, the CMI shift would reduce net patient revenue by $2.5 million.

For example, suppose the chief financial officer (CFO) of UMC Hospital is concerned because the Medicare inpatient revenue is significantly below budget for the third quarter of 2010. The Medicare CMI is one of the key performance indicators tracked by the UMC Hospital management team. The CMI for the last 36 months is presented in figure 6.6.

The CMI is further broken down into clinical areas. The largest drop during the period of interest occurred in the cardiovascular surgery area. Since this is one of the few areas where the facility has a positive margin with Medicare patients, the CFO is concerned about this trend. The CFO questions the medical director about this trend and finds out that the second-highest-volume cardiovascular surgeon was lured away to a competing facility.

In this case, the shift in CMI is due not to documentation and coding issues but to a change in the referral pattern in UMC Hospital's service area. At this point the CFO may choose to recruit another surgeon to rebuild the business, try to regain the surgeon's business, or build another equally profitable product line such as orthopedics.

Commercial Payer Contracts

Unlike typical government payer contracts, providers are able to negotiate contract terms with **commercial payers.** The array of services that must be covered in a health insurance plan is defined and enforced by each state's department of insurance. This protects the consumers or enrollees of the plan but does

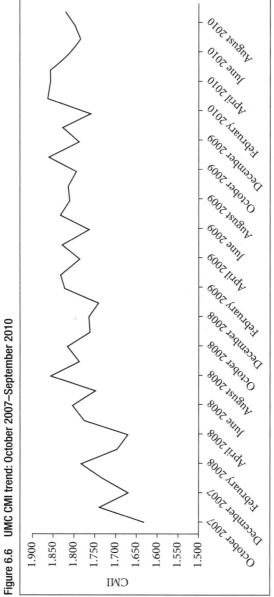

Figure 6.6   UMC CMI trend: October 2007–September 2010

not address the provider–insurance company relationship. The amount that the insurer pays to each provider is negotiated individually and is typically protected by confidentiality clauses in the contract. The operating margin for acute care hospitals has been negative for Medicare services since 2003 (Med-PAC 2010a). Figure 6.7 shows a comparison of hospital overall Medicare and all-payer margins from 1997 to 2008. To ensure the financial viability of the organization, it is imperative that the provider negotiate commercial contracts with a positive margin.

The payment methods for commercial contracts fall into four broad categories:

1. Prospective payment
2. Fee schedule and per diem
3. Percentage of charge
4. **Capitated rates**

Many contracts are actually some combination of these payment methods. The contracts typically also include some terms that limit the risk of financial loss for both the provider and the payer. Providers are at somewhat of a disadvantage in these negotiations. Since much of the charge and estimated cost of care is available at the provider–level in various public data sets, the payer may already know if the provider is high or low cost in comparison to the local competitors. Provider representatives should prepare for negotiations by acquiring as much comparative information as possible to be prepared to address any concerns from the payer regarding cost or quality of care. Providers should also be prepared to highlight their accomplishments and prove that they are providing a valuable product to the payer's enrollees.

Figure 6.7   Comparison of all-payer and Medicare margin

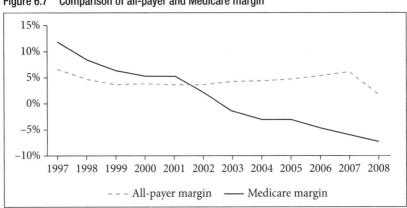

Prospective Payment

Commercial payers historically follow Medicare's lead in determining the payment to providers. The Medicare program is a special case of the more general category of prospective payment systems. In prospective payment, the payment is determined prior to the delivery of care to a patient. Many private payers now use MS-DRGs to pay in the inpatient setting and are beginning to adopt an APC-based system in the hospital outpatient setting.

Payments based on case rates would also be considered prospective payment. The predetermined payment is typically based on the expected resource intensity of the typical patient treated. For instance, case rates for cardiovascular surgery are typically higher than those assigned to medical cases such as pneumonia. In IPPS and OPPS, the resource intensity is reflected as that base rate for each MS-DRG and APC, respectively. These base rates are calibrated so that the payment covers the cost of the typical patient treated for the MS-DRG or APC to which they are assigned.

The Medicare-based payment systems do not always translate to the all-patient situation. The MS-DRG system includes categories for all types of patients, but there are very few Medicare trauma patients and hardly any Medicare obstetrics cases. This lack of data results in relative weights that are not scaled appropriately for the amount of resources required to treat these patients. Managed care payers that adopt the Medicare weights for MS-DRGs will typically include a separate set of payment rules for obstetric cases. The payment terms are either case rates or a per diem rate.

Prospective payment systems usually include an outlier or stop-loss term to limit the amount of risk to the provider. Without an outlier term, a provider would have to absorb the cost of an unusually sick patient where the variables used to determine the case rate are not adequate to reflect the resources required to treat the patient. An outlier term typically adds an amount to the fixed prospective payment. A **stop-loss** term shifts the prospective payment into a percentage of charge payment after the charge reaches a fixed threshold. The threshold for a stop-loss for inpatient admissions may be as high as $100,000 or more.

Commercial payers often implement MS-DRG payments without including the statutory adjustments afforded by the Medicare payment system. The base rates are typically higher for commercial payers but do not allow additional payments for providers that are eligible for Medicare payment adjustments like **disproportionate share payments** or **indirect medical education payments.**

This is likely because the administration of these adjustments would require additional effort on the part of the payer. The unfortunate side effect of this practice is that payments are likely less aligned with the cost and resource intensity used in the treatment of patients.

Fee Schedules and Per Diem Payment

Fee schedules are payment terms that are based on the service provided. Typical fee schedules are based on HCPCS codes. Each HCPCS procedure code is assigned a fee or payment amount. The calculation of payment under a fee schedule is fairly straightforward. The number of units of service provided is multiplied by the fee for that service to determine the payment.

CMS uses fee schedule payments for physician services, laboratory services, physical therapy, occupational therapy, and speech therapy. An extract from the 2011 Medicare Clinical Laboratory Fee Schedule is presented in table 6.3. Fee schedule contracts are easy to administer for both the provider and the payer, but they do not include any incentive for lowering utilization. As long as the fee amount is adequate to cover the cost of delivering the service, the incentive is actually to provide more services. Managed care plans typically implement strict medical necessity reviews along with fee schedules to maintain cost control.

Fee schedule payments may be implemented so payments are the lesser of the provider's charge and the fee amount. If the contract includes a lesser-of provision, then the provider must ensure that its charge is at least the fee schedule amount in order to receive full fee schedule reimbursement.

Per diems are payments that are made based on the length of stay for inpatient admissions. They are essentially a special case of fee schedules. The fee is a per-day payment as opposed to a per-procedure or per-code payment. The incentives are the same, though. There is really no incentive for a provider to reduce the length of stay as long as the net revenue for each day exceeds the cost of the patient remaining in the hospital. Commercial payers that pay via a per diem rate implement aggressive utilization review programs to ensure that the number of days is clinically appropriate for inpatient admissions.

Percentage of Charge

Pure percentage of charge contracts are rare in managed care contracting and are typically invoked for indemnity plans. Portions of managed care contracts may be based on a percentage of charges. These terms are referred to as carve-outs and allow for separate payment for unusually costly items in a pro-spective payment system. A carve-out for high-cost drugs or devices is often negotiated into contracts. The high-cost items may be identified by a particu-lar **revenue code** or charge threshold. If that threshold is met, then the addi-tional payment may be based on a percentage of the charge for that item. For example, UMC has a contract with a payer that pays a case rate of $3,500 for cardiovascular surgery. The payment terms also include payment of 50 percent of charges for devices with a charge of more than $10,000. If a patient received a defibrillator implant and the charge for that implant was $11,500, then the payment for the case would be the case rate plus 50 percent of the charge for the implant, or $3,500 + (0.50 \times 11,500) = \$9,250$.

Percentage of charge contracts do not have an incentive for providers to reduce their cost or utilization. Indemnity plans have little or no control over where their enrollees seek care, and enrollees may choose the highest-cost provider in the market. The plans may implement some level of utilization review or place a ceiling on the charges for particular items based on a usual and customary charge.

Capitated Rates

Capitated payment rates are based on the number of enrollees in the health plan. A provider receives a fixed payment amount for providing healthcare to enroll-ees for a fixed fee. The fixed fee is typically defined as **per member per month** (PMPM). To fully participate in a capitated payment system, a hospital must partner with a group of physicians or employ a staff of physicians. **Physician–hospital organization**s (PHOs) are uniquely positioned to take on capitated contracts because of the close relationship between the physicians and the hospital.

Under a capitated payment system, the provider is incented to carefully manage the resource use of the enrollees so that the cost of care is below the PMPM. If the cost of care is above the PMPM, then the provider must absorb the excess cost. If the cost of care is below the PMPM, then the provider keeps the unexpended portion of the PMPM.

Capitated payment rates are typically used by HMOs. Since HMOs restrict their members to a particular network of providers and requires enrollees to obtain a referral prior to visiting a specialist or obtaining outpatient diagnos-tic services, they can hold the PCP accountable for the care provided to the patient. Since the PCP controls all aspects of the enrollee's healthcare, a capi-tated payment provides a financial incentive to the PCP for controlling costs.

Commercial Contract Management

Commercial or private health plans are classified as either indemnity plans or managed care plans. Indemnity plans or fee-for-service plans do not limit the choice of provider that the patient may use. Managed care plans can be of a number of distinct designs, including HMOs, PPOs, or point of service (POS). Managed care plans limit the choice of provider as a cost-control measure. An insurance company that offers an indemnity plan does not have as much negotiating leverage with providers as one offering a managed care plan. Since managed care plans limit the choice of providers to those in their network, they can offer an increase in market share to the providers. This potential increase in volume may motivate a provider to accept a lower per-service payment rate from a managed care plan than an indemnity plan. Because of this, indemnity plans often pay providers on a percentage of charge basis. A detailed financial analysis should be performed before and during contract negotiation.

In the article "3 Steps to Profitable Managed Care Contracts," the authors discuss three types of analysis that should be performed to ensure optimal financial performance (Wilson et al. 2004):

1. Internal analysis—comparing the terms and results of a contract among the provider's other contracts, and comparing those terms to the historical cost of care provided to that payer's enrollees
2. External analysis—comparing the contract with those of other providers and payers in the market
3. Payment performance—is the payer paying the correct amount according to the negotiated contract?

Providers often have a contract matrix that summarizes the terms of each major payer. That matrix is the first step in the internal analysis of a managed care contract. An example of a contract matrix is displayed in table 6.4.

Example 1: This example includes only three commercial contracts and Medicare. A typical provider would have many more commercial payers and perhaps other government payers such as Medicaid or worker's compensation. The contract matrix should include the data elements in table 6.4 at a minimum. The fee schedule amounts and weights associated with each case category (MS-DRG or surgical case rate) should be available electronically to allow the calculation of the impact of any changes in contract terms. It is sometimes difficult to compare contracts that have different types of payment terms. This example demonstrates one method of comparing the payment across the plans found in the example contract matrix.

Table 6.4　Memorial Hospital contract matrix

Payer	Plan Type	Start Date	End Date	Inpatient Terms	Outpatient Terms
Insurance Company 1	PPO	1/1/2010	12/31/2011	MS-DRG base rate $6,500 Carve-out: 50% of charge for high-cost drugs	Fee schedule: Lab/Rad Case rate: Ambulatory surgery
Insurance Company 2	HMO	7/1/2009	6/30/2011	Per diem: $2,200 Stop loss: 60% of charges over 20 days	Fee schedule: All services Second procedure discount: Ambulatory surgery
Insurance Company 3	Indemnity	7/1/2010	Auto renew annually	65% of charges	65% of charges
Medicare	FFS	Inpatient: 10/1/2010 Outpatient: 1/1/2010	Inpatient: 9/30/2011 Outpatient: 12/31/2011	MS-DRG base rate $5,700 with outlier	Fee schedule: Lab, PT, OT, ST APC: OPPS payable services

Suppose the CFO of Memorial Hospital wishes to compare the three commercial plans listed in the example contract matrix. The analysis starts with the collection of some historical financial information about the patients served at Memorial Hospital. Projecting payment for the same set of patients across all three plans will give an idea of which provides the better payment terms. The statistics from table 6.5 may be combined with the contract terms displayed in table 6.4 to compare the financial performance of the various contracts.

Insurance Company 1 (C1) pays based on MS-DRG with a base rate of $6,500 and a 50 percent of charge rate for high-cost drugs. High-cost drugs are typically identified by revenue code 636 appearing on the claim. The expected payment for C1 is as follows:

C1 Payment = Total MS-DRG Payment + Total High-Cost Drug Payment

Total MS-DRG Payment = Volume × CMI × Base Rate = 1,695 × 1.86 × 6,500
= $20,492,550

Total High-Cost Drug Payment = Volume × Percentage of cases with high-cost drugs × Average charge for high-cost drugs × High-cost drug payment rate =
1,695 × 0.05 × 25,000 × .50 = $1,059,375

C1 Payment = $20,492,550 + $1,059,375 = $21,551,925

Table 6.5   Memorial Hospital patient statistics

Statistic	Value
Number of discharges	1,695
Case-mix index	1.86
Average length of stay (LOS)	5.2 days
Average charge	$20,790
Percentage of cases with high-cost drugs	5%
Average charge for high-cost drugs	$25,000
Percentage of cases with LOS over 20 days	1%
Average charge for cases with LOS over 20 days	$132,540
Average LOS for cases with LOS < 20 days	4.9 days

Insurance Company 2 (C2) pays based on a per diem amount of $2,200 and includes a stop-loss that provides payment of 60 percent of charges for any patients staying longer than 20 days. The estimated payment for C2 is as follows:

$$\text{C2 Payment} = \text{Per diem payment} + \text{Stop-loss payment}$$

$$\begin{aligned} \text{Per diem payment} &= \text{Volume} \times \text{Percentage of cases with LOS} < 20 \text{ days} \times \\ &\quad \text{LOS for patients} < 20 \text{ days} \times \text{per diem} \\ &= 1{,}695 \times 0.99 \times 4.9 \times 2{,}200 = \$18{,}089{,}379 \end{aligned}$$

$$\begin{aligned} \text{Stop-loss payment} &= \text{Volume} \times \text{Percentage of cases with LOS over} \\ &\quad 20 \text{ days} \times \text{Average charge for cases with LOS over} \\ &\quad 20 \text{ days} \times 0.60 \\ &= 1{,}695 \times 0.01 \times 132{,}540 \times 0.60 = \$1{,}347{,}932 \end{aligned}$$

$$\text{C2 Payment} = 18{,}089{,}379 + 1{,}347{,}932 = \$19{,}437{,}311$$

Insurance Company 3 (C3) pays at a percentage of charge. The estimated payment for C3 is as follows:

$$\text{C3 Payment} = \text{Volume} \times \text{Average Charge per Case} \times \text{Percentage of charge rate}$$
$$\text{C3 Payment} = 1{,}695 \times 20{,}790 \times 0.65 = \$22{,}905{,}383$$

The total charge is estimated as the volume times the average charge per case from table 6.5. From the summary table it is clear that C3 has the best payment terms for the inpatient portion of the business. Since the additional payment amounts for high-cost drugs in C1 and long-stay patients in C2 are less predictable than the base payment, a comparison should also be made between the base payments. In comparing the base payments in table 6.6, C2 is slightly higher than C1.

Table 6.6   Memorial Hospital inpatient contracted payment amounts

Plan	Inpatient Base Payment	Inpatient Additional Payment	Inpatient Total Payment	Total Charge	Ratio of Net Revenue to Gross Revenue
Insurance Company 1	$20,492,550	$1,059,375	$21,551,925	$35,239,050	61%
Insurance Company 2	$18,272,100	$1,347,932	$19,437,311	$35,239,050	56%
Insurance Company 3	$22,905,383	$0	$22,905,383	$35,239,050	65%

If C2 would like to stay with the per-diem term, it may be interesting to determine the **per-diem rate** that makes the base payment in that contract closer to C1. That value may be calculated by taking the base payment for C1 and dividing by the total days for patients with stays shorter than 20 days (average LOS times volume): $20,492,550/(4.9 \times 1,695) = \$2,467$. If the contract were up for renegotiation, then the negotiation target for C2 should be a per diem of $2,467.

Understanding the basic payment terms and combining that with statistics regarding the provider's claims history can provide valuable information for contract negotiations. These data are also critical in managing the expense portion of the margin equation. Recall that the numerator of the operating margin is operating revenues minus expenses. If there is no opportunity to improve the revenue for a particular payer, then this analysis will allow the development of expense targets that can be used to improve the financial performance of the organization or explain budget variances. In comparing the rates of the three insurance companies listed in table 6.6, C1 clearly pays the higher amount. What if the cost per case was approximately $13,000? Would the payment from C1 cover the cost of care? The average base payment per case is $20,492,550/1,695 = \$12,090$. Memorial Hospital is losing nearly $1,000 per case on C1. The terms of C1 look good compared to C2, but at this time neither of these contracts is covering the cost of care.

This internal analysis of the contract terms makes comparing the performance straightforward. This type of information is invaluable when entering into a contract negotiation with a commercial insurance company.

External analysis is far more difficult to perform. Most commercial insurance plan provider contracts include very strict confidentiality statements and are designed to prevent external comparisons. A few consulting firms may provide these data in aggregate, but they typically are blinded to conform to nondisclosure agreements. One external comparison that is available to all providers is the Medicare payment terms. Negotiating terms that are similar to Medicare allows a direct comparison to that plan and simplifies the estimation process required to predict the net revenue to be received under the contract.

External benchmarks may be used to determine if the payment rates are keeping up with the Consumer Price Index (CPI) or the medical inflation rate. Both figures are maintained by the Bureau of Labor Statistics. Any trends found in premium rate changes may also be used as a proxy for the level of rate changes a provider should target in negotiating a contract renewal.

Monitoring the payment performance of managed care contracts is a step that providers often overlook. Putting a significant amount of effort into ensuring that the best contract terms possible are negotiated may be all for naught if the payer is not paying according to the contract terms. The first step in monitoring payment performance is ensuring that contracts are structured in a way that allows the accurate modeling of the expected payment. Contracts that are vague and do not explicitly state the criteria for terms like "high-cost drug" or "usual and customary" cannot be accurately modeled.

The expected payment for contracts should be compared to the actual payment on a regular basis. If the patient accounting or decision support system includes the functionality of modeling the expected payment based on the primary payer assigned to an account, then reports making a comparison of the expected to actual payment should be a part of regular reporting. Identification of any variances should be tracked to the plan and patient type.

Example 2: Memorial Hospital recently purchased a new contract management system that allowed the staff to compare the expected and actual payment for all government and commercial contracts in effect at the hospital. The revenue cycle manager at Memorial Hospital noted that the actual payment was significantly below the expected payment for MMP, a Medicaid managed care plan. The actual payment varied between 30 percent and 60 percent of the expected payment for the last 12 months. She created a graph of the ratio of the actual to expected payment by patient type to try to isolate where the difference was occurring. Figure 6.8 shows the results of the trend analysis.

The lowest percentage of actual to expected payment appeared in the emergency setting. According to the contract in effect for this period of time, MMP should have paid emergency claims as a case rate based on the level of the emergency evaluation and management CPT code submitted on the claim. The payment for Emergency Visit Level 3, the most commonly billed code,

Figure 6.8   Actual/expected payment from MMP

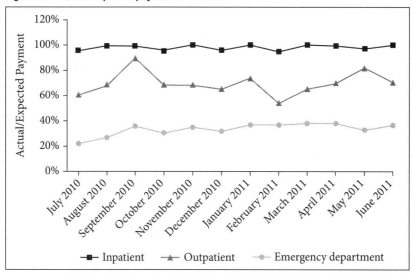

was $2,150 per case. The payment for Emergency Visit Level 3 varied from $230 to $572. The manager requested a listing of the actual and expected payment for Level 3 emergency claims during March 2011. The payment rate for the claims was 72 percent of the charge. The manager then checked the other emergency level codes and determined that MMP had applied a provision that paid the lesser of 72 percent of the charges or the case rate. Using this logic, the case rate was paid for only a small percentage of the Level 4 claims. Memorial Hospital representatives were able to recover $2.2 million in underpayments.

Case Study: Renegotiating a Poorly Performing Contract

Memorial Hospital is beginning the process of renegotiating its contract with BPPO. The current contract terms with BPPO are outlined in table 6.7.

The contracting manager knows that the outpatient contract terms are favorable. The average ratio of cost to charge at Memorial is 0.42. The margin on outpatient services may be calculated using this formula:

Table 6.7   BPPO inpatient and outpatient contract terms

Inpatient Payment	
Base payment	Medicare MS-DRG weights with base rate of $6,000
Outlier provision	62% of difference between total allowed charge and $100,000 if the total allowed charge is in excess of $100,000
Outpatient Payment	
All services	62% of charge

$$\text{BPPO Outpatient Margin} = \frac{\text{BPPO Revenue} - \text{BPPO Expense}}{\text{BPPO Revenue}}$$

$$\text{BPPO Outpatient Margin} = \frac{0.62 \times \text{BPPO Charge} - 0.42 \text{ BPPO Charge}}{0.62 \times \text{BPPO Charge}}$$

$$\text{BPPO Outpatient Margin} = \frac{0.62 \times \cancel{\text{BPPO Charge}} - 0.42 \cancel{\text{BPPO Charge}}}{0.62 \times \cancel{\text{BPPO Charge}}}$$

$$= \frac{0.62 - 0.42}{0.62} = 32\%$$

The margin on the inpatient side of the contract is less favorable. Memorial submitted claims for 2,527 inpatient admissions to BPPO. The CMI was 1.75. None of the accounts was in excess of $100,000, so the outlier provision is not included in the estimates. The average charge per claim was $27,580. Using the average ratio of cost to charge, the average cost per claim is $27{,}580 \times 0.42 = 11{,}584$. The average payment per claim is the CMI multiplied by the base rate, or $1.75 \times 6{,}000 = 10{,}500$. The margin on inpatient services may be calculated using this formula:

$$\text{BPPO Inpatient Margin} = \frac{\text{BPPO Revenue} - \text{BPPO Expense}}{\text{BPPO Revenue}}$$

$$\text{BPPO Inpatient Margin} = \frac{10{,}500 - 11{,}584}{10{,}500} = -10\%$$

Before concluding that the outpatient margin offsets the inpatient margin, the manager knows that she needs to take the mix of inpatient and outpatient services to determine the overall margin. The percentage of revenue received for inpatient services for BPPO claims is 85 percent. The overall margin is then as follows:

$$\text{BPPO Overall Margin} = 0.85 \times (-0.10) + 0.15 \times 0.32 = -0.037$$

The resulting –3.7 percent overall margin for BPPO is surprising to the manager. The formula for the overall margin reveals two potential strategies for achieving a positive margin for BPPO. The first strategy is to increase the proportion of services and therefore revenue coming from the outpatient setting. The second strategy is to increase the revenue per case on the inpatient side.

The manager wants to go into the negotiation knowing exactly how much of an increase in the inpatient rate is required to get to breakeven if the proportion of inpatient and outpatient revenue does not change. She puts together the following formula:

$$\text{BPPO Overall Margin} = 0.85 \times (\text{ip margin}) + 0.15 \times 0.32 = 0$$

$$\text{BPPO Inpatient Margin} = \frac{-0.15 \times 0.32}{0.85} = -0.056$$

The inpatient payment per claim required to achieve the –5.6 percent inpatient margin is as follows:

$$\text{BPPO Inpatient Margin} = \frac{\text{BPPO Revenue} - 11,584}{\text{BPPO Revenue}} = -0.056$$

$$\text{BPPO Revenue} - 11,584 = -0.056 \times \text{BPPO Revenue}$$

$$\text{BPPO Revenue} + 0.056 \times \text{BPPO Revenue} = 11,584$$

$$\text{BPPO Revenue} = \frac{11,584}{1 + 0.056} = \frac{11,584}{1.056} = 10,960$$

Based on this calculation, the manager must negotiate a contract so that the average payment per inpatient claim is at least $10,960. The CMI for Memorial is 1.75. If we assume the CMI will stay at least that high next year, then the base rate needs to be renegotiated to be 10,960/1.75 = $6,263. This represents a 4.5 percent increase over the previous base rate of $6,000. The manager now has a good "worst case" for her negotiation. She knows that she may need to reduce the outpatient percentage of charge rate to improve the inpatient case rate. She puts together a spreadsheet to help her understand the relationship between the two payment figures. The relationship between the outpatient percentage of charge and the inpatient base rate required to produce a break-even margin for the BPPO contract appears in figure 6.9.

Figure 6.9   Relationship between outpatient and inpatient payment terms at break-even margin

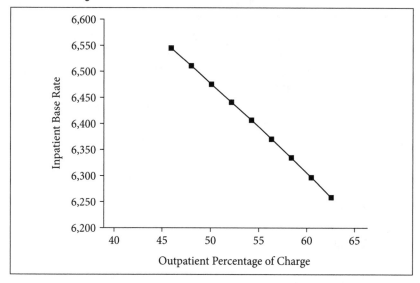

The current scenario is the point at the right-hand end of the line with 62 percent of charges in the outpatient setting and the previously calculated breakeven inpatient base rate of $6,263. This graph will be a valuable tool for the manager to have as a personal reference during the negotiation process. The manager knows that if she can negotiate rates with values above this line, the overall margin will be positive for the BPPO book of business.

Summary

Effective financial management requires a thorough understanding of the methods that the provider may use to collect revenue for treating patients. The provider has far more control over the payment received for treating patients with private or commercial insurance than with government payers. These contracts are negotiated on a regular basis. Understanding the nature of the terms of the contract and the estimated cost of treating the patients who may subscribe to that insurance plan will allow the provider to negotiate an appropriate rate of payment.

Providers are not able to negotiate payment rates with government payers. Managing financial performance under those contracts requires analysis of the payment drivers and diligent tracking of those drivers to ensure that proper payment is received for services.

CHECK YOUR UNDERSTANDING

1. A contractual allowance is the amount of payment received from a payer for services provided to a patient. (True/False)
2. The case-mix index may be used to measure the average resource intensity required to treat the typical Medicare inpatient admission. (True/False)
3. Medicare inpatient payment rates are adjusted for the cost of living in the location of the provider. (True/False)
4. A stop-loss protects the payer from significant financial loss if a patient requires more resources than expected. (True/False)
5. A state Medicaid plan must cover nursing facility services for individuals over 21 years of age. (True/False)
6. Which of the following is not a prospective payment system?
   a. Percentage of charge
   b. MS-DRG
   c. Fee schedule
   d. Case rate

7. Most Medicare beneficiaries receive their prescription drug coverage from:
   a. Medicare Advantage plan with drug coverage
   b. Stand-alone prescription drug plans
   c. Medicare retiree drug subsidy
   d. Other prescription drug coverage
8. If a provider's Medicare base rate is $5,000 and its Medicare case-mix index shifts from 1.75 to 1.65, how will this affect its average Medicare payment per inpatient case?
   a. Reduce the payment by $250
   b. Increase the payment by $500
   c. Reduce the payment by $500
   d. The case-mix index has no relationship to average Medicare payment
9. Which of the following is not an element in a typical contract matrix?
   a. Plan type
   b. Contract start and end dates
   c. Payment terms
   d. All of the above
10. Contract negotiations may impact what portions of the financial statement?
    a. Patient accounts receivable in the income statement
    b. Accumulated depreciation in the balance sheet
    c. Long-term debt in the balance sheet
    d. None of these

References

American Hospital Association. 2010. American Hospital Association underpayment by Medicare and Medicaid fact sheet. http://www.aha.org/aha/content/2010/pdf/10medunderpayment.pdf.

Casto, A., and E. Layman. 2011. *Principles of Healthcare Reimbursement,* 3rd ed. Chicago: AHIMA Press.

Centers for Medicare and Medicaid Services. 2009. Roadmap for implementing value driven healthcare in the traditional Medicare fee-for-service program. https://www.cms.gov/QualityInitiativesGenInfo/downloads/VBPRoadmap_OEA_1-16_508.pdf.

Centers for Medicare and Medicaid Services. 2010a. Medicaid managed care enrollment report. https://www.cms.gov/MedicaidDataSourcesGenInfo/downloads/09ENROLLMENT.pdf.

Centers for Medicare and Medicaid Services. 2010b. Your guide to Medicare Special Needs Plans (SNPs). Baltimore: Department of Health and Human Services.

Centers for Medicare and Medicaid Services. 2011a. Fee schedules—general information. https://www.cms.gov/feeschedulegeninfo.

Centers for Medicare and Medicaid Services. 2011b. FY 2011 IPPS Final Rule home page. http://www.cms.gov/AcuteInpatientPPS.

Centers for Medicare and Medicaid Services. 2011c. Medicare and you. http://www.medicare.gov/publications/pubs/pdf/10050.pdf.

Centers for Medicare and Medicaid Services. 2011d. Medicare program general information. http://www.cms.gov/MedicareGenInfo.

Centers for Medicare and Medicaid Services. 2011e. Prescription drug coverage overview. https://www.cms.gov/PrescriptionDrugCovGenIn/Downloads/2010_Enrollment_Release.zip.

MedPAC. 2010a. A data book: Healthcare spending and the Medicare program. http://www.medpac.gov/documents/jun10databookentirereport.pdf.

MedPAC. 2010b. Hospital acute inpatient payment system. http://www.medpac.gov/documents/MedPAC_Payment_Basics_10_hospital.pdf.

MedPAC. 2010c. Medicare Advantage Program payment system. http://www.medpac.gov/documents/MedPAC_Payment_Basics_10_MA.pdf.

Wilson, D., M. Malloy, J. McCoy, and M. Turner. 2004. 3 steps to profitable managed care contracts. *Health Financial Management* 58(5):34–38.

Appendix 6.1: MS-DRG Weight Table—Federal Fiscal Year 2011

MS-DRG	MDC	Type	MS-DRG Title	Weight	Geometric Mean LOS	Arithmetic Mean LOS
001	PRE	SURG	HEART TRANSPLANT OR IMPLANT OF HEART ASSIST SYSTEM W MCC	26.344	31.6	41.9
002	PRE	SURG	HEART TRANSPLANT OR IMPLANT OF HEART ASSIST SYSTEM W/O MCC	13.613	17.6	22.6
003	PRE	SURG	ECMO OR TRACH W MV 96+ HRS OR PDX EXC FACE, MOUTH & NECK W MAJ O.R.	18.124	30.1	36.6
004	PRE	SURG	TRACH W MV 96+ HRS OR PDX EXC FACE, MOUTH & NECK W/O MAJ O.R.	11.240	22.2	27.1
005	PRE	SURG	LIVER TRANSPLANT W MCC OR INTESTINAL TRANSPLANT	10.177	14.9	19.9
006	PRE	SURG	LIVER TRANSPLANT W/O MCC	4.835	8.3	9.3
007	PRE	SURG	LUNG TRANSPLANT	9.335	15.4	18.6
008	PRE	SURG	SIMULTANEOUS PANCREAS/KIDNEY TRANSPLANT	4.963	10.1	11.7
010	PRE	SURG	PANCREAS TRANSPLANT	3.783	8.6	9.7
011	PRE	SURG	TRACHEOSTOMY FOR FACE, MOUTH & NECK DIAGNOSES W MCC	4.767	12.3	15.5
012	PRE	SURG	TRACHEOSTOMY FOR FACE, MOUTH & NECK DIAGNOSES W CC	3.131	8.5	10.1
013	PRE	SURG	TRACHEOSTOMY FOR FACE, MOUTH & NECK DIAGNOSES W/O CC/MCC	1.951	5.7	6.8
014	PRE	SURG	ALLOGENEIC BONE MARROW TRANSPLANT	11.595	21.1	28.2
015	PRE	SURG	AUTOLOGOUS BONE MARROW TRANSPLANT	5.950	16.7	19.3
020	01	SURG	INTRACRANIAL VASCULAR PROCEDURES W PDX HEMORRHAGE W MCC	8.248	14.1	17.3
021	01	SURG	INTRACRANIAL VASCULAR PROCEDURES W PDX HEMORRHAGE W CC	6.289	12.1	13.9
022	01	SURG	INTRACRANIAL VASCULAR PROCEDURES W PDX HEMORRHAGE W/O CC/MCC	4.158	6.7	8.4
023	01	SURG	CRANIO W MAJOR DEV IMPL/ACUTE COMPLEX CNS PDX W MCC OR CHEMO IMPLANT	5.088	8.2	11.8
024	01	SURG	CRANIO W MAJOR DEV IMPL/ACUTE COMPLEX CNS PDX W/O MCC	3.495	5.7	8.1
025	01	SURG	CRANIOTOMY & ENDOVASCULAR INTRACRANIAL PROCEDURES W MCC	4.758	8.8	11.5
026	01	SURG	CRANIOTOMY & ENDOVASCULAR INTRACRANIAL PROCEDURES W CC	2.983	5.8	7.3
027	01	SURG	CRANIOTOMY & ENDOVASCULAR INTRACRANIAL PROCEDURES W/O CC/MCC	2.131	3.0	3.9
028	01	SURG	SPINAL PROCEDURES W MCC	5.355	10.1	13.1
029	01	SURG	SPINAL PROCEDURES W CC OR SPINAL NEUROSTIMULATORS	2.874	4.7	6.6
030	01	SURG	SPINAL PROCEDURES W/O CC/MCC	1.643	2.5	3.3
031	01	SURG	VENTRICULAR SHUNT PROCEDURES W MCC	4.126	8.6	12.3
032	01	SURG	VENTRICULAR SHUNT PROCEDURES W CC	1.922	3.6	5.3
033	01	SURG	VENTRICULAR SHUNT PROCEDURES W/O CC/MCC	1.363	2.1	2.6
034	01	SURG	CAROTID ARTERY STENT PROCEDURE W MCC	3.524	4.7	7.0

MS-DRG	MDC	Type	MS-DRG Title	Weight	Geometric Mean LOS	Arithmetic Mean LOS
035	01	SURG	CAROTID ARTERY STENT PROCEDURE W CC	2.144	2.2	3.2
036	01	SURG	CAROTID ARTERY STENT PROCEDURE W/O CC/MCC	1.639	1.3	1.5
037	01	SURG	EXTRACRANIAL PROCEDURES W MCC	3.154	5.7	8.4
038	01	SURG	EXTRACRANIAL PROCEDURES W CC	1.546	2.4	3.5
039	01	SURG	EXTRACRANIAL PROCEDURES W/O CC/MCC	1.019	1.4	1.7
040	01	SURG	PERIPH/CRANIAL NERVE & OTHER NERV SYST PROC W MCC	3.935	9.0	12.1
041	01	SURG	PERIPH/CRANIAL NERVE & OTHER NERV SYST PROC W CC OR PERIPH NEUROSTIM	2.143	5.0	6.7
042	01	SURG	PERIPH/CRANIAL NERVE & OTHER NERV SYST PROC W/O CC/MCC	1.691	2.4	3.2
052	01	MED	SPINAL DISORDERS & INJURIES W CC/MCC	1.611	4.5	6.7
053	01	MED	SPINAL DISORDERS & INJURIES W/O CC/MCC	0.844	2.9	3.6
054	01	MED	NERVOUS SYSTEM NEOPLASMS W MCC	1.486	4.6	6.3
055	01	MED	NERVOUS SYSTEM NEOPLASMS W/O MCC	1.065	3.5	4.6
056	01	MED	DEGENERATIVE NERVOUS SYSTEM DISORDERS W MCC	1.675	5.5	7.1
057	01	MED	DEGENERATIVE NERVOUS SYSTEM DISORDERS W/O MCC	0.935	3.7	4.8
058	01	MED	MULTIPLE SCLEROSIS & CEREBELLAR ATAXIA W MCC	1.586	5.4	7.2
059	01	MED	MULTIPLE SCLEROSIS & CEREBELLAR ATAXIA W CC	0.981	4.1	4.9
060	01	MED	MULTIPLE SCLEROSIS & CEREBELLAR ATAXIA W/O CC/MCC	0.758	3.2	3.8
061	01	MED	ACUTE ISCHEMIC STROKE W USE OF THROMBOLYTIC AGENT W MCC	2.957	6.4	8.4
062	01	MED	ACUTE ISCHEMIC STROKE W USE OF THROMBOLYTIC AGENT W CC	1.948	4.8	5.6
063	01	MED	ACUTE ISCHEMIC STROKE W USE OF THROMBOLYTIC AGENT W/O CC/MCC	1.525	3.4	3.9
064	01	MED	INTRACRANIAL HEMORRHAGE OR CEREBRAL INFARCTION W MCC	1.867	5.1	6.9
065	01	MED	INTRACRANIAL HEMORRHAGE OR CEREBRAL INFARCTION W CC	1.167	4.0	4.8
066	01	MED	INTRACRANIAL HEMORRHAGE OR CEREBRAL INFARCTION W/O CC/MCC	0.820	2.7	3.3
067	01	MED	NONSPECIFIC CVA & PRECEREBRAL OCCLUSION W/O INFARCT W MCC	1.423	4.2	5.5
068	01	MED	NONSPECIFIC CVA & PRECEREBRAL OCCLUSION W/O INFARCT W/O MCC	0.875	2.7	3.3
069	01	MED	TRANSIENT ISCHEMIA	0.731	2.3	2.8
070	01	MED	NONSPECIFIC CEREBROVASCULAR DISORDERS W MCC	1.842	5.6	7.3
071	01	MED	NONSPECIFIC CEREBROVASCULAR DISORDERS W CC	1.105	4.1	5.1
072	01	MED	NONSPECIFIC CEREBROVASCULAR DISORDERS W/O CC/MCC	0.750	2.5	3.1

MS-DRG	MDC	Type	MS-DRG Title	Weight	Geometric Mean LOS	Arithmetic Mean LOS
073	01	MED	CRANIAL & PERIPHERAL NERVE DISORDERS W MCC	1.291	4.2	5.6
074	01	MED	CRANIAL & PERIPHERAL NERVE DISORDERS W/O MCC	0.861	3.2	4.1
075	01	MED	VIRAL MENINGITIS W CC/MCC	1.657	5.5	7.0
076	01	MED	VIRAL MENINGITIS W/O CC/MCC	0.905	3.3	3.9
077	01	MED	HYPERTENSIVE ENCEPHALOPATHY W MCC	1.738	5.1	6.4
078	01	MED	HYPERTENSIVE ENCEPHALOPATHY W CC	1.015	3.5	4.4
079	01	MED	HYPERTENSIVE ENCEPHALOPATHY W/O CC/MCC	0.753	2.6	3.1
080	01	MED	NONTRAUMATIC STUPOR & COMA W MCC	1.191	3.6	4.9
081	01	MED	NONTRAUMATIC STUPOR & COMA W/O MCC	0.739	2.7	3.4
082	01	MED	TRAUMATIC STUPOR & COMA, COMA >1 HR W MCC	2.013	3.5	6.1
083	01	MED	TRAUMATIC STUPOR & COMA, COMA >1 HR W CC	1.326	3.4	4.7
084	01	MED	TRAUMATIC STUPOR & COMA, COMA >1 HR W/O CC/MCC	0.896	2.2	2.8
085	01	MED	TRAUMATIC STUPOR & COMA, COMA <1 HR W MCC	2.142	5.2	7.2
086	01	MED	TRAUMATIC STUPOR & COMA, COMA <1 HR W CC	1.205	3.7	4.6
087	01	MED	TRAUMATIC STUPOR & COMA, COMA <1 HR W/O CC/MCC	0.793	2.3	2.9
088	01	MED	CONCUSSION W MCC	1.487	4.2	5.5
089	01	MED	CONCUSSION W CC	0.967	2.9	3.7
090	01	MED	CONCUSSION W/O CC/MCC	0.693	1.9	2.3
091	01	MED	OTHER DISORDERS OF NERVOUS SYSTEM W MCC	1.632	4.4	6.2
092	01	MED	OTHER DISORDERS OF NERVOUS SYSTEM W CC	0.940	3.3	4.2
093	01	MED	OTHER DISORDERS OF NERVOUS SYSTEM W/O CC/MCC	0.683	2.4	2.9
094	01	MED	BACTERIAL & TUBERCULOUS INFECTIONS OF NERVOUS SYSTEM W MCC	3.677	8.9	11.7
095	01	MED	BACTERIAL & TUBERCULOUS INFECTIONS OF NERVOUS SYSTEM W CC	2.398	6.6	8.4
096	01	MED	BACTERIAL & TUBERCULOUS INFECTIONS OF NERVOUS SYSTEM W/O CC/MCC	1.925	4.6	5.6
097	01	MED	NON-BACTERIAL INFECT OF NERVOUS SYS EXC VIRAL MENINGITIS W MCC	3.219	9.0	11.6
098	01	MED	NON-BACTERIAL INFECT OF NERVOUS SYS EXC VIRAL MENINGITIS W CC	1.911	6.4	7.9
099	01	MED	NON-BACTERIAL INFECT OF NERVOUS SYS EXC VIRAL MENINGITIS W/O CC/MCC	1.208	4.1	5.2
100	01	MED	SEIZURES W MCC	1.511	4.5	6.0
101	01	MED	SEIZURES W/O MCC	0.762	2.8	3.4

MS-DRG	MDC	Type	MS-DRG Title	Weight	Geometric Mean LOS	Arithmetic Mean LOS
102	01	MED	HEADACHES W MCC	1.029	3.1	4.3
103	01	MED	HEADACHES W/O MCC	0.670	2.4	3.0
113	02	SURG	ORBITAL PROCEDURES W CC/MCC	1.831	3.9	5.6
114	02	SURG	ORBITAL PROCEDURES W/O CC/MCC	0.899	2.0	2.6
115	02	SURG	EXTRAOCULAR PROCEDURES EXCEPT ORBIT	1.208	3.5	4.6
116	02	SURG	INTRAOCULAR PROCEDURES W CC/MCC	1.268	3.0	4.4
117	02	SURG	INTRAOCULAR PROCEDURES W/O CC/MCC	0.731	1.6	2.0
121	02	MED	ACUTE MAJOR EYE INFECTIONS W CC/MCC	0.910	4.1	5.1
122	02	MED	ACUTE MAJOR EYE INFECTIONS W/O CC/MCC	0.652	3.3	4.0
123	02	MED	NEUROLOGICAL EYE DISORDERS	0.714	2.2	2.7
124	02	MED	OTHER DISORDERS OF THE EYE W MCC	1.190	3.8	5.3
125	02	MED	OTHER DISORDERS OF THE EYE W/O MCC	0.686	2.7	3.4
129	03	SURG	MAJOR HEAD & NECK PROCEDURES W CC/MCC OR MAJOR DEVICE	2.235	3.7	5.2
130	03	SURG	MAJOR HEAD & NECK PROCEDURES W/O CC/MCC	1.230	2.3	2.9
131	03	SURG	CRANIAL/FACIAL PROCEDURES W CC/MCC	2.092	4.1	5.6
132	03	SURG	CRANIAL/FACIAL PROCEDURES W/O CC/MCC	1.245	2.1	2.7
133	03	SURG	OTHER EAR, NOSE, MOUTH & THROAT O.R. PROCEDURES W CC/MCC	1.700	3.6	5.4
134	03	SURG	OTHER EAR, NOSE, MOUTH & THROAT O.R. PROCEDURES W/O CC/MCC	0.851	1.7	2.1
135	03	SURG	SINUS & MASTOID PROCEDURES W CC/MCC	1.908	4.3	6.4
136	03	SURG	SINUS & MASTOID PROCEDURES W/O CC/MCC	0.975	1.7	2.3
137	03	SURG	MOUTH PROCEDURES W CC/MCC	1.301	3.6	5.0
138	03	SURG	MOUTH PROCEDURES W/O CC/MCC	0.784	1.9	2.5
139	03	SURG	SALIVARY GLAND PROCEDURES	0.876	1.4	1.8
146	03	MED	EAR, NOSE, MOUTH & THROAT MALIGNANCY W MCC	2.189	6.5	9.1
147	03	MED	EAR, NOSE, MOUTH & THROAT MALIGNANCY W CC	1.241	4.1	5.7
148	03	MED	EAR, NOSE, MOUTH & THROAT MALIGNANCY W/O CC/MCC	0.807	2.4	3.3
149	03	MED	DYSEQUILIBRIUM	0.639	2.2	2.6
150	03	MED	EPISTAXIS W MCC	1.281	3.7	5.0
151	03	MED	EPISTAXIS W/O MCC	0.639	2.3	2.9

MS-DRG	MDC	Type	MS-DRG Title	Weight	Geometric Mean LOS	Arithmetic Mean LOS
152	03	MED	OTITIS MEDIA & URI W MCC	0.958	3.3	4.3
153	03	MED	OTITIS MEDIA & URI W/O MCC	0.629	2.5	3.1
154	03	MED	OTHER EAR, NOSE, MOUTH & THROAT DIAGNOSES W MCC	1.397	4.3	5.8
155	03	MED	OTHER EAR, NOSE, MOUTH & THROAT DIAGNOSES W CC	0.902	3.3	4.2
156	03	MED	OTHER EAR, NOSE, MOUTH & THROAT DIAGNOSES W/O CC/MCC	0.623	2.4	2.9
157	03	MED	DENTAL & ORAL DISEASES W MCC	1.579	4.8	6.7
158	03	MED	DENTAL & ORAL DISEASES W CC	0.903	3.4	4.4
159	03	MED	DENTAL & ORAL DISEASES W/O CC/MCC	0.590	2.2	2.7
163	04	SURG	MAJOR CHEST PROCEDURES W MCC	5.083	11.5	14.0
164	04	SURG	MAJOR CHEST PROCEDURES W CC	2.624	6.2	7.4
165	04	SURG	MAJOR CHEST PROCEDURES W/O CC/MCC	1.776	3.7	4.4
166	04	SURG	OTHER RESP SYSTEM O.R. PROCEDURES W MCC	3.738	9.5	11.9
167	04	SURG	OTHER RESP SYSTEM O.R. PROCEDURES W CC	2.057	5.8	7.4
168	04	SURG	OTHER RESP SYSTEM O.R. PROCEDURES W/O CC/MCC	1.301	3.3	4.3
175	04	MED	PULMONARY EMBOLISM W MCC	1.610	5.7	6.8
176	04	MED	PULMONARY EMBOLISM W/O MCC	1.071	4.2	4.9
177	04	MED	RESPIRATORY INFECTIONS & INFLAMMATIONS W MCC	2.067	6.8	8.5
178	04	MED	RESPIRATORY INFECTIONS & INFLAMMATIONS W CC	1.489	5.6	6.8
179	04	MED	RESPIRATORY INFECTIONS & INFLAMMATIONS W/O CC/MCC	0.986	4.1	5.0
180	04	MED	RESPIRATORY NEOPLASMS W MCC	1.736	5.7	7.5
181	04	MED	RESPIRATORY NEOPLASMS W CC	1.218	4.2	5.4
182	04	MED	RESPIRATORY NEOPLASMS W/O CC/MCC	0.810	2.8	3.7
183	04	MED	MAJOR CHEST TRAUMA W MCC	1.494	5.2	6.5
184	04	MED	MAJOR CHEST TRAUMA W CC	0.976	3.6	4.3
185	04	MED	MAJOR CHEST TRAUMA W/O CC/MCC	0.680	2.6	3.0
186	04	MED	PLEURAL EFFUSION W MCC	1.564	5.3	6.7
187	04	MED	PLEURAL EFFUSION W CC	1.103	3.9	4.9
188	04	MED	PLEURAL EFFUSION W/O CC/MCC	0.768	2.8	3.5
189	04	MED	PULMONARY EDEMA & RESPIRATORY FAILURE	1.281	4.3	5.5

MS-DRG	MDC	Type	MS-DRG Title	Weight	Geometric Mean LOS	Arithmetic Mean LOS
190	04	MED	CHRONIC OBSTRUCTIVE PULMONARY DISEASE W MCC	1.192	4.5	5.5
191	04	MED	CHRONIC OBSTRUCTIVE PULMONARY DISEASE W CC	0.974	3.8	4.6
192	04	MED	CHRONIC OBSTRUCTIVE PULMONARY DISEASE W/O CC/MCC	0.722	3.1	3.7
193	04	MED	SIMPLE PNEUMONIA & PLEURISY W MCC	1.480	5.3	6.5
194	04	MED	SIMPLE PNEUMONIA & PLEURISY W CC	1.015	4.2	5.0
195	04	MED	SIMPLE PNEUMONIA & PLEURISY W/O CC/MCC	0.710	3.1	3.7
196	04	MED	INTERSTITIAL LUNG DISEASE W MCC	1.606	5.6	6.9
197	04	MED	INTERSTITIAL LUNG DISEASE W CC	1.118	4.2	5.1
198	04	MED	INTERSTITIAL LUNG DISEASE W/O CC/MCC	0.820	3.1	3.8
199	04	MED	PNEUMOTHORAX W MCC	1.790	6.3	8.0
200	04	MED	PNEUMOTHORAX W CC	1.025	3.7	4.8
201	04	MED	PNEUMOTHORAX W/O CC/MCC	0.721	2.8	3.6
202	04	MED	BRONCHITIS & ASTHMA W CC/MCC	0.842	3.4	4.1
203	04	MED	BRONCHITIS & ASTHMA W/O CC/MCC	0.608	2.6	3.2
204	04	MED	RESPIRATORY SIGNS & SYMPTOMS	0.671	2.1	2.7
205	04	MED	OTHER RESPIRATORY SYSTEM DIAGNOSES W MCC	1.297	3.9	5.3
206	04	MED	OTHER RESPIRATORY SYSTEM DIAGNOSES W/O MCC	0.758	2.6	3.3
207	04	MED	RESPIRATORY SYSTEM DIAGNOSIS W VENTILATOR SUPPORT 96+ HOURS	5.207	12.6	14.7
208	04	MED	RESPIRATORY SYSTEM DIAGNOSIS W VENTILATOR SUPPORT <96 HOURS	2.263	5.1	7.0
215	05	SURG	OTHER HEART ASSIST SYSTEM IMPLANT	12.609	6.9	12.2
216	05	SURG	CARDIAC VALVE & OTH MAJ CARDIOTHORACIC PROC W CARD CATH W MCC	10.024	14.6	17.0
217	05	SURG	CARDIAC VALVE & OTH MAJ CARDIOTHORACIC PROC W CARD CATH W CC	6.804	9.8	10.9
218	05	SURG	CARDIAC VALVE & OTH MAJ CARDIOTHORACIC PROC W CARD CATH W/O CC/MCC	5.329	7.2	8.0
219	05	SURG	CARDIAC VALVE & OTH MAJ CARDIOTHORACIC PROC W/O CARD CATH W MCC	8.083	10.8	13.1
220	05	SURG	CARDIAC VALVE & OTH MAJ CARDIOTHORACIC PROC W/O CARD CATH W CC	5.379	7.2	8.0
221	05	SURG	CARDIAC VALVE & OTH MAJ CARDIOTHORACIC PROC W/O CARD CATH W/O CC/MCC	4.480	5.6	6.0
222	05	SURG	CARDIAC DEFIB IMPLANT W CARDIAC CATH W AMI/HF/SHOCK W MCC	8.523	9.4	11.8
223	05	SURG	CARDIAC DEFIB IMPLANT W CARDIAC CATH W AMI/HF/SHOCK W/O MCC	6.425	4.5	6.2
224	05	SURG	CARDIAC DEFIB IMPLANT W CARDIAC CATH W/O AMI/HF/SHOCK W MCC	7.582	7.7	9.7

MS-DRG	MDC	Type	MS-DRG Title	Weight	Geometric Mean LOS	Arithmetic Mean LOS
225	05	SURG	CARDIAC DEFIB IMPLANT W CARDIAC CATH W/O AMI/HF/SHOCK W/O MCC	6.020	4.2	5.3
226	05	SURG	CARDIAC DEFIBRILLATOR IMPLANT W/O CARDIAC CATH W MCC	6.451	5.0	7.7
227	05	SURG	CARDIAC DEFIBRILLATOR IMPLANT W/O CARDIAC CATH W/O MCC	5.194	2.0	3.1
228	05	SURG	OTHER CARDIOTHORACIC PROCEDURES W MCC	7.588	11.8	14.2
229	05	SURG	OTHER CARDIOTHORACIC PROCEDURES W CC	4.775	7.2	8.3
230	05	SURG	OTHER CARDIOTHORACIC PROCEDURES W/O CC/MCC	3.545	4.6	5.5
231	05	SURG	CORONARY BYPASS W PTCA W MCC	7.858	10.9	12.9
232	05	SURG	CORONARY BYPASS W PTCA W/O MCC	5.818	8.5	9.4
233	05	SURG	CORONARY BYPASS W CARDIAC CATH W MCC	7.208	12.1	13.7
234	05	SURG	CORONARY BYPASS W CARDIAC CATH W/O MCC	4.828	8.2	8.9
235	05	SURG	CORONARY BYPASS W/O CARDIAC CATH W MCC	5.853	9.3	10.8
236	05	SURG	CORONARY BYPASS W/O CARDIAC CATH W/O MCC	3.771	6.0	6.5
237	05	SURG	MAJOR CARDIOVASC PROCEDURES W MCC OR THORACIC AORTIC ANEURYSM REPAIR	5.190	7.1	10.1
238	05	SURG	MAJOR CARDIOVASC PROCEDURES W/O MCC	3.083	2.9	4.2
239	05	SURG	AMPUTATION FOR CIRC SYS DISORDERS EXC UPPER LIMB & TOE W MCC	4.554	11.2	14.3
240	05	SURG	AMPUTATION FOR CIRC SYS DISORDERS EXC UPPER LIMB & TOE W CC	2.659	7.8	9.6
241	05	SURG	AMPUTATION FOR CIRC SYS DISORDERS EXC UPPER LIMB & TOE W/O CC/MCC	1.463	5.0	6.0
242	05	SURG	PERMANENT CARDIAC PACEMAKER IMPLANT W MCC	3.728	6.3	8.1
243	05	SURG	PERMANENT CARDIAC PACEMAKER IMPLANT W CC	2.651	3.9	4.9
244	05	SURG	PERMANENT CARDIAC PACEMAKER IMPLANT W/O CC/MCC	2.040	2.2	2.8
245	05	SURG	AICD GENERATOR PROCEDURES	4.249	2.5	3.8
246	05	SURG	PERC CARDIOVASC PROC W DRUG-ELUTING STENT W MCC OR 4+ VESSELS/STENTS	3.180	3.5	5.0
247	05	SURG	PERC CARDIOVASC PROC W DRUG-ELUTING STENT W/O MCC	1.969	1.8	2.3
248	05	SURG	PERC CARDIOVASC PROC W NON-DRUG-ELUTING STENT W MCC OR 4+ VES/STENTS	2.925	4.4	6.0
249	05	SURG	PERC CARDIOVASC PROC W NON-DRUG-ELUTING STENT W/O MCC	1.773	2.2	2.8
250	05	SURG	PERC CARDIOVASC PROC W/O CORONARY ARTERY STENT W MCC	2.884	5.0	7.0
251	05	SURG	PERC CARDIOVASC PROC W/O CORONARY ARTERY STENT W/O MCC	1.799	2.2	3.0
252	05	SURG	OTHER VASCULAR PROCEDURES W MCC	2.975	5.2	7.9
253	05	SURG	OTHER VASCULAR PROCEDURES W CC	2.401	4.4	6.0

MS-DRG	MDC	Type	MS-DRG Title	Weight	Geometric Mean LOS	Arithmetic Mean LOS
254	05	SURG	OTHER VASCULAR PROCEDURES W/O CC/MCC	1.615	2.0	2.7
255	05	SURG	UPPER LIMB & TOE AMPUTATION FOR CIRC SYSTEM DISORDERS W MCC	2.504	7.0	9.2
256	05	SURG	UPPER LIMB & TOE AMPUTATION FOR CIRC SYSTEM DISORDERS W CC	1.597	5.6	7.0
257	05	SURG	UPPER LIMB & TOE AMPUTATION FOR CIRC SYSTEM DISORDERS W/O CC/MCC	0.975	3.4	4.3
258	05	SURG	CARDIAC PACEMAKER DEVICE REPLACEMENT W MCC	2.888	5.2	7.0
259	05	SURG	CARDIAC PACEMAKER DEVICE REPLACEMENT W/O MCC	1.833	2.4	3.2
260	05	SURG	CARDIAC PACEMAKER REVISION EXCEPT DEVICE REPLACEMENT W MCC	3.550	7.7	10.7
261	05	SURG	CARDIAC PACEMAKER REVISION EXCEPT DEVICE REPLACEMENT W CC	1.647	3.2	4.5
262	05	SURG	CARDIAC PACEMAKER REVISION EXCEPT DEVICE REPLACEMENT W/O CC/MCC	1.125	2.0	2.6
263	05	SURG	VEIN LIGATION & STRIPPING	1.757	3.5	5.6
264	05	SURG	OTHER CIRCULATORY SYSTEM O.R. PROCEDURES	2.531	5.5	8.2
265	05	SURG	AICD LEAD PROCEDURES	2.316	2.3	3.4
280	05	MED	ACUTE MYOCARDIAL INFARCTION, DISCHARGED ALIVE W MCC	1.850	5.2	6.6
281	05	MED	ACUTE MYOCARDIAL INFARCTION, DISCHARGED ALIVE W CC	1.191	3.6	4.4
282	05	MED	ACUTE MYOCARDIAL INFARCTION, DISCHARGED ALIVE W/O CC/MCC	0.806	2.2	2.8
283	05	MED	ACUTE MYOCARDIAL INFARCTION, EXPIRED W MCC	1.715	3.2	5.1
284	05	MED	ACUTE MYOCARDIAL INFARCTION, EXPIRED W CC	0.889	2.1	3.0
285	05	MED	ACUTE MYOCARDIAL INFARCTION, EXPIRED W/O CC/MCC	0.571	1.4	1.8
286	05	MED	CIRCULATORY DISORDERS EXCEPT AMI, W CARD CATH W MCC	2.001	4.8	6.5
287	05	MED	CIRCULATORY DISORDERS EXCEPT AMI, W CARD CATH W/O MCC	1.088	2.5	3.2
288	05	MED	ACUTE & SUBACUTE ENDOCARDITIS W MCC	2.940	8.6	10.8
289	05	MED	ACUTE & SUBACUTE ENDOCARDITIS W CC	1.849	6.4	7.8
290	05	MED	ACUTE & SUBACUTE ENDOCARDITIS W/O CC/MCC	1.296	4.4	5.6
291	05	MED	HEART FAILURE & SHOCK W MCC	1.494	4.8	6.2
292	05	MED	HEART FAILURE & SHOCK W CC	1.030	4.0	4.9
293	05	MED	HEART FAILURE & SHOCK W/O CC/MCC	0.685	2.8	3.3
294	05	MED	DEEP VEIN THROMBOPHLEBITIS W CC/MCC	1.037	4.4	5.4
295	05	MED	DEEP VEIN THROMBOPHLEBITIS W/O CC/MCC	0.640	3.4	4.0
296	05	MED	CARDIAC ARREST, UNEXPLAINED W MCC	1.169	1.8	2.8

MS-DRG	MDC	Type	MS-DRG Title	Weight	Geometric Mean LOS	Arithmetic Mean LOS
297	05	MED	CARDIAC ARREST, UNEXPLAINED W CC	0.679	1.4	1.7
298	05	MED	CARDIAC ARREST, UNEXPLAINED W/O CC/MCC	0.450	1.1	1.2
299	05	MED	PERIPHERAL VASCULAR DISORDERS W MCC	1.407	4.7	6.1
300	05	MED	PERIPHERAL VASCULAR DISORDERS W CC	0.978	3.9	4.9
301	05	MED	PERIPHERAL VASCULAR DISORDERS W/O CC/MCC	0.662	2.8	3.5
302	05	MED	ATHEROSCLEROSIS W MCC	0.976	3.0	4.0
303	05	MED	ATHEROSCLEROSIS W/O MCC	0.583	2.0	2.4
304	05	MED	HYPERTENSION W MCC	1.026	3.5	4.6
305	05	MED	HYPERTENSION W/O MCC	0.614	2.2	2.8
306	05	MED	CARDIAC CONGENITAL & VALVULAR DISORDERS W MCC	1.467	4.4	5.9
307	05	MED	CARDIAC CONGENITAL & VALVULAR DISORDERS W/O MCC	0.797	2.7	3.4
308	05	MED	CARDIAC ARRHYTHMIA & CONDUCTION DISORDERS W MCC	1.234	4.0	5.2
309	05	MED	CARDIAC ARRHYTHMIA & CONDUCTION DISORDERS W CC	0.839	3.0	3.7
310	05	MED	CARDIAC ARRHYTHMIA & CONDUCTION DISORDERS W/O CC/MCC	0.571	2.1	2.5
311	05	MED	ANGINA PECTORIS	0.507	1.8	2.2
312	05	MED	SYNCOPE & COLLAPSE	0.717	2.4	2.9
313	05	MED	CHEST PAIN	0.550	1.7	2.1
314	05	MED	OTHER CIRCULATORY SYSTEM DIAGNOSES W MCC	1.815	5.0	6.8
315	05	MED	OTHER CIRCULATORY SYSTEM DIAGNOSES W CC	0.968	3.3	4.2
316	05	MED	OTHER CIRCULATORY SYSTEM DIAGNOSES W/O CC/MCC	0.615	2.1	2.6
326	06	SURG	STOMACH, ESOPHAGEAL & DUODENAL PROC W MCC	5.814	12.6	16.2
327	06	SURG	STOMACH, ESOPHAGEAL & DUODENAL PROC W CC	2.723	6.9	8.8
328	06	SURG	STOMACH, ESOPHAGEAL & DUODENAL PROC W/O CC/MCC	1.430	2.9	3.8
329	06	SURG	MAJOR SMALL & LARGE BOWEL PROCEDURES W MCC	5.281	12.5	15.4
330	06	SURG	MAJOR SMALL & LARGE BOWEL PROCEDURES W CC	2.583	7.8	9.1
331	06	SURG	MAJOR SMALL & LARGE BOWEL PROCEDURES W/O CC/MCC	1.627	4.8	5.3
332	06	SURG	RECTAL RESECTION W MCC	4.864	11.8	14.2
333	06	SURG	RECTAL RESECTION W CC	2.496	7.1	8.1
334	06	SURG	RECTAL RESECTION W/O CC/MCC	1.598	4.2	4.9

MS-DRG	MDC	Type	MS-DRG Title	Weight	Geometric Mean LOS	Arithmetic Mean LOS
335	06	SURG	PERITONEAL ADHESIOLYSIS W MCC	4.278	11.4	13.7
336	06	SURG	PERITONEAL ADHESIOLYSIS W CC	2.346	7.2	8.8
337	06	SURG	PERITONEAL ADHESIOLYSIS W/O CC/MCC	1.479	4.0	5.1
338	06	SURG	APPENDECTOMY W COMPLICATED PRINCIPAL DIAG W MCC	3.212	8.3	10.0
339	06	SURG	APPENDECTOMY W COMPLICATED PRINCIPAL DIAG W CC	1.866	5.6	6.5
340	06	SURG	APPENDECTOMY W COMPLICATED PRINCIPAL DIAG W/O CC/MCC	1.239	3.2	3.7
341	06	SURG	APPENDECTOMY W/O COMPLICATED PRINCIPAL DIAG W MCC	2.264	4.9	6.6
342	06	SURG	APPENDECTOMY W/O COMPLICATED PRINCIPAL DIAG W CC	1.325	3.0	3.8
343	06	SURG	APPENDECTOMY W/O COMPLICATED PRINCIPAL DIAG W/O CC/MCC	0.957	1.7	2.0
344	06	SURG	MINOR SMALL & LARGE BOWEL PROCEDURES W MCC	3.159	8.9	11.2
345	06	SURG	MINOR SMALL & LARGE BOWEL PROCEDURES W CC	1.704	6.0	7.0
346	06	SURG	MINOR SMALL & LARGE BOWEL PROCEDURES W/O CC/MCC	1.188	4.2	4.6
347	06	SURG	ANAL & STOMAL PROCEDURES W MCC	2.418	6.3	8.8
348	06	SURG	ANAL & STOMAL PROCEDURES W CC	1.371	4.1	5.4
349	06	SURG	ANAL & STOMAL PROCEDURES W/O CC/MCC	0.798	2.3	2.9
350	06	SURG	INGUINAL & FEMORAL HERNIA PROCEDURES W MCC	2.488	5.6	7.9
351	06	SURG	INGUINAL & FEMORAL HERNIA PROCEDURES W CC	1.354	3.5	4.5
352	06	SURG	INGUINAL & FEMORAL HERNIA PROCEDURES W/O CC/MCC	0.863	1.9	2.4
353	06	SURG	HERNIA PROCEDURES EXCEPT INGUINAL & FEMORAL W MCC	2.751	6.3	8.4
354	06	SURG	HERNIA PROCEDURES EXCEPT INGUINAL & FEMORAL W CC	1.552	4.0	5.0
355	06	SURG	HERNIA PROCEDURES EXCEPT INGUINAL & FEMORAL W/O CC/MCC	1.033	2.3	2.8
356	06	SURG	OTHER DIGESTIVE SYSTEM O.R. PROCEDURES W MCC	4.029	9.2	12.7
357	06	SURG	OTHER DIGESTIVE SYSTEM O.R. PROCEDURES W CC	2.147	5.7	7.4
358	06	SURG	OTHER DIGESTIVE SYSTEM O.R. PROCEDURES W/O CC/MCC	1.301	3.0	4.0
368	06	MED	MAJOR ESOPHAGEAL DISORDERS W MCC	1.758	5.1	6.7
369	06	MED	MAJOR ESOPHAGEAL DISORDERS W CC	1.077	3.7	4.5
370	06	MED	MAJOR ESOPHAGEAL DISORDERS W/O CC/MCC	0.755	2.6	3.1
371	06	MED	MAJOR GASTROINTESTINAL DISORDERS & PERITONEAL INFECTIONS W MCC	2.099	6.8	8.8
372	06	MED	MAJOR GASTROINTESTINAL DISORDERS & PERITONEAL INFECTIONS W CC	1.294	5.3	6.5

MS-DRG	MDC	Type	MS-DRG Title	Weight	Geometric Mean LOS	Arithmetic Mean LOS
373	06	MED	MAJOR GASTROINTESTINAL DISORDERS & PERITONEAL INFECTIONS W/O CC/MCC	0.860	3.9	4.6
374	06	MED	DIGESTIVE MALIGNANCY W MCC	2.067	6.3	8.4
375	06	MED	DIGESTIVE MALIGNANCY W CC	1.280	4.4	5.8
376	06	MED	DIGESTIVE MALIGNANCY W/O CC/MCC	0.848	2.8	3.6
377	06	MED	G.I. HEMORRHAGE W MCC	1.754	5.0	6.4
378	06	MED	G.I. HEMORRHAGE W CC	1.027	3.5	4.2
379	06	MED	G.I. HEMORRHAGE W/O CC/MCC	0.715	2.6	3.0
380	06	MED	COMPLICATED PEPTIC ULCER W MCC	1.966	5.8	7.6
381	06	MED	COMPLICATED PEPTIC ULCER W CC	1.121	3.9	4.8
382	06	MED	COMPLICATED PEPTIC ULCER W/O CC/MCC	0.813	2.9	3.5
383	06	MED	UNCOMPLICATED PEPTIC ULCER W MCC	1.198	4.2	5.3
384	06	MED	UNCOMPLICATED PEPTIC ULCER W/O MCC	0.833	3.0	3.6
385	06	MED	INFLAMMATORY BOWEL DISEASE W MCC	1.910	6.3	8.4
386	06	MED	INFLAMMATORY BOWEL DISEASE W CC	1.044	4.2	5.3
387	06	MED	INFLAMMATORY BOWEL DISEASE W/O CC/MCC	0.781	3.2	3.9
388	06	MED	G.I. OBSTRUCTION W MCC	1.646	5.5	7.2
389	06	MED	G.I. OBSTRUCTION W CC	0.934	3.9	4.8
390	06	MED	G.I. OBSTRUCTION W/O CC/MCC	0.637	2.8	3.3
391	06	MED	ESOPHAGITIS, GASTROENT & MISC DIGEST DISORDERS W MCC	1.155	3.9	5.1
392	06	MED	ESOPHAGITIS, GASTROENT & MISC DIGEST DISORDERS W/O MCC	0.717	2.8	3.4
393	06	MED	OTHER DIGESTIVE SYSTEM DIAGNOSES W MCC	1.659	4.9	6.8
394	06	MED	OTHER DIGESTIVE SYSTEM DIAGNOSES W CC	0.994	3.7	4.7
395	06	MED	OTHER DIGESTIVE SYSTEM DIAGNOSES W/O CC/MCC	0.675	2.5	3.1
405	07	SURG	PANCREAS, LIVER & SHUNT PROCEDURES W MCC	5.574	12.0	15.8
406	07	SURG	PANCREAS, LIVER & SHUNT PROCEDURES W CC	2.779	6.5	8.4
407	07	SURG	PANCREAS, LIVER & SHUNT PROCEDURES W/O CC/MCC	1.867	4.2	5.2
408	07	SURG	BILIARY TRACT PROC EXCEPT ONLY CHOLECYST W OR W/O C.D.E. W MCC	3.937	11.0	13.5
409	07	SURG	BILIARY TRACT PROC EXCEPT ONLY CHOLECYST W OR W/O C.D.E. W CC	2.488	7.4	8.9
410	07	SURG	BILIARY TRACT PROC EXCEPT ONLY CHOLECYST W OR W/O C.D.E. W/O CC/MCC	1.611	4.9	5.8

MS-DRG	MDC	Type	MS-DRG Title	Weight	Geometric Mean LOS	Arithmetic Mean LOS
411	07	SURG	CHOLECYSTECTOMY W C.D.E. W MCC	3.682	9.9	11.8
412	07	SURG	CHOLECYSTECTOMY W C.D.E. W CC	2.491	7.0	8.3
413	07	SURG	CHOLECYSTECTOMY W C.D.E. W/O CC/MCC	1.718	4.5	5.4
414	07	SURG	CHOLECYSTECTOMY EXCEPT BY LAPAROSCOPE W/O C.D.E. W MCC	3.668	9.3	11.4
415	07	SURG	CHOLECYSTECTOMY EXCEPT BY LAPAROSCOPE W/O C.D.E. W CC	2.090	6.2	7.3
416	07	SURG	CHOLECYSTECTOMY EXCEPT BY LAPAROSCOPE W/O C.D.E. W/O CC/MCC	1.308	3.7	4.4
417	07	SURG	LAPAROSCOPIC CHOLECYSTECTOMY W/O C.D.E. W MCC	2.503	6.2	7.8
418	07	SURG	LAPAROSCOPIC CHOLECYSTECTOMY W/O C.D.E. W CC	1.700	4.4	5.4
419	07	SURG	LAPAROSCOPIC CHOLECYSTECTOMY W/O C.D.E. W/O CC/MCC	1.170	2.4	3.0
420	07	SURG	HEPATOBILIARY DIAGNOSTIC PROCEDURES W MCC	3.644	9.2	13.0
421	07	SURG	HEPATOBILIARY DIAGNOSTIC PROCEDURES W CC	1.891	5.1	7.0
422	07	SURG	HEPATOBILIARY DIAGNOSTIC PROCEDURES W/O CC/MCC	1.274	3.0	4.1
423	07	SURG	OTHER HEPATOBILIARY OR PANCREAS O.R. PROCEDURES W MCC	4.458	10.9	14.4
424	07	SURG	OTHER HEPATOBILIARY OR PANCREAS O.R. PROCEDURES W CC	2.434	7.1	9.1
425	07	SURG	OTHER HEPATOBILIARY OR PANCREAS O.R. PROCEDURES W/O CC/MCC	1.627	4.4	5.7
432	07	MED	CIRRHOSIS & ALCOHOLIC HEPATITIS W MCC	1.700	5.0	6.5
433	07	MED	CIRRHOSIS & ALCOHOLIC HEPATITIS W CC	0.955	3.6	4.6
434	07	MED	CIRRHOSIS & ALCOHOLIC HEPATITIS W/O CC/MCC	0.615	2.5	3.2
435	07	MED	MALIGNANCY OF HEPATOBILIARY SYSTEM OR PANCREAS W MCC	1.802	5.6	7.4
436	07	MED	MALIGNANCY OF HEPATOBILIARY SYSTEM OR PANCREAS W CC	1.222	4.2	5.5
437	07	MED	MALIGNANCY OF HEPATOBILIARY SYSTEM OR PANCREAS W/O CC/MCC	0.900	2.8	3.7
438	07	MED	DISORDERS OF PANCREAS EXCEPT MALIGNANCY W MCC	1.834	5.4	7.5
439	07	MED	DISORDERS OF PANCREAS EXCEPT MALIGNANCY W CC	1.009	4.0	5.0
440	07	MED	DISORDERS OF PANCREAS EXCEPT MALIGNANCY W/O CC/MCC	0.689	2.9	3.5
441	07	MED	DISORDERS OF LIVER EXCEPT MALIG,CIRR,ALC HEPA W MCC	1.824	5.1	7.1
442	07	MED	DISORDERS OF LIVER EXCEPT MALIG,CIRR,ALC HEPA W CC	0.986	3.7	4.8
443	07	MED	DISORDERS OF LIVER EXCEPT MALIG,CIRR,ALC HEPA W/O CC/MCC	0.662	2.7	3.3
444	07	MED	DISORDERS OF THE BILIARY TRACT W MCC	1.559	4.8	6.2
445	07	MED	DISORDERS OF THE BILIARY TRACT W CC	1.069	3.6	4.5

MS-DRG	MDC	Type	MS-DRG Title	Weight	Geometric Mean LOS	Arithmetic Mean LOS
446	07	MED	DISORDERS OF THE BILIARY TRACT W/O CC/MCC	0.741	2.5	3.1
453	08	SURG	COMBINED ANTERIOR/POSTERIOR SPINAL FUSION W MCC	10.265	10.7	13.5
454	08	SURG	COMBINED ANTERIOR/POSTERIOR SPINAL FUSION W CC	7.256	5.5	6.7
455	08	SURG	COMBINED ANTERIOR/POSTERIOR SPINAL FUSION W/O CC/MCC	5.431	3.1	3.7
456	08	SURG	SPINAL FUS EXC CERV W SPINAL CURV/MALIG/INFEC OR 9+ FUS W MCC	9.289	10.8	13.4
457	08	SURG	SPINAL FUS EXC CERV W SPINAL CURV/MALIG/INFEC OR 9+ FUS W CC	6.202	5.9	7.0
458	08	SURG	SPINAL FUS EXC CERV W SPINAL CURV/MALIG/INFEC OR 9+ FUS W/O CC/MCC	4.938	3.5	4.0
459	08	SURG	SPINAL FUSION EXCEPT CERVICAL W MCC	6.507	7.4	9.1
460	08	SURG	SPINAL FUSION EXCEPT CERVICAL W/O MCC	3.871	3.3	3.9
461	08	SURG	BILATERAL OR MULTIPLE MAJOR JOINT PROCS OF LOWER EXTREMITY W MCC	4.939	6.7	8.2
462	08	SURG	BILATERAL OR MULTIPLE MAJOR JOINT PROCS OF LOWER EXTREMITY W/O MCC	3.343	3.7	4.1
463	08	SURG	WND DEBRID & SKN GRFT EXC HAND, FOR MUSCULO-CONN TISS DIS W MCC	4.998	11.0	15.1
464	08	SURG	WND DEBRID & SKN GRFT EXC HAND, FOR MUSCULO-CONN TISS DIS W CC	2.853	6.9	8.9
465	08	SURG	WND DEBRID & SKN GRFT EXC HAND, FOR MUSCULO-CONN TISS DIS W/O CC/MCC	1.791	4.1	5.3
466	08	SURG	REVISION OF HIP OR KNEE REPLACEMENT W MCC	4.914	7.3	9.0
467	08	SURG	REVISION OF HIP OR KNEE REPLACEMENT W CC	3.232	4.3	5.0
468	08	SURG	REVISION OF HIP OR KNEE REPLACEMENT W/O CC/MCC	2.573	3.3	3.6
469	08	SURG	MAJOR JOINT REPLACEMENT OR REATTACHMENT OF LOWER EXTREMITY W MCC	3.472	6.7	8.0
470	08	SURG	MAJOR JOINT REPLACEMENT OR REATTACHMENT OF LOWER EXTREMITY W/O MCC	2.104	3.4	3.7
471	08	SURG	CERVICAL SPINAL FUSION W MCC	4.730	6.6	9.3
472	08	SURG	CERVICAL SPINAL FUSION W CC	2.772	2.6	3.8
473	08	SURG	CERVICAL SPINAL FUSION W/O CC/MCC	2.077	1.5	1.8
474	08	SURG	AMPUTATION FOR MUSCULOSKELETAL SYS & CONN TISSUE DIS W MCC	3.491	9.1	11.9
475	08	SURG	AMPUTATION FOR MUSCULOSKELETAL SYS & CONN TISSUE DIS W CC	1.959	6.1	7.7
476	08	SURG	AMPUTATION FOR MUSCULOSKELETAL SYS & CONN TISSUE DIS W/O CC/MCC	0.992	3.2	4.1
477	08	SURG	BIOPSIES OF MUSCULOSKELETAL SYSTEM & CONNECTIVE TISSUE W MCC	3.329	8.9	11.1
478	08	SURG	BIOPSIES OF MUSCULOSKELETAL SYSTEM & CONNECTIVE TISSUE W CC	2.255	5.3	6.8
479	08	SURG	BIOPSIES OF MUSCULOSKELETAL SYSTEM & CONNECTIVE TISSUE W/O CC/MCC	1.637	2.4	3.4
480	08	SURG	HIP & FEMUR PROCEDURES EXCEPT MAJOR JOINT W MCC	3.094	7.7	9.0

MS-DRG	MDC	Type	MS-DRG Title	Weight	Geometric Mean LOS	Arithmetic Mean LOS
481	08	SURG	HIP & FEMUR PROCEDURES EXCEPT MAJOR JOINT W CC	1.889	5.1	5.6
482	08	SURG	HIP & FEMUR PROCEDURES EXCEPT MAJOR JOINT W/O CC/MCC	1.537	4.1	4.5
483	08	SURG	MAJOR JOINT & LIMB REATTACHMENT PROC OF UPPER EXTREMITY W CC/MCC	2.402	3.0	3.7
484	08	SURG	MAJOR JOINT & LIMB REATTACHMENT PROC OF UPPER EXTREMITY W/O CC/MCC	1.955	2.0	2.2
485	08	SURG	KNEE PROCEDURES W PDX OF INFECTION W MCC	3.213	9.0	11.0
486	08	SURG	KNEE PROCEDURES W PDX OF INFECTION W CC	2.034	6.1	7.2
487	08	SURG	KNEE PROCEDURES W PDX OF INFECTION W/O CC/MCC	1.472	4.4	5.1
488	08	SURG	KNEE PROCEDURES W/O PDX OF INFECTION W CC/MCC	1.722	3.8	4.7
489	08	SURG	KNEE PROCEDURES W/O PDX OF INFECTION W/O CC/MCC	1.214	2.5	2.9
490	08	SURG	BACK & NECK PROC EXC SPINAL FUSION W CC/MCC OR DISC DEVICE/NEUROSTIM	1.792	3.0	4.3
491	08	SURG	BACK & NECK PROC EXC SPINAL FUSION W/O CC/MCC	0.991	1.7	2.1
492	08	SURG	LOWER EXTREM & HUMER PROC EXCEPT HIP, FOOT, FEMUR W MCC	3.067	6.8	8.6
493	08	SURG	LOWER EXTREM & HUMER PROC EXCEPT HIP, FOOT, FEMUR W CC	1.852	4.2	5.0
494	08	SURG	LOWER EXTREM & HUMER PROC EXCEPT HIP, FOOT, FEMUR W/O CC/MCC	1.314	2.7	3.2
495	08	SURG	LOCAL EXCISION & REMOVAL INT FIX DEVICES EXC HIP & FEMUR W MCC	2.868	7.6	10.2
496	08	SURG	LOCAL EXCISION & REMOVAL INT FIX DEVICES EXC HIP & FEMUR W CC	1.621	4.1	5.4
497	08	SURG	LOCAL EXCISION & REMOVAL INT FIX DEVICES EXC HIP & FEMUR W/O CC/MCC	1.077	2.0	2.6
498	08	SURG	LOCAL EXCISION & REMOVAL INT FIX DEVICES OF HIP & FEMUR W CC/MCC	1.991	5.4	7.3
499	08	SURG	LOCAL EXCISION & REMOVAL INT FIX DEVICES OF HIP & FEMUR W/O CC/MCC	0.992	2.2	3.0
500	08	SURG	SOFT TISSUE PROCEDURES W MCC	3.029	7.6	10.3
501	08	SURG	SOFT TISSUE PROCEDURES W CC	1.585	4.6	6.0
502	08	SURG	SOFT TISSUE PROCEDURES W/O CC/MCC	1.031	2.3	2.8
503	08	SURG	FOOT PROCEDURES W MCC	2.281	6.5	8.5
504	08	SURG	FOOT PROCEDURES W CC	1.569	5.0	6.2
505	08	SURG	FOOT PROCEDURES W/O CC/MCC	1.077	2.5	3.1
506	08	SURG	MAJOR THUMB OR JOINT PROCEDURES	1.182	2.7	3.8
507	08	SURG	MAJOR SHOULDER OR ELBOW JOINT PROCEDURES W CC/MCC	1.871	3.4	4.5
508	08	SURG	MAJOR SHOULDER OR ELBOW JOINT PROCEDURES W/O CC/MCC	1.396	1.7	2.1
509	08	SURG	ARTHROSCOPY	1.315	2.3	3.5

MS-DRG	MDC	Type	MS-DRG Title	Weight	Geometric Mean LOS	Arithmetic Mean LOS
510	08	SURG	SHOULDER, ELBOW OR FOREARM PROC, EXC MAJOR JOINT PROC W MCC	2.170	5.0	6.3
511	08	SURG	SHOULDER, ELBOW OR FOREARM PROC, EXC MAJOR JOINT PROC W CC	1.469	3.2	3.9
512	08	SURG	SHOULDER, ELBOW OR FOREARM PROC, EXC MAJOR JOINT PROC W/O CC/MCC	1.046	1.8	2.1
513	08	SURG	HAND OR WRIST PROC, EXCEPT MAJOR THUMB OR JOINT PROC W CC/MCC	1.301	3.5	4.8
514	08	SURG	HAND OR WRIST PROC, EXCEPT MAJOR THUMB OR JOINT PROC W/O CC/MCC	0.821	2.1	2.7
515	08	SURG	OTHER MUSCULOSKELET SYS & CONN TISS O.R. PROC W MCC	3.189	7.7	9.8
516	08	SURG	OTHER MUSCULOSKELET SYS & CONN TISS O.R. PROC W CC	1.924	4.7	5.9
517	08	SURG	OTHER MUSCULOSKELET SYS & CONN TISS O.R. PROC W/O CC/MCC	1.480	2.6	3.4
533	08	MED	FRACTURES OF FEMUR W MCC	1.566	4.9	6.5
534	08	MED	FRACTURES OF FEMUR W/O MCC	0.760	3.1	3.9
535	08	MED	FRACTURES OF HIP & PELVIS W MCC	1.353	4.5	5.8
536	08	MED	FRACTURES OF HIP & PELVIS W/O MCC	0.719	3.2	3.7
537	08	MED	SPRAINS, STRAINS, & DISLOCATIONS OF HIP, PELVIS & THIGH W CC/MCC	0.828	3.5	4.1
538	08	MED	SPRAINS, STRAINS, & DISLOCATIONS OF HIP, PELVIS & THIGH W/O CC/MCC	0.611	2.6	3.1
539	08	MED	OSTEOMYELITIS W MCC	2.047	7.1	9.4
540	08	MED	OSTEOMYELITIS W CC	1.313	5.4	6.8
541	08	MED	OSTEOMYELITIS W/O CC/MCC	0.871	3.7	4.7
542	08	MED	PATHOLOGICAL FRACTURES & MUSCULOSKELET & CONN TISS MALIG W MCC	1.952	6.3	8.3
543	08	MED	PATHOLOGICAL FRACTURES & MUSCULOSKELET & CONN TISS MALIG W CC	1.160	4.5	5.6
544	08	MED	PATHOLOGICAL FRACTURES & MUSCULOSKELET & CONN TISS MALIG W/O CC/MCC	0.778	3.4	4.1
545	08	MED	CONNECTIVE TISSUE DISORDERS W MCC	2.547	6.4	9.0
546	08	MED	CONNECTIVE TISSUE DISORDERS W CC	1.171	4.2	5.4
547	08	MED	CONNECTIVE TISSUE DISORDERS W/O CC/MCC	0.735	2.9	3.6
548	08	MED	SEPTIC ARTHRITIS W MCC	1.965	6.7	8.8
549	08	MED	SEPTIC ARTHRITIS W CC	1.204	4.8	6.1
550	08	MED	SEPTIC ARTHRITIS W/O CC/MCC	0.828	3.3	4.0
551	08	MED	MEDICAL BACK PROBLEMS W MCC	1.640	5.2	6.8
552	08	MED	MEDICAL BACK PROBLEMS W/O MCC	0.820	3.3	4.0
553	08	MED	BONE DISEASES & ARTHROPATHIES W MCC	1.136	4.3	5.5

MS-DRG	MDC	Type	MS-DRG Title	Weight	Geometric Mean LOS	Arithmetic Mean LOS
554	08	MED	BONE DISEASES & ARTHROPATHIES W/O MCC	0.681	3.0	3.7
555	08	MED	SIGNS & SYMPTOMS OF MUSCULOSKELETAL SYSTEM & CONN TISSUE W MCC	1.095	3.6	4.9
556	08	MED	SIGNS & SYMPTOMS OF MUSCULOSKELETAL SYSTEM & CONN TISSUE W/O MCC	0.657	2.6	3.2
557	08	MED	TENDONITIS, MYOSITIS & BURSITIS W MCC	1.602	5.4	6.8
558	08	MED	TENDONITIS, MYOSITIS & BURSITIS W/O MCC	0.882	3.6	4.4
559	08	MED	AFTERCARE, MUSCULOSKELETAL SYSTEM & CONNECTIVE TISSUE W MCC	1.772	5.2	7.2
560	08	MED	AFTERCARE, MUSCULOSKELETAL SYSTEM & CONNECTIVE TISSUE W CC	1.002	3.6	4.6
561	08	MED	AFTERCARE, MUSCULOSKELETAL SYSTEM & CONNECTIVE TISSUE W/O CC/MCC	0.621	2.1	2.6
562	08	MED	FX, SPRN, STRN & DISL EXCEPT FEMUR, HIP, PELVIS & THIGH W MCC	1.394	4.5	5.8
563	08	MED	FX, SPRN, STRN & DISL EXCEPT FEMUR, HIP, PELVIS & THIGH W/O MCC	0.715	3.0	3.6
564	08	MED	OTHER MUSCULOSKELETAL SYS & CONNECTIVE TISSUE DIAGNOSES W MCC	1.470	4.9	6.5
565	08	MED	OTHER MUSCULOSKELETAL SYS & CONNECTIVE TISSUE DIAGNOSES W CC	0.910	3.8	4.7
566	08	MED	OTHER MUSCULOSKELETAL SYS & CONNECTIVE TISSUE DIAGNOSES W/O CC/MCC	0.663	2.8	3.4
573	09	SURG	SKIN GRAFT &/OR DEBRID FOR SKN ULCER OR CELLULITIS W MCC	3.246	9.1	12.5
574	09	SURG	SKIN GRAFT &/OR DEBRID FOR SKN ULCER OR CELLULITIS W CC	1.868	6.7	8.5
575	09	SURG	SKIN GRAFT &/OR DEBRID FOR SKN ULCER OR CELLULITIS W/O CC/MCC	1.090	4.2	5.2
576	09	SURG	SKIN GRAFT &/OR DEBRID EXC FOR SKIN ULCER OR CELLULITIS W MCC	3.925	9.1	13.0
577	09	SURG	SKIN GRAFT &/OR DEBRID EXC FOR SKIN ULCER OR CELLULITIS W CC	1.704	4.1	6.2
578	09	SURG	SKIN GRAFT &/OR DEBRID EXC FOR SKIN ULCER OR CELLULITIS W/O CC/MCC	1.042	2.4	3.3
579	09	SURG	OTHER SKIN, SUBCUT TISS & BREAST PROC W MCC	2.958	7.7	10.4
580	09	SURG	OTHER SKIN, SUBCUT TISS & BREAST PROC W CC	1.496	3.8	5.4
581	09	SURG	OTHER SKIN, SUBCUT TISS & BREAST PROC W/O CC/MCC	0.922	1.8	2.4
582	09	SURG	MASTECTOMY FOR MALIGNANCY W CC/MCC	1.057	2.0	2.7
583	09	SURG	MASTECTOMY FOR MALIGNANCY W/O CC/MCC	0.845	1.5	1.7
584	09	SURG	BREAST BIOPSY, LOCAL EXCISION & OTHER BREAST PROCEDURES W CC/MCC	1.515	3.5	5.0
585	09	SURG	BREAST BIOPSY, LOCAL EXCISION & OTHER BREAST PROCEDURES W/O CC/MCC	1.041	1.7	2.2
592	09	MED	SKIN ULCERS W MCC	1.767	6.2	8.2
593	09	MED	SKIN ULCERS W CC	1.071	4.8	5.8
594	09	MED	SKIN ULCERS W/O CC/MCC	0.759	3.6	4.6

MS-DRG	MDC	Type	MS-DRG Title	Weight	Geometric Mean LOS	Arithmetic Mean LOS
595	09	MED	MAJOR SKIN DISORDERS W MCC	1.869	5.9	7.8
596	09	MED	MAJOR SKIN DISORDERS W/O MCC	0.878	3.7	4.6
597	09	MED	MALIGNANT BREAST DISORDERS W MCC	1.560	5.5	7.5
598	09	MED	MALIGNANT BREAST DISORDERS W CC	1.061	4.1	5.4
599	09	MED	MALIGNANT BREAST DISORDERS W/O CC/MCC	0.627	2.5	3.2
600	09	MED	NON-MALIGNANT BREAST DISORDERS W CC/MCC	0.960	4.1	4.9
601	09	MED	NON-MALIGNANT BREAST DISORDERS W/O CC/MCC	0.673	3.0	3.6
602	09	MED	CELLULITIS W MCC	1.475	5.3	6.7
603	09	MED	CELLULITIS W/O MCC	0.838	3.8	4.5
604	09	MED	TRAUMA TO THE SKIN, SUBCUT TISS & BREAST W MCC	1.236	3.9	5.2
605	09	MED	TRAUMA TO THE SKIN, SUBCUT TISS & BREAST W/O MCC	0.718	2.7	3.3
606	09	MED	MINOR SKIN DISORDERS W MCC	1.308	4.3	6.0
607	09	MED	MINOR SKIN DISORDERS W/O MCC	0.686	2.8	3.7
614	10	SURG	ADRENAL & PITUITARY PROCEDURES W CC/MCC	2.455	4.7	6.5
615	10	SURG	ADRENAL & PITUITARY PROCEDURES W/O CC/MCC	1.397	2.5	3.0
616	10	SURG	AMPUTAT OF LOWER LIMB FOR ENDOCRINE, NUTRIT, & METABOL DIS W MCC	4.493	12.4	15.6
617	10	SURG	AMPUTAT OF LOWER LIMB FOR ENDOCRINE, NUTRIT, & METABOL DIS W CC	2.001	6.5	7.9
618	10	SURG	AMPUTAT OF LOWER LIMB FOR ENDOCRINE, NUTRIT, & METABOL DIS W/O CC/MCC	1.201	4.1	5.1
619	10	SURG	O.R. PROCEDURES FOR OBESITY W MCC	3.521	4.6	7.4
620	10	SURG	O.R. PROCEDURES FOR OBESITY W CC	1.863	2.6	3.4
621	10	SURG	O.R. PROCEDURES FOR OBESITY W/O CC/MCC	1.475	1.6	1.9
622	10	SURG	SKIN GRAFTS & WOUND DEBRID FOR ENDOC, NUTRIT & METAB DIS W MCC	3.417	9.4	12.5
623	10	SURG	SKIN GRAFTS & WOUND DEBRID FOR ENDOC, NUTRIT & METAB DIS W CC	1.856	6.1	7.6
624	10	SURG	SKIN GRAFTS & WOUND DEBRID FOR ENDOC, NUTRIT & METAB DIS W/O CC/MCC	1.012	3.8	4.7
625	10	SURG	THYROID, PARATHYROID & THYROGLOSSAL PROCEDURES W MCC	2.242	4.6	6.9
626	10	SURG	THYROID, PARATHYROID & THYROGLOSSAL PROCEDURES W CC	1.170	2.1	3.0
627	10	SURG	THYROID, PARATHYROID & THYROGLOSSAL PROCEDURES W/O CC/MCC	0.782	1.2	1.4
628	10	SURG	OTHER ENDOCRINE, NUTRIT & METAB O.R. PROC W MCC	3.382	7.2	10.6
629	10	SURG	OTHER ENDOCRINE, NUTRIT & METAB O.R. PROC W CC	2.265	6.5	8.0

MS-DRG	MDC	Type	MS-DRG Title	Weight	Geometric Mean LOS	Arithmetic Mean LOS
630	10	SURG	OTHER ENDOCRINE, NUTRIT & METAB O.R. PROC W/O CC/MCC	1.416	3.4	4.5
637	10	MED	DIABETES W MCC	1.446	4.5	5.9
638	10	MED	DIABETES W CC	0.831	3.2	4.0
639	10	MED	DIABETES W/O CC/MCC	0.554	2.3	2.8
640	10	MED	NUTRITIONAL & MISC METABOLIC DISORDERS W MCC	1.140	3.6	5.1
641	10	MED	NUTRITIONAL & MISC METABOLIC DISORDERS W/O MCC	0.692	2.9	3.6
642	10	MED	INBORN ERRORS OF METABOLISM	1.029	3.4	4.7
643	10	MED	ENDOCRINE DISORDERS W MCC	1.816	6.0	7.6
644	10	MED	ENDOCRINE DISORDERS W CC	1.066	4.2	5.2
645	10	MED	ENDOCRINE DISORDERS W/O CC/MCC	0.720	2.9	3.6
652	11	SURG	KIDNEY TRANSPLANT	3.044	6.3	7.4
653	11	SURG	MAJOR BLADDER PROCEDURES W MCC	6.093	13.6	16.6
654	11	SURG	MAJOR BLADDER PROCEDURES W CC	3.005	8.2	9.3
655	11	SURG	MAJOR BLADDER PROCEDURES W/O CC/MCC	1.957	4.8	5.6
656	11	SURG	KIDNEY & URETER PROCEDURES FOR NEOPLASM W MCC	3.571	7.7	10.0
657	11	SURG	KIDNEY & URETER PROCEDURES FOR NEOPLASM W CC	2.000	4.9	5.9
658	11	SURG	KIDNEY & URETER PROCEDURES FOR NEOPLASM W/O CC/MCC	1.422	3.0	3.4
659	11	SURG	KIDNEY & URETER PROCEDURES FOR NON-NEOPLASM W MCC	3.499	7.9	10.8
660	11	SURG	KIDNEY & URETER PROCEDURES FOR NON-NEOPLASM W CC	1.903	4.5	6.0
661	11	SURG	KIDNEY & URETER PROCEDURES FOR NON-NEOPLASM W/O CC/MCC	1.264	2.4	2.9
662	11	SURG	MINOR BLADDER PROCEDURES W MCC	3.016	7.5	10.7
663	11	SURG	MINOR BLADDER PROCEDURES W CC	1.472	3.6	5.2
664	11	SURG	MINOR BLADDER PROCEDURES W/O CC/MCC	1.107	1.5	1.9
665	11	SURG	PROSTATECTOMY W MCC	2.865	8.7	11.3
666	11	SURG	PROSTATECTOMY W CC	1.644	4.5	6.4
667	11	SURG	PROSTATECTOMY W/O CC/MCC	0.792	1.8	2.4
668	11	SURG	TRANSURETHRAL PROCEDURES W MCC	2.518	6.6	8.9
669	11	SURG	TRANSURETHRAL PROCEDURES W CC	1.260	3.2	4.4
670	11	SURG	TRANSURETHRAL PROCEDURES W/O CC/MCC	0.777	1.8	2.3

MS-DRG	MDC	Type	MS-DRG Title	Weight	Geometric Mean LOS	Arithmetic Mean LOS
671	11	SURG	URETHRAL PROCEDURES W CC/MCC	1.440	4.1	5.6
672	11	SURG	URETHRAL PROCEDURES W/O CC/MCC	0.789	1.8	2.2
673	11	SURG	OTHER KIDNEY & URINARY TRACT PROCEDURES W MCC	2.926	5.9	9.5
674	11	SURG	OTHER KIDNEY & URINARY TRACT PROCEDURES W CC	2.093	4.6	6.7
675	11	SURG	OTHER KIDNEY & URINARY TRACT PROCEDURES W/O CC/MCC	1.338	1.6	2.1
682	11	MED	RENAL FAILURE W MCC	1.641	5.1	6.8
683	11	MED	RENAL FAILURE W CC	1.024	4.0	4.9
684	11	MED	RENAL FAILURE W/O CC/MCC	0.659	2.8	3.4
685	11	MED	ADMIT FOR RENAL DIALYSIS	0.894	2.5	3.4
686	11	MED	KIDNEY & URINARY TRACT NEOPLASMS W MCC	1.824	5.8	7.8
687	11	MED	KIDNEY & URINARY TRACT NEOPLASMS W CC	1.084	3.8	5.0
688	11	MED	KIDNEY & URINARY TRACT NEOPLASMS W/O CC/MCC	0.648	2.2	2.8
689	11	MED	KIDNEY & URINARY TRACT INFECTIONS W MCC	1.219	4.6	5.8
690	11	MED	KIDNEY & URINARY TRACT INFECTIONS W/O MCC	0.786	3.4	4.1
691	11	MED	URINARY STONES W ESW LITHOTRIPSY W CC/MCC	1.616	3.3	4.3
692	11	MED	URINARY STONES W ESW LITHOTRIPSY W/O CC/MCC	1.119	1.8	2.3
693	11	MED	URINARY STONES W/O ESW LITHOTRIPSY W MCC	1.351	3.9	5.2
694	11	MED	URINARY STONES W/O ESW LITHOTRIPSY W/O MCC	0.710	2.1	2.6
695	11	MED	KIDNEY & URINARY TRACT SIGNS & SYMPTOMS W MCC	1.208	4.3	5.7
696	11	MED	KIDNEY & URINARY TRACT SIGNS & SYMPTOMS W/O MCC	0.659	2.6	3.2
697	11	MED	URETHRAL STRICTURE	0.777	2.4	3.1
698	11	MED	OTHER KIDNEY & URINARY TRACT DIAGNOSES W MCC	1.610	5.2	6.8
699	11	MED	OTHER KIDNEY & URINARY TRACT DIAGNOSES W CC	1.000	3.7	4.7
700	11	MED	OTHER KIDNEY & URINARY TRACT DIAGNOSES W/O CC/MCC	0.676	2.6	3.2
707	12	SURG	MAJOR MALE PELVIC PROCEDURES W CC/MCC	1.775	3.2	4.2
708	12	SURG	MAJOR MALE PELVIC PROCEDURES W/O CC/MCC	1.258	1.6	1.9
709	12	SURG	PENIS PROCEDURES W CC/MCC	1.863	3.4	5.7
710	12	SURG	PENIS PROCEDURES W/O CC/MCC	1.271	1.4	1.7
711	12	SURG	TESTES PROCEDURES W CC/MCC	1.764	5.2	7.3

MS-DRG	MDC	Type	MS-DRG Title	Weight	Geometric Mean LOS	Arithmetic Mean LOS
712	12	SURG	TESTES PROCEDURES W/O CC/MCC	0.808	2.1	2.7
713	12	SURG	TRANSURETHRAL PROSTATECTOMY W CC/MCC	1.180	2.9	4.1
714	12	SURG	TRANSURETHRAL PROSTATECTOMY W/O CC/MCC	0.654	1.6	1.8
715	12	SURG	OTHER MALE REPRODUCTIVE SYSTEM O.R. PROC FOR MALIGNANCY W CC/MCC	1.743	4.1	6.0
716	12	SURG	OTHER MALE REPRODUCTIVE SYSTEM O.R. PROC FOR MALIGNANCY W/O CC/MCC	0.997	1.2	1.4
717	12	SURG	OTHER MALE REPRODUCTIVE SYSTEM O.R. PROC EXC MALIGNANCY W CC/MCC	1.614	4.6	6.4
718	12	SURG	OTHER MALE REPRODUCTIVE SYSTEM O.R. PROC EXC MALIGNANCY W/O CC/MCC	0.804	2.0	2.6
722	12	MED	MALIGNANCY, MALE REPRODUCTIVE SYSTEM W MCC	1.689	5.4	7.7
723	12	MED	MALIGNANCY, MALE REPRODUCTIVE SYSTEM W CC	1.019	3.9	5.1
724	12	MED	MALIGNANCY, MALE REPRODUCTIVE SYSTEM W/O CC/MCC	0.621	2.1	2.7
725	12	MED	BENIGN PROSTATIC HYPERTROPHY W MCC	1.274	4.7	6.1
726	12	MED	BENIGN PROSTATIC HYPERTROPHY W/O MCC	0.701	2.8	3.5
727	12	MED	INFLAMMATION OF THE MALE REPRODUCTIVE SYSTEM W MCC	1.366	4.9	6.4
728	12	MED	INFLAMMATION OF THE MALE REPRODUCTIVE SYSTEM W/O MCC	0.761	3.3	4.1
729	12	MED	OTHER MALE REPRODUCTIVE SYSTEM DIAGNOSES W CC/MCC	0.989	3.6	4.7
730	12	MED	OTHER MALE REPRODUCTIVE SYSTEM DIAGNOSES W/O CC/MCC	0.641	2.3	2.9
734	13	SURG	PELVIC EVISCERATION, RAD HYSTERECTOMY & RAD VULVECTOMY W CC/MCC	2.436	5.2	7.0
735	13	SURG	PELVIC EVISCERATION, RAD HYSTERECTOMY & RAD VULVECTOMY W/O CC/MCC	1.168	2.2	2.7
736	13	SURG	UTERINE & ADNEXA PROC FOR OVARIAN OR ADNEXAL MALIGNANCY W MCC	4.394	11.5	14.0
737	13	SURG	UTERINE & ADNEXA PROC FOR OVARIAN OR ADNEXAL MALIGNANCY W CC	2.038	5.7	6.6
738	13	SURG	UTERINE & ADNEXA PROC FOR OVARIAN OR ADNEXAL MALIGNANCY W/O CC/MCC	1.232	3.2	3.6
739	13	SURG	UTERINE,ADNEXA PROC FOR NON-OVARIAN/ADNEXAL MALIG W MCC	3.430	7.4	9.8
740	13	SURG	UTERINE,ADNEXA PROC FOR NON-OVARIAN/ADNEXAL MALIG W CC	1.528	3.8	4.7
741	13	SURG	UTERINE,ADNEXA PROC FOR NON-OVARIAN/ADNEXAL MALIG W/O CC/MCC	1.098	2.2	2.6
742	13	SURG	UTERINE & ADNEXA PROC FOR NON-MALIGNANCY W CC/MCC	1.388	3.2	4.1
743	13	SURG	UTERINE & ADNEXA PROC FOR NON-MALIGNANCY W/O CC/MCC	0.908	1.8	2.1
744	13	SURG	D&C, CONIZATION, LAPAROSCOPY & TUBAL INTERRUPTION W CC/MCC	1.515	4.0	5.5
745	13	SURG	D&C, CONIZATION, LAPAROSCOPY & TUBAL INTERRUPTION W/O CC/MCC	0.805	2.0	2.4
746	13	SURG	VAGINA, CERVIX & VULVA PROCEDURES W CC/MCC	1.337	3.0	4.2

MS-DRG	MDC	Type	MS-DRG Title	Weight	Geometric Mean LOS	Arithmetic Mean LOS
747	13	SURG	VAGINA, CERVIX & VULVA PROCEDURES W/O CC/MCC	0.885	1.5	1.8
748	13	SURG	FEMALE REPRODUCTIVE SYSTEM RECONSTRUCTIVE PROCEDURES	0.917	1.4	1.7
749	13	SURG	OTHER FEMALE REPRODUCTIVE SYSTEM O.R. PROCEDURES W CC/MCC	2.528	6.2	8.5
750	13	SURG	OTHER FEMALE REPRODUCTIVE SYSTEM O.R. PROCEDURES W/O CC/MCC	0.937	2.2	2.8
754	13	MED	MALIGNANCY, FEMALE REPRODUCTIVE SYSTEM W MCC	2.030	6.4	8.8
755	13	MED	MALIGNANCY, FEMALE REPRODUCTIVE SYSTEM W CC	1.144	4.0	5.3
756	13	MED	MALIGNANCY, FEMALE REPRODUCTIVE SYSTEM W/O CC/MCC	0.636	2.3	3.1
757	13	MED	INFECTIONS, FEMALE REPRODUCTIVE SYSTEM W MCC	1.657	6.0	7.8
758	13	MED	INFECTIONS, FEMALE REPRODUCTIVE SYSTEM W CC	1.096	4.7	5.7
759	13	MED	INFECTIONS, FEMALE REPRODUCTIVE SYSTEM W/O CC/MCC	0.737	3.3	4.0
760	13	MED	MENSTRUAL & OTHER FEMALE REPRODUCTIVE SYSTEM DISORDERS W CC/MCC	0.839	2.9	3.8
761	13	MED	MENSTRUAL & OTHER FEMALE REPRODUCTIVE SYSTEM DISORDERS W/O CC/MCC	0.522	1.8	2.2
765	14	SURG	CESAREAN SECTION W CC/MCC	1.127	3.9	4.9
766	14	SURG	CESAREAN SECTION W/O CC/MCC	0.800	2.9	3.1
767	14	SURG	VAGINAL DELIVERY W STERILIZATION &/OR D&C	0.911	2.4	2.7
768	14	SURG	VAGINAL DELIVERY W O.R. PROC EXCEPT STERIL &/OR D&C	1.811	4.7	5.8
769	14	SURG	POSTPARTUM & POST ABORTION DIAGNOSES W O.R. PROCEDURE	2.063	3.5	5.7
770	14	SURG	ABORTION W D&C, ASPIRATION CURETTAGE OR HYSTEROTOMY	0.702	1.6	2.1
774	14	MED	VAGINAL DELIVERY W COMPLICATING DIAGNOSES	0.685	2.6	3.2
775	14	MED	VAGINAL DELIVERY W/O COMPLICATING DIAGNOSES	0.526	2.1	2.3
776	14	MED	POSTPARTUM & POST ABORTION DIAGNOSES W/O O.R. PROCEDURE	0.651	2.6	3.4
777	14	MED	ECTOPIC PREGNANCY	0.741	1.7	2.1
778	14	MED	THREATENED ABORTION	0.494	2.1	3.2
779	14	MED	ABORTION W/O D&C	0.531	1.6	2.1
780	14	MED	FALSE LABOR	0.228	1.2	1.6
781	14	MED	OTHER ANTEPARTUM DIAGNOSES W MEDICAL COMPLICATIONS	0.681	2.7	3.9
782	14	MED	OTHER ANTEPARTUM DIAGNOSES W/O MEDICAL COMPLICATIONS	0.474	1.9	2.6
789	15	MED	NEONATES, DIED OR TRANSFERRED TO ANOTHER ACUTE CARE FACILITY	1.488	1.8	1.8
790	15	MED	EXTREME IMMATURITY OR RESPIRATORY DISTRESS SYNDROME, NEONATE	4.906	17.9	17.9

MS-DRG	MDC	Type	MS-DRG Title	Weight	Geometric Mean LOS	Arithmetic Mean LOS
791	15	MED	PREMATURITY W MAJOR PROBLEMS	3.351	13.3	13.3
792	15	MED	PREMATURITY W/O MAJOR PROBLEMS	2.022	8.6	8.6
793	15	MED	FULL TERM NEONATE W MAJOR PROBLEMS	3.442	4.7	4.7
794	15	MED	NEONATE W OTHER SIGNIFICANT PROBLEMS	1.218	3.4	3.4
795	15	MED	NORMAL NEWBORN	0.165	3.1	3.1
799	16	SURG	SPLENECTOMY W MCC	4.943	10.4	13.5
800	16	SURG	SPLENECTOMY W CC	2.587	5.9	7.5
801	16	SURG	SPLENECTOMY W/O CC/MCC	1.559	3.1	3.9
802	16	SURG	OTHER O.R. PROC OF THE BLOOD & BLOOD FORMING ORGANS W MCC	3.617	8.5	12.1
803	16	SURG	OTHER O.R. PROC OF THE BLOOD & BLOOD FORMING ORGANS W CC	1.891	4.8	6.5
804	16	SURG	OTHER O.R. PROC OF THE BLOOD & BLOOD FORMING ORGANS W/O CC/MCC	1.045	2.3	3.0
808	16	MED	MAJOR HEMATOL/IMMUN DIAG EXC SICKLE CELL CRISIS & COAGUL W MCC	2.148	6.3	8.2
809	16	MED	MAJOR HEMATOL/IMMUN DIAG EXC SICKLE CELL CRISIS & COAGUL W CC	1.195	4.0	5.1
810	16	MED	MAJOR HEMATOL/IMMUN DIAG EXC SICKLE CELL CRISIS & COAGUL W/O CC/MCC	0.923	3.0	3.7
811	16	MED	RED BLOOD CELL DISORDERS W MCC	1.254	3.8	5.2
812	16	MED	RED BLOOD CELL DISORDERS W/O MCC	0.796	2.8	3.6
813	16	MED	COAGULATION DISORDERS	1.437	3.6	5.0
814	16	MED	RETICULOENDOTHELIAL & IMMUNITY DISORDERS W MCC	1.643	5.0	6.9
815	16	MED	RETICULOENDOTHELIAL & IMMUNITY DISORDERS W CC	1.002	3.6	4.6
816	16	MED	RETICULOENDOTHELIAL & IMMUNITY DISORDERS W/O CC/MCC	0.682	2.6	3.2
820	17	SURG	LYMPHOMA & LEUKEMIA W MAJOR O.R. PROCEDURE W MCC	5.711	13.1	17.2
821	17	SURG	LYMPHOMA & LEUKEMIA W MAJOR O.R. PROCEDURE W CC	2.400	5.3	7.4
822	17	SURG	LYMPHOMA & LEUKEMIA W MAJOR O.R. PROCEDURE W/O CC/MCC	1.225	2.3	3.1
823	17	SURG	LYMPHOMA & NON-ACUTE LEUKEMIA W OTHER O.R. PROC W MCC	4.564	12.2	15.9
824	17	SURG	LYMPHOMA & NON-ACUTE LEUKEMIA W OTHER O.R. PROC W CC	2.306	6.6	8.7
825	17	SURG	LYMPHOMA & NON-ACUTE LEUKEMIA W OTHER O.R. PROC W/O CC/MCC	1.242	2.8	4.0
826	17	SURG	MYELOPROLIF DISORD OR POORLY DIFF NEOPL W MAJ O.R. PROC W MCC	4.867	11.2	14.7
827	17	SURG	MYELOPROLIF DISORD OR POORLY DIFF NEOPL W MAJ O.R. PROC W CC	2.146	5.3	6.9
828	17	SURG	MYELOPROLIF DISORD OR POORLY DIFF NEOPL W MAJ O.R. PROC W/O CC/MCC	1.386	3.1	3.8

MS-DRG	MDC	Type	MS-DRG Title	Weight	Geometric Mean LOS	Arithmetic Mean LOS
829	17	SURG	MYELOPROLIF DISORD OR POORLY DIFF NEOPL W OTHER O.R. PROC W CC/MCC	2.709	6.3	9.4
830	17	SURG	MYELOPROLIF DISORD OR POORLY DIFF NEOPL W OTHER O.R. PROC W/O CC/MCC	1.098	2.4	3.2
834	17	MED	ACUTE LEUKEMIA W/O MAJOR O.R. PROCEDURE W MCC	4.928	10.1	16.2
835	17	MED	ACUTE LEUKEMIA W/O MAJOR O.R. PROCEDURE W CC	2.428	5.7	9.2
836	17	MED	ACUTE LEUKEMIA W/O MAJOR O.R. PROCEDURE W/O CC/MCC	1.139	3.0	4.5
837	17	MED	CHEMO W ACUTE LEUKEMIA AS SDX OR W HIGH DOSE CHEMO AGENT W MCC	6.660	17.8	23.5
838	17	MED	CHEMO W ACUTE LEUKEMIA AS SDX W CC OR HIGH DOSE CHEMO AGENT	3.143	8.1	12.2
839	17	MED	CHEMO W ACUTE LEUKEMIA AS SDX W/O CC/MCC	1.282	4.6	5.7
840	17	MED	LYMPHOMA & NON-ACUTE LEUKEMIA W MCC	2.932	7.8	10.6
841	17	MED	LYMPHOMA & NON-ACUTE LEUKEMIA W CC	1.638	5.1	6.8
842	17	MED	LYMPHOMA & NON-ACUTE LEUKEMIA W/O CC/MCC	1.039	3.2	4.2
843	17	MED	OTHER MYELOPROLIF DIS OR POORLY DIFF NEOPL DIAG W MCC	1.836	6.0	8.0
844	17	MED	OTHER MYELOPROLIF DIS OR POORLY DIFF NEOPL DIAG W CC	1.194	4.3	5.6
845	17	MED	OTHER MYELOPROLIF DIS OR POORLY DIFF NEOPL DIAG W/O CC/MCC	0.803	2.9	3.7
846	17	MED	CHEMOTHERAPY W/O ACUTE LEUKEMIA AS SECONDARY DIAGNOSIS W MCC	2.196	5.4	8.0
847	17	MED	CHEMOTHERAPY W/O ACUTE LEUKEMIA AS SECONDARY DIAGNOSIS W CC	0.986	2.8	3.4
848	17	MED	CHEMOTHERAPY W/O ACUTE LEUKEMIA AS SECONDARY DIAGNOSIS W/O CC/MCC	0.808	2.4	3.0
849	17	MED	RADIOTHERAPY	1.263	4.4	6.1
853	18	SURG	INFECTIOUS & PARASITIC DISEASES W O.R. PROCEDURE W MCC	5.524	12.0	15.6
854	18	SURG	INFECTIOUS & PARASITIC DISEASES W O.R. PROCEDURE W CC	2.788	8.2	10.0
855	18	SURG	INFECTIOUS & PARASITIC DISEASES W O.R. PROCEDURE W/O CC/MCC	1.380	3.9	5.3
856	18	SURG	POSTOPERATIVE OR POST-TRAUMATIC INFECTIONS W O.R. PROC W MCC	5.130	11.2	15.0
857	18	SURG	POSTOPERATIVE OR POST-TRAUMATIC INFECTIONS W O.R. PROC W CC	2.098	6.2	7.9
858	18	SURG	POSTOPERATIVE OR POST-TRAUMATIC INFECTIONS W O.R. PROC W/O CC/MCC	1.305	4.1	5.1
862	18	MED	POSTOPERATIVE & POST-TRAUMATIC INFECTIONS W MCC	1.951	5.8	7.7
863	18	MED	POSTOPERATIVE & POST-TRAUMATIC INFECTIONS W/O MCC	0.979	4.0	4.9
864	18	MED	FEVER	0.828	3.0	3.8
865	18	MED	VIRAL ILLNESS W MCC	1.565	4.5	6.5
866	18	MED	VIRAL ILLNESS W/O MCC	0.746	2.8	3.5

MS-DRG	MDC	Type	MS-DRG Title	Weight	Geometric Mean LOS	Arithmetic Mean LOS
867	18	MED	OTHER INFECTIOUS & PARASITIC DISEASES DIAGNOSES W MCC	2.471	6.7	9.2
868	18	MED	OTHER INFECTIOUS & PARASITIC DISEASES DIAGNOSES W CC	1.161	4.3	5.4
869	18	MED	OTHER INFECTIOUS & PARASITIC DISEASES DIAGNOSES W/O CC/MCC	0.721	3.0	3.6
870	18	MED	SEPTICEMIA OR SEVERE SEPSIS W MV 96+ HOURS	5.831	12.8	15.1
871	18	MED	SEPTICEMIA OR SEVERE SEPSIS W/O MV 96+ HOURS W MCC	1.907	5.4	7.2
872	18	MED	SEPTICEMIA OR SEVERE SEPSIS W/O MV 96+ HOURS W/O MCC	1.155	4.5	5.4
876	19	SURG	O.R. PROCEDURE W PRINCIPAL DIAGNOSES OF MENTAL ILLNESS	2.814	8.1	12.7
880	19	MED	ACUTE ADJUSTMENT REACTION & PSYCHOSOCIAL DYSFUNCTION	0.616	2.3	3.0
881	19	MED	DEPRESSIVE NEUROSES	0.618	3.1	4.2
882	19	MED	NEUROSES EXCEPT DEPRESSIVE	0.628	3.1	4.3
883	19	MED	DISORDERS OF PERSONALITY & IMPULSE CONTROL	1.069	4.9	7.7
884	19	MED	ORGANIC DISTURBANCES & MENTAL RETARDATION	0.931	4.0	5.3
885	19	MED	PSYCHOSES	0.904	5.4	7.4
886	19	MED	BEHAVIORAL & DEVELOPMENTAL DISORDERS	0.790	3.8	5.9
887	19	MED	OTHER MENTAL DISORDER DIAGNOSES	0.789	2.9	4.1
894	20	MED	ALCOHOL/DRUG ABUSE OR DEPENDENCE, LEFT AMA	0.407	2.1	3.0
895	20	MED	ALCOHOL/DRUG ABUSE OR DEPENDENCE W REHABILITATION THERAPY	1.028	8.5	10.9
896	20	MED	ALCOHOL/DRUG ABUSE OR DEPENDENCE W/O REHABILITATION THERAPY W MCC	1.457	4.7	6.5
897	20	MED	ALCOHOL/DRUG ABUSE OR DEPENDENCE W/O REHABILITATION THERAPY W/O MCC	0.651	3.2	4.0
901	21	SURG	WOUND DEBRIDEMENTS FOR INJURIES W MCC	3.904	9.1	14.0
902	21	SURG	WOUND DEBRIDEMENTS FOR INJURIES W CC	1.792	5.4	7.5
903	21	SURG	WOUND DEBRIDEMENTS FOR INJURIES W/O CC/MCC	1.062	3.3	4.4
904	21	SURG	SKIN GRAFTS FOR INJURIES W CC/MCC	2.934	7.2	10.9
905	21	SURG	SKIN GRAFTS FOR INJURIES W/O CC/MCC	1.171	3.4	4.5
906	21	SURG	HAND PROCEDURES FOR INJURIES	1.036	2.1	3.1
907	21	SURG	OTHER O.R. PROCEDURES FOR INJURIES W MCC	3.827	7.8	11.1
908	21	SURG	OTHER O.R. PROCEDURES FOR INJURIES W CC	1.925	4.7	6.3
909	21	SURG	OTHER O.R. PROCEDURES FOR INJURIES W/O CC/MCC	1.155	2.6	3.4
913	21	MED	TRAUMATIC INJURY W MCC	1.344	4.0	5.6

MS-DRG	MDC	Type	MS-DRG Title	Weight	Geometric Mean LOS	Arithmetic Mean LOS
914	21	MED	TRAUMATIC INJURY W/O MCC	0.699	2.6	3.2
915	21	MED	ALLERGIC REACTIONS W MCC	1.425	3.6	5.1
916	21	MED	ALLERGIC REACTIONS W/O MCC	0.487	1.7	2.1
917	21	MED	POISONING & TOXIC EFFECTS OF DRUGS W MCC	1.487	3.7	5.1
918	21	MED	POISONING & TOXIC EFFECTS OF DRUGS W/O MCC	0.627	2.1	2.7
919	21	MED	COMPLICATIONS OF TREATMENT W MCC	1.590	4.4	6.2
920	21	MED	COMPLICATIONS OF TREATMENT W CC	0.979	3.2	4.3
921	21	MED	COMPLICATIONS OF TREATMENT W/O CC/MCC	0.622	2.2	2.8
922	21	MED	OTHER INJURY, POISONING & TOXIC EFFECT DIAG W MCC	1.348	3.8	5.4
923	21	MED	OTHER INJURY, POISONING & TOXIC EFFECT DIAG W/O MCC	0.681	2.3	3.2
927	22	SURG	EXTENSIVE BURNS OR FULL THICKNESS BURNS W MV 96+ HRS W SKIN GRAFT	12.665	21.8	28.5
928	22	SURG	FULL THICKNESS BURN W SKIN GRAFT OR INHAL INJ W CC/MCC	4.772	10.8	14.8
929	22	SURG	FULL THICKNESS BURN W SKIN GRAFT OR INHAL INJ W/O CC/MCC	2.056	5.2	7.7
933	22	MED	EXTENSIVE BURNS OR FULL THICKNESS BURNS W MV 96+ HRS W/O SKIN GRAFT	2.198	2.3	5.1
934	22	MED	FULL THICKNESS BURN W/O SKIN GRFT OR INHAL INJ	1.356	4.1	5.8
935	22	MED	NON-EXTENSIVE BURNS	1.292	3.5	5.2
939	23	SURG	O.R. PROC W DIAGNOSES OF OTHER CONTACT W HEALTH SERVICES W MCC	2.870	6.9	10.0
940	23	SURG	O.R. PROC W DIAGNOSES OF OTHER CONTACT W HEALTH SERVICES W CC	1.680	3.6	5.4
941	23	SURG	O.R. PROC W DIAGNOSES OF OTHER CONTACT W HEALTH SERVICES W/O CC/MCC	1.146	2.0	2.6
945	23	MED	REHABILITATION W CC/MCC	1.280	8.2	10.1
946	23	MED	REHABILITATION W/O CC/MCC	1.127	6.6	7.5
947	23	MED	SIGNS & SYMPTOMS W MCC	1.095	3.7	4.9
948	23	MED	SIGNS & SYMPTOMS W/O MCC	0.687	2.7	3.4
949	23	MED	AFTERCARE W CC/MCC	1.001	2.6	4.4
950	23	MED	AFTERCARE W/O CC/MCC	0.504	2.2	2.8
951	23	MED	OTHER FACTORS INFLUENCING HEALTH STATUS	0.659	2.2	4.0
955	24	SURG	CRANIOTOMY FOR MULTIPLE SIGNIFICANT TRAUMA	5.534	8.9	12.6
956	24	SURG	LIMB REATTACHMENT, HIP & FEMUR PROC FOR MULTIPLE SIGNIFICANT TRAUMA	3.370	7.0	8.5
957	24	SURG	OTHER O.R. PROCEDURES FOR MULTIPLE SIGNIFICANT TRAUMA W MCC	6.252	10.1	14.2

MS-DRG	MDC	Type	MS-DRG Title	Weight	Geometric Mean LOS	Arithmetic Mean LOS
958	24	SURG	OTHER O.R. PROCEDURES FOR MULTIPLE SIGNIFICANT TRAUMA W CC	3.769	7.5	9.6
959	24	SURG	OTHER O.R. PROCEDURES FOR MULTIPLE SIGNIFICANT TRAUMA W/O CC/MCC	2.321	4.7	5.9
963	24	MED	OTHER MULTIPLE SIGNIFICANT TRAUMA W MCC	2.812	6.0	8.7
964	24	MED	OTHER MULTIPLE SIGNIFICANT TRAUMA W CC	1.490	4.5	5.6
965	24	MED	OTHER MULTIPLE SIGNIFICANT TRAUMA W/O CC/MCC	0.939	3.1	3.8
969	25	SURG	HIV W EXTENSIVE O.R. PROCEDURE W MCC	5.507	12.0	17.1
970	25	SURG	HIV W EXTENSIVE O.R. PROCEDURE W/O MCC	2.676	6.3	8.6
974	25	MED	HIV W MAJOR RELATED CONDITION W MCC	2.585	6.8	9.6
975	25	MED	HIV W MAJOR RELATED CONDITION W CC	1.364	5.1	6.6
976	25	MED	HIV W MAJOR RELATED CONDITION W/O CC/MCC	0.898	3.5	4.4
977	25	MED	HIV W OR W/O OTHER RELATED CONDITION	1.049	3.7	4.9
981		SURG	EXTENSIVE O.R. PROCEDURE UNRELATED TO PRINCIPAL DIAGNOSIS W MCC	5.063	11.0	14.1
982		SURG	EXTENSIVE O.R. PROCEDURE UNRELATED TO PRINCIPAL DIAGNOSIS W CC	2.940	6.8	8.7
983		SURG	EXTENSIVE O.R. PROCEDURE UNRELATED TO PRINCIPAL DIAGNOSIS W/O CC/MCC	1.777	3.1	4.3
984		SURG	PROSTATIC O.R. PROCEDURE UNRELATED TO PRINCIPAL DIAGNOSIS W MCC	3.324	10.5	13.3
985		SURG	PROSTATIC O.R. PROCEDURE UNRELATED TO PRINCIPAL DIAGNOSIS W CC	2.151	6.8	9.0
986		SURG	PROSTATIC O.R. PROCEDURE UNRELATED TO PRINCIPAL DIAGNOSIS W/O CC/MCC	1.114	2.7	4.0
987		SURG	NON-EXTENSIVE O.R. PROC UNRELATED TO PRINCIPAL DIAGNOSIS W MCC	3.450	9.3	12.1
988		SURG	NON-EXTENSIVE O.R. PROC UNRELATED TO PRINCIPAL DIAGNOSIS W CC	1.874	5.6	7.4
989		SURG	NON-EXTENSIVE O.R. PROC UNRELATED TO PRINCIPAL DIAGNOSIS W/O CC/MCC	1.059	2.5	3.5
998		**	PRINCIPAL DIAGNOSIS INVALID AS DISCHARGE DIAGNOSIS	0.000	0.0	0.0
999		**	UNGROUPABLE	0.000	0.0	0.0

MS-DRGs 998 and 999 contain cases that could not be assigned to valid DRGs.
Note: If there is no value in either the geometric mean LOS or the arithmetic mean LOS column, the volume of cases is insufficient to determine a meaningful computation of these statistics.

Appendix 6.2: Hospital Acute Inpatient Services Payment System

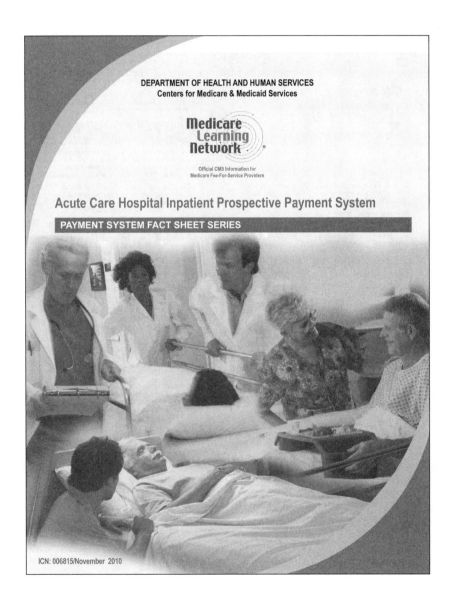

DEPARTMENT OF HEALTH AND HUMAN SERVICES
Centers for Medicare & Medicaid Services

Medicare Learning Network

Official CMS Information for
Medicare Fee-For-Service Providers

Acute Care Hospital Inpatient Prospective Payment System

PAYMENT SYSTEM FACT SHEET SERIES

ICN: 006815/November 2010

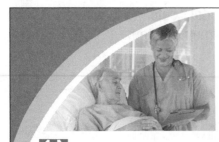

his publication provides the following information about the Acute Care Hospital Inpatient Prospective Payment System (IPPS):

❖ Basis for IPPS payment;

❖ Payment rates:

❖ How payment rates are set; and

❖ Resources.

Facilities contract with Medicare to furnish acute hospital inpatient care and agree to accept predetermined acute IPPS rates as payment in full.

The inpatient hospital benefit covers beneficiaries for 90 days of care per episode of illness with an additional 60 day lifetime reserve. Illness episodes begin when beneficiaries are admitted and end after they have been out of the hospital or Skilled Nursing Facility (SNF) for 60 consecutive days.

Basis for Payment

Generally, hospitals receive Medicare IPPS payment on a per discharge or per case basis for Medicare beneficiaries with inpatient stays. Related therapeutic outpatient department services provided within three days prior to admission are included in the payment for the inpatient stay and may not be separately billed.

Discharges are assigned to diagnosis-related groups (DRG), a classification system that groups similar clinical conditions (diagnoses) and the procedures furnished by the hospital during the stay. The beneficiary's principal diagnosis and up to eight secondary diagnoses that indicate comorbidities and complications will determine the DRG assignment. Similarly, DRG assignment can be affected by up to six procedures furnished during the stay. The Centers for Medicare & Medicaid Services (CMS) reviews the DRG definitions annually to ensure that each group continues to include cases with clinically similar conditions that require comparable amounts of inpatient resources. When the review shows that subsets of clinically similar cases within a DRG consume significantly different amounts of resources, they may be assigned to a different DRG with comparable resource use or a new DRG may be created.

For discharges occurring on or after October 1, 2007, a new DRG system called Medicare Severity (MS)-DRG is being

used to better account for severity of illness and resource consumption for Medicare beneficiaries. Use of MS-DRGs was transitioned during a two-year period. For the period October 1, 2007, through September 30, 2008, payment was based on a 50/50 blend of MS-DRGs and the previous DRG system. Beginning October 1, 2008 (fiscal year [FY] 2009) and after, payment is based solely on the MS-DRGs.

There are three levels of severity in the MS-DRGs based on secondary diagnosis codes:

1) MCC – Major Complication/Comorbidity, which reflect the highest level of severity;

2) CC – Complication/Comorbidity, which is the next level of severity; and

3) Non-CC – Non-Complication/Comorbidity, which do not significantly affect severity of illness and resource use.

Payment Rates

The IPPS per-discharge payment is based on two national base payment rates or "standardized amounts:" one that provides for operating expenses and another for capital expenses. These payment rates are adjusted to account for:

❖ The costs associated with the beneficiary's clinical condition and related treatment relative to the costs of the average Medicare case (i.e., the DRG relative weight, as described in the "How Payment Rates Are Set" section below); and

❖ Market conditions in the facility's location relative to national conditions (i.e., the wage index, as described in the "How Payment Rates Are Set" section below).

In addition to these adjusted per discharge base payment rates, hospitals can qualify for outlier payments for cases that are extremely costly and receive additional payments per discharge for the indirect costs of graduate medical education (IME) if they train residents in approved graduate medical education (GME) programs, treating a disproportionate share of low-income patients, and the use of certain new technologies. Hospitals that train residents in approved GME programs receive a payment separate from the IPPS for the direct costs of GME, while the operating and capital payment rates for these hospitals are increased to reflect the higher indirect patient care costs of teaching hospitals relative to non-teaching hospitals or IME. Operating and capital payment rates are also increased for facilities that treat a disproportionate share of low-income patients. In addition, hospitals may be paid an additional amount for treating patients with certain approved technologies that are new and costly and offer a substantial clinical improvement over existing treatments available to Medicare beneficiaries. Finally, payment is reduced when a beneficiary has a short length of stay (LOS) and is transferred to another acute care hospital or, in some circumstances, to a post-acute care setting.

The steps for determining an IPPS payment are as follows:

1) The hospital submits a bill to the Medicare Administrative Contractor for each Medicare

patient they treat. Based on the information on the bill, the case is categorized into a DRG.

2) The base payment rate, or standardized amount (a dollar figure), includes a labor-related and non-labor related share. The labor-related share is adjusted by a wage index to reflect area differences in the cost of labor. If the area wage index is greater than or equal to 1.0, the labor share equals 68.8 percent. The law requires the labor share to equal 62 percent if the area wage index is less than 1.0. The non-labor related share is adjusted by a cost-of-living adjustment (COLA) factor, which equals 1.0 for all states except Alaska and Hawaii.

3) The wage-adjusted standardized amount is multiplied by a relative weight for the DRG. The relative weight is specific to each of 747 DRGs (for FY 2011) and represents the relative average costs associated with one DRG.

4) If applicable, additional amounts will be added to the IPPS payment for hospitals engaged in teaching medical residents to reflect the higher indirect patient care costs of teaching hospitals relative to non-teaching hospitals, hospitals that treat a disproportionate share of low-income patients, cases that involve certain approved new technologies, and for high cost outlier cases.

The chart below shows the formula for calculating Medicare's IPPS operating rate, and the chart on page 4 shows the formula for calculating Medicare's capital payment rate.

How Payment Rates Are Set

IPPS payments are derived through a series of adjustments applied to separate operating and capital base payment rates. The base rates are updated annually and unless there are other policy changes, the update raises all payment rates proportionately.

BASE PAYMENT AMOUNTS

Discharge base rates, also known as standardized payment amounts, for operating payments and the Federal rate for capital payments are set for the operating and capital costs that efficient facilities would be expected to incur in furnishing covered inpatient services. Some costs, such as direct costs of operating GME programs and organ acquisition costs, are excluded from the IPPS and paid separately. For FY 2011, the national IPPS operating base rate is $5,164.11. Capital payments cover costs for depreciation, interest, rent, and property-related insurance and taxes. For FY 2011, the national IPPS capital base rate is $420.01. Hospitals in Puerto Rico receive a 75 percent/25 percent blend of the Federal base payment amount and a Puerto Rico-specific rate, respectively, for both operating and capital payments.

DIAGNOSIS-RELATED GROUP RELATIVE WEIGHTS

A weight is assigned to each MS-DRG that reflects the average relative costliness of cases in that group compared with the costliness for the average Medicare case. The same MS-DRG weights are used to set operating and capital payment

Acute Care Hospital Inpatient Prospective Payment System
Operating Base Payment Rate

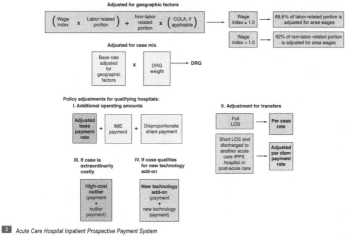

Acute Care Hospital Inpatient Prospective Payment System

Acute Care Hospital Inpatient Prospective Payment System
Capital Base Payment Rate

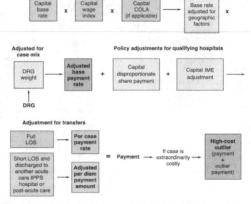

rates. The MS-DRG weights are recalibrated annually, without affecting overall payments, based on standardized charges and costs for all IPPS cases in each MS-DRG. Hospitals' billed charges are standardized to improve comparability, which involves adjusting charges to remove differences associated with hospital wage rates across labor markets, the size and intensity of hospitals' resident training activities, and the number of low-income patients treated by a hospital. The charges are reduced to costs by using national average ratios of hospital costs to charges for 15 different hospital departments.

ADJUSTMENT FOR MARKET CONDITIONS

Base operating and capital rates are adjusted by an area wage index to reflect the expected differences in local market prices for labor, which is intended to measure differences in hospital wage rates among labor markets by comparing the average hourly wage for hospital workers in each urban or statewide rural area to the nationwide average. CMS uses the Office of Management and Budget's Core Based Statistical Area definitions (with some modifications) to define each labor market area. The wage index is revised each year based on wage data reported by IPPS hospitals. Hospitals may request geographic reclassification if they believe that they compete for labor with a different area than the one in which they are located. A COLA, which reflects the higher costs of supplies and other non-labor resources, is also applied to the base operating and capital rates of IPPS hospitals in Hawaii and Alaska. The wage index is applied to the labor-related portion or labor share of the operating base rate, which reflects an estimated portion of costs affected by local wage rates and fringe benefits. Additionally, the wage index is applied to the whole capital base rate. The current estimate of the national operating labor share is 68.8 percent, which is applied to hospitals with a wage index greater than or equal to 1.0. The national operating labor share is 62 percent for areas with a wage index less than 1.0. There are alternative labor shares that are applicable to hospitals

located in Puerto Rico. The wage index applied to the capital base rate is raised to a fractional power, which narrows the geographic variation in wage index values among market areas.

BAD DEBTS

Acute care hospitals are reimbursed for 70 percent of bad debts resulting from beneficiaries' nonpayment of copayments and deductibles after a reasonable effort has been made to collect the unpaid amounts.

POLICY ADJUSTMENTS

Additional operating and capital amounts are paid as follows:

❖ Teaching hospitals or hospitals that train residents in approved medical allopathic, osteopathic, dental, or podiatry residency programs receive direct GME payments that reflect the direct costs of operating approved residency training programs and are paid separately from the IPPS. Direct GME payments are generally based on the product of:

  • Updated hospital-specific costs per resident in a historical base year; and

  • The number of residents a hospital trains; and

  • The hospital's Medicare patient load (the proportion of Medicare inpatient days to total inpatient days).

❖ Teaching hospitals or hospitals that train residents in approved medical, osteopathic, dental, or podiatry residency programs also receive IME adjustments to reflect the higher indirect patient care costs of teaching hospitals relative to non-teaching hospitals. The size of the IME adjustment depends on the hospital's teaching

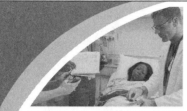

intensity. For operating payments, teaching intensity is measured by the hospital's number of residents trained per inpatient bed (i.e., the resident-to-bed ratio). In FYs 2008, 2009, and 2010, the operating IME adjustment increased per-case payments by 5.5 percent for approximately every 10 percent increase in the resident-to-bed ratio. In FY 2011, the rate is still 5.5 percent.

❖ Hospitals that treat a disproportionate share of low-income patients receive additional operating and capital payments. A hospital can qualify for the Medicare operating disproportionate share hospital (DSH) adjustment by using one of the following methods:

• Primary method – The hospital's DSH patient percentage exceeds an amount specified in statute. The DSH patient percentage equals the sum of the percentage of Medicare inpatient days attributable to patients entitled to both Medicare Part A and Supplemental Security Income benefits and the percentage of total inpatient days attributable to patients eligible for Medicaid but not eligible for Medicare Part A.

• Alternate method (known as the Pickle methodology) – Large urban hospitals qualify for DSH if they can demonstrate that more than 30 percent of their total net inpatient care revenues come from State and local governments for indigent care (other than Medicare or Medicaid).

For hospitals with a DSH patient percentage that exceeds 15 percent, operating DSH payments are based on a statutory formula. The DSH payment add-on rate is capped at 12 percent of base inpatient payments for rural hospitals with fewer than 500 beds and for urban hospitals with fewer than 100 beds. Rural Referral Center payments are based on a separate formula. Hospitals that qualify for a DSH payment under the Pickle methodology (i.e., they receive at least 30 percent of inpatient revenue from State and local government subsidies) have a 35 percent adjustment rate. Urban hospitals with 100 or more beds and all hospitals that receive at least 30 percent of inpatient revenue from State and local government subsidies are eligible for capital DSH payments (regardless of their DSH patient percentage). The capital DSH add-on payment is based on the empirically estimated cost effect of treating low-income patients.

❖ Sole Community Hospitals (SCH) and Medicare Dependent Hospitals (MDH) can receive operating payments based on their hospital-specific payment rate as follows, while their capital payments are solely based on the capital base rate (i.e., like all other IPPS hospitals):

• SCHs receive the higher of either the IPPS payment rate or a payment based on the hospital's costs in a base year updated to the current year

and adjusted for changes in their case mix for IPPS operating payments. To qualify as a SCH, a hospital must meet one of the following criteria:

1) The hospital is located at least 35 miles from other like hospitals;

2) The hospital is rural, located between 25 and 35 miles from other like hospitals, AND meets ONE of the following criteria:

• No more than 25 percent of residents who become hospital inpatients or no more than 25 percent of the Medicare beneficiaries who become hospital inpatients in the hospital's service area are admitted to other like hospitals located within a 35-mile radius of the hospital or, if larger, within its service area; or

• The hospital has fewer than 50 beds and would meet the 25 percent criterion above were it not for the fact that some beneficiaries or residents were forced to seek specialized care outside of the service area due to the unavailability of necessary specialty services at the hospital;

3) The hospital is rural and located between 15 and 25 miles from other like hospitals but because of local topography or periods of prolonged severe weather conditions, the other like hospitals are inaccessible for at least 30 days in each of two out of three years; or

4) The hospital is rural and because of distance, posted speed limits, and predictable weather conditions, the travel time between the hospital and the nearest hospital is at least 45 minutes.

SCHs may also qualify for a low-volume hospital payment adjustment.

Certain Essential Access Community Hospitals are also treated as SCHs for payment purposes under the IPPS.

• MDHs receive the higher of either the IPPS payment rate or the IPPS payment rate plus 75 percent of the difference between the IPPS payment rate and a payment based on the hospital's costs in a base year updated to the current year adjusted for changes in their case mix for operating IPPS payments.

MDHs are small hospitals (not more than 100 beds) located in a rural area, are not a SCH, and have a high percentage of Medicare discharges (not less than 60 percent of its inpatient days or discharges based on a specified cost reporting period).

❖ Under the Affordable Care Act, the payment adjustment for low-volume hospitals was amended such that qualifying hospitals will receive add-on payments in FYs 2011 and 2012 as follows:

• Those with 200 or fewer Medicare discharges will receive an adjustment of an additional 25 percent for each discharge; and

• Those with more than 200 and fewer than 1,600 Medicare discharges will receive an adjustment of an additional percentage for each discharge that is calculated using the formula [(4/14) − (Medicare discharges/5600)].

To qualify as a low-volume hospital, the hospital must:

- Be more than 15 road miles from the nearest subsection (d) hospital; and

- Have fewer than 1,600 Medicare discharges based on the latest available Medicare Provider Analysis and Review (MedPAR) data.

❖ Under Section 1109 of Public Law 111-152, qualifying hospitals will receive annual add-on payments in FYs 2011 and 2012. A qualifying hospital is located in a county that ranks per enrollee within the lowest quartile of such counties in the United States based on its ranking in age, sex, and race adjusted spending for benefits under Medicare Parts A and B.

OUTLIER PAYMENTS

To promote access to high quality inpatient care for seriously ill beneficiaries, additional payments are made for outlier or extremely costly cases. These cases are identified by comparing their estimated operating and capital costs to a fixed loss threshold. The fixed loss amount is set each year, which is adjusted to reflect labor costs in the hospital's local market. The fixed loss amount for FY 2008 was $22,185; for FY 2009, it was $20,045; and for FY 2010, it was $23,140 for discharges on or after October 1, 2010, through discharges on or before March 31, 2010, and $23,135 for discharges on or after April 1, 2010, through discharges on or before September 30, 2010. For FY 2011, the fixed loss amount is $23,075.

Hospitals are paid 80 percent of their costs above their fixed loss thresholds and 90 percent of costs above the outlier threshold for burn cases. Outliers are financed by offsetting reductions in the operating and capital base rates (i.e., there is a reduction to the rates paid to all cases so that the amount paid as outliers does not increase or decrease estimated aggregate Medicare spending). The national fixed loss amount is established at the level that will result in estimated outlier payments equaling 5.1 percent of total payments for the FY.

TRANSFER POLICY

DRG payments are reduced when:

❖ The beneficiary's LOS is at least one day less than the geometric mean LOS for the DRG;

❖ The beneficiary is transferred to another hospital covered by the Acute Care Hospital IPPS or, for certain MS-DRGs, discharged to a post-acute setting;

❖ The beneficiary is transferred to a hospital that does not have an agreement to participate in the Medicare Program (effective October 1, 2010); and

❖ The beneficiary is transferred to a Critical Access Hospital (CAH) (effective October 1, 2010).

The following post-acute care settings are included in the transfer policy:

❖ Long-term care hospitals;

❖ Rehabilitation facilities;

❖ Psychiatric facilities;

❖ SNFs;

❖ Home health care when the beneficiary receives clinically related care that begins within three days after the hospital stay;

❖ Rehabilitation distinct part (DP) units located in an acute care hospital or a CAH;

❖ Psychiatric DP units located in an acute care hospital or a CAH;

❖ Cancer hospitals; and

❖ Children's hospitals.

PAYMENT UPDATES

The operating and capital payment rates are updated annually. The operating update is set by Congress, considering the projected increase in the market basket index. The market basket index measures the price increases of goods and services hospitals buy to produce patient care. For FY 2011, the applicable percentage increase for IPPS hospitals equals the rate-of-increase in the hospital market basket for IPPS hospitals in all areas reduced by 0.25 percentage point. The Secretary of the Department of Health and Human Services (HHS) determines the capital update based on an update framework.

Hospitals that report specific quality data to HHS receive the full operating update set by Congress. In 2011, if a hospital does not report the quality data, it will receive the operating update of the rate-of-increase in the hospital market basket for IPPS hospitals in all areas reduced by 0.25 percentage point less an additional 2.0 percentage points. (Currently there is no adjustment to the capital update based on the reporting of quality data.)

Resources

To find additional information about the Acute Care Hospital IPPS, visit *http://www.cms.gov/Acute InpatientPPS/01_overview.asp* on the CMS website.

Medicare
Learning
Network

Official CMS Information for
Medicare Fee-For-Service Providers

Appendix 6.3: Medicare Advantage Program Payment System

MEDICARE ADVANTAGE PROGRAM PAYMENT SYSTEM

*payment**basics***

Revised:
October 2010

The Medicare Advantage (MA) program allows Medicare beneficiaries to receive their Medicare benefits from private plans rather than from the traditional fee-for-service (FFS) program. Under some MA plans, beneficiaries may receive additional benefits beyond those offered under traditional Medicare and may pay additional premiums for them. Medicare pays plans a capitated rate for the 25 percent of beneficiaries enrolled in MA plans in 2010. These payments amounted to $109 billion in 2009, 25 percent of total Medicare spending.

Available MA plans include health maintenance organizations (HMOs), preferred provider organizations (PPOs), private fee-for-service (PFFS) plans, and special needs plans (SNPs). For payment purposes, there are two different categories of MA plans: local plans and regional plans. Local plans may be any of the available plan types and may serve one or more counties. Medicare pays them based on their enrollees' counties of residence. Regional plans, however, must be PPOs and must serve all of one of the 26 regions established by the Centers for Medicare & Medicaid Services (CMS) (Figure 1). Each region comprises one or more entire states.

Defining the Medicare Advantage products Medicare buys

This document does not reflect proposed legislation or regulatory actions.

MEDPAC

601 New Jersey Ave., NW
Suite 9000
Washington, DC 20001
ph: 202-220-3700
fax: 202-220-3759
www.medpac.gov

Under the MA program, Medicare buys insurance coverage for its beneficiaries from private plans with payments made monthly. The coverage must include all Medicare Part A and Part B benefits except hospice. All plans, except PFFS plans, must also offer an option that includes the Part D drug benefit. Plans may limit enrollees' choices of providers more narrowly than under the traditional fee-for-service program. Plans may supplement Medicare benefits by reducing

cost-sharing requirements, providing coverage of non-Medicare benefits, or providing a rebate of all or part of the Part B or Part D premium. To pay for these additional benefits, plans must use their cost savings in providing the Medicare benefit and may charge a supplemental premium.

Determining Medicare payment for local MA plans

Beginning in 2006, plan bids partially determine the Medicare payments they receive (Figure 2). Plans bid to offer Parts A and B (Part D coverage is handled separately) coverage to Medicare beneficiaries. The bid here is presented as the bid to cover an average, or standard, beneficiary. The bid will include plan administrative cost and profit. CMS bases the Medicare payment for a private plan on the relationship between its bid and benchmark.

The benchmark is a bidding target. The local MA benchmarks are based on the county-level payment rates used to pay MA plans before 2006. (Those payment rates were at least as high as per capita FFS Medicare spending in each county and often substantially higher because the Congress set floors to raise the lowest rates to stimulate plan growth in areas where plans historically had not found it profitable to enter.) Generally, CMS updates the local benchmarks each year by the national growth rate in per capita Medicare spending. Regional benchmarks are based on the local benchmarks and are discussed in detail later in this document.

If a plan's standard bid is above the benchmark, then the plan receives a base rate equal to the benchmark and the enrollees have to pay an additional premium that equals the difference between the bid and the benchmark. If

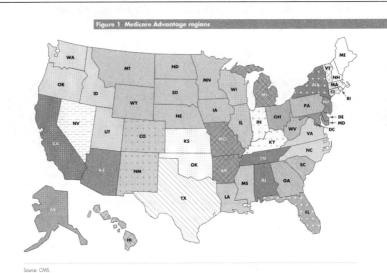

Figure 1 Medicare Advantage regions

Source: CMS.

a plan bid falls below the benchmark, the plan receives a base rate equal to its standard bid.

Medicare payments are also based on enrolled beneficiaries' demographics and health risk characteristics. Medicare uses beneficiaries' characteristics, such as age and prior health conditions, and a risk-adjustment model—the CMS–hierarchical condition category (CMS–HCC)—to develop a measure of their expected relative risk for covered Medicare spending. The base payment for an enrollee is the base rate for the enrollee's county of residence, multiplied by the enrollee's risk measure, also referred to as the CMS–HCC weight.

Plans that bid below the benchmark also receive payment from Medicare in the form of a "rebate." The law defines the rebate as 75 percent of the difference between the plan's actual bid (not standardized) and its casemix-adjusted benchmark. The plan must then return the rebate to its enrollees in the form of supplemental benefits or lower premiums. The plan can apply any premium savings to the Part B premium (in which case the government retains the amount for that use), to the Part D premium, or to the premium for the total package that may include supplemental benefits. For example, if a local plan bid $700 per month in a county with an $800 benchmark (for simplicity, assume that the plan assumes an average casemix in its bid), the

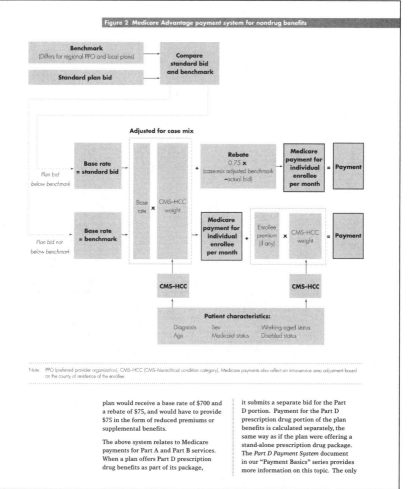

Figure 2 Medicare Advantage payment system for nondrug benefits

Note. PPO (preferred provider organization). CMS–HCC (CMS–hierarchical condition category). Medicare payments also reflect an intra-service area adjustment based on the county of residence of the enrollee.

plan would receive a base rate of $700 and a rebate of $75, and would have to provide $75 in the form of reduced premiums or supplemental benefits.

The above system relates to Medicare payments for Part A and Part B services. When a plan offers Part D prescription drug benefits as part of its package,

it submits a separate bid for the Part D portion. Payment for the Part D prescription drug portion of the plan benefits is calculated separately, the same way as if the plan were offering a stand-alone prescription drug package. The *Part D Payment System* document in our "Payment Basics" series provides more information on this topic. The only

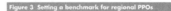

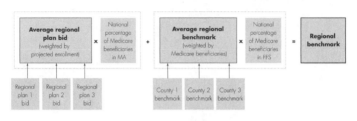

Figure 3   Setting a benchmark for regional PPOs

| Average regional plan bid (weighted by projected enrollment) | × | National percentage of Medicare beneficiaries in MA | + | Average regional benchmark (weighted by Medicare beneficiaries) | × | National percentage of Medicare beneficiaries in FFS | = | Regional benchmark |

Regional plan 1 bid | Regional plan 2 bid | Regional plan 3 bid

County 1 benchmark | County 2 benchmark | County 3 benchmark

Note: MA (Medicare Advantage), FFS (fee-for-service).

difference from stand-alone prescription drug plans is that the MA plan may choose to apply some of its rebate payments to lower the Part D premium that enrollees would otherwise be required to pay.

Determining Medicare payment for regional MA plans

Aside from a few special payment incentives, payment for regional MA plans is determined like payment for local plans, except that the benchmarks are calculated differently (Figure 3).

CMS determines the benchmarks for the MA regional plans by using a more complicated formula that incorporates the plan bids. A region's benchmark is a weighted average of the average county rate and the average plan bid. As directed by law, CMS computes the average county rate as the individual county rates weighted by the number of Medicare beneficiaries who live in each county. The average plan bid is each plan's bid weighted by each plan's projected number of enrollees. CMS then combines the average county rate and the average bid into an overall average. In calculating the overall average, the average bid is weighted by the number of enrollees in all private plans across the country, and the average county rate is weighted by the number of all Medicare beneficiaries who remain in FFS Medicare. ∎

Appendix 6.4: Outpatient Hospital Services Payment System

OUTPATIENT HOSPITAL SERVICES
PAYMENT SYSTEM

*payment**basics***

Revised:
October 2010

Medicare beneficiaries receive a wide range of services in hospital outpatient departments, from injections to complex procedures that require anesthesia. Spending for these services has grown rapidly, largely because of changes in technology and medical practice that have led to new services and encouraged shifts in care from inpatient to ambulatory care settings. Outpatient hospital care accounted for $28 billion of total Medicare spending in 2009.

Medicare originally based payments for outpatient care on hospitals' costs, but the Centers for Medicare & Medicaid Services (CMS) began using the outpatient prospective payment system (OPPS) in August 2000. In 2009, about 3,900 hospitals provided OPPS services, and about 46 percent of fee-for-service beneficiaries received at least one OPPS service.

Under the cost-based system that preceded the OPPS, copayments had become nearly 50 percent of Medicare payments to hospitals for outpatient care. Under the OPPS, copayments are declining each year as a share of total OPPS payments until they reach 20 percent. In 2009, beneficiaries' copayments accounted for 23 percent of total payments under the OPPS.

The OPPS is largely a fee schedule. It sets payments for individual services using a set of relative weights, a conversion factor, and adjustments for geographic differences in input prices. Hospitals also can receive additional payments in the form of outlier adjustments for extraordinarily high-cost services and pass-through payments for some new technologies.

When CMS began using the OPPS, the new payment system had the potential to substantially reduce hospital payments below the amounts under the cost-based system. In response, the Congress partially

protected hospitals that experienced financial losses by providing "transitional corridor" and "hold harmless" provisions. The Congress has legislated permanent hold-harmless status to cancer and children's hospitals. In addition, beginning in 2006 rural sole community hospitals (SCHs) receive an additional 7.1 percent above standard payment rates on all OPPS services except drugs and biologicals. Finally, small rural hospitals and SCHs receive 85 percent of their full hold-harmless payments in 2010.

Defining the outpatient hospital products that Medicare buys

The unit of payment under the OPPS is the individual service as identified by Healthcare Common Procedure Coding System codes. CMS classifies services into ambulatory payment classifications (APCs) on the basis of clinical and cost similarity. All services within an APC have the same payment rate. In addition, CMS assigns some new services to "new technology" APCs based only on similarity of resource use. CMS chose to establish new technology APCs because some services were too new to be represented in the data the agency used to develop the initial payment rates for the OPPS. Services remain in these APCs for two to three years, while CMS collects the data necessary to develop payment rates for them. Each year CMS determines which new services, if any, should be placed in new technology APCs. Payments for new technology APCs are not subject to budget neutrality adjustments, so they increase total OPPS spending.

Within each APC, CMS packages integral services and items with the primary service. In deciding which services to package, CMS considers comments from hospitals, hospital suppliers, and others.

This document does not reflect proposed legislation or regulatory actions.

MEDPAC

601 New Jersey Ave., NW
Suite 9000
Washington, DC 20001
ph: 202-220-3700
fax: 202-220-3759
www.medpac.gov

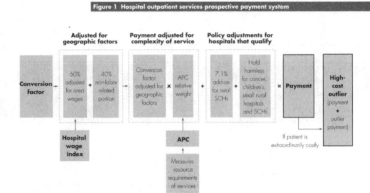

Figure 1 Hospital outpatient services prospective payment system

Note: APC (ambulatory payment classification), SCH (sole community hospital). The APC is the service classification system for the outpatient prospective payment system. Small rural hospitals and SCHs receive 85 percent of full hold-harmless payments in 2010.

In response to these comments, CMS pays separately for:

- corneal tissue acquisition costs,
- blood and blood products, and
- many drugs.

In 2008, CMS expanded the list of services—including observation services—that are packaged into the payment for the associated primary service. The intent of this expanded packaging was to give hospitals more incentive to consider the cost of the package of services used to treat a patient during an outpatient visit. Under greater packaging, hospitals whose costs exceed the payment rate for a package of services have an incentive to evaluate their treatment methods to identify lower cost alternatives for providing care. Consequently, expanded packaging can help slow the growth of Medicare spending in the OPPS.

While CMS makes most OPPS payments on a per service basis, CMS pays for partial hospitalizations on a per diem basis. The per diem rate represents the expected costs for a day of care in the facilities that provide these services, hospital outpatient departments and community mental health centers.

Setting the payment rates

CMS determines the payment rate for each service by multiplying the relative weight for the service's APC by a conversion factor (Figure 1). The relative weight for an APC measures the resource requirements of the service and is based on the median cost of services in that APC. CMS pays separately for professional services, such as physician services.

The conversion factor translates the relative weights into dollar payment rates. To account for geographic differences in input prices, CMS adjusts the labor portion of the conversion factor (60 percent) by the hospital wage index. CMS does not adjust the remaining 40 percent.

CMS initially set the conversion factor so that projected total payments—including beneficiary copayments—would equal the estimated amount that would have been spent under the old payment system, after correcting for some anomalies in statutory formulas.

One exception to CMS's method for setting payment rates is the new technology APCs. Each new technology APC encompasses a cost range, the lowest being for services that cost $0 to $10, the highest for services that cost $9,500 to $10,000. CMS assigns services to new technology APCs on the basis of cost information collected from applications for new technology status. CMS sets the payment rate for a new technology APC at the midpoint of its cost range.

Hospitals can receive three payments in addition to the standard OPPS payments:

- pass-through payments for new technologies,
- outlier payments for unusually costly services, and
- hold-harmless payments for cancer hospitals, children's hospitals, rural hospitals with 100 or fewer beds, and SCHs.

In addition to new technology APCs, pass-through payments are another way that the OPPS accounts for new technologies. In contrast to new technology APCs—which are payments for individual services—pass-through payments are for specific drugs, biologicals, and devices that providers use in the delivery of services. The purpose of pass-through payments is to help ensure beneficiaries' access to technologies that are too new to be well represented in the data that CMS uses to set OPPS payment rates. For pass-through devices, CMS bases payments on each hospital's costs, determined by adjusting charges to costs using a cost-to-charge ratio.

Total pass-through payments cannot be more than 2 percent of total OPPS

payments in 2004 and beyond. Before the start of each calendar year, CMS estimates total pass-through spending. If this estimate exceeds 2 percent of estimated total OPPS payments, the agency must reduce all pass-through payments in that year by a uniform percentage to meet the 2 percent threshold.[1] Also, CMS adjusts the conversion factor to make pass-through payments budget neutral.

CMS makes outlier payments for individual services that cost hospitals much more than the payment rates for the services' APC groups. In 2010, CMS defines an outlier as a service with costs that exceed 1.75 times the APC payment rate and exceed the APC payment rate by at least $2,175. For a service meeting both thresholds, CMS will reimburse the hospital for 50 percent of the difference between the cost of furnishing the service and 1.75 times the APC rate. For 2010, CMS is limiting aggregate outlier payments to 1 percent of total OPPS payments. CMS will make the outlier payments budget neutral by reducing the conversion factor in the OPPS by 1 percent.

The OPPS has permanent hold-harmless status for cancer and children's hospitals. In addition, rural hospitals with 100 or fewer beds and SCHs have hold-harmless payments that are 85 percent of full hold-harmless payments in 2010. If PPS payments for these hospitals are lower than those they would have received under previous policies, CMS provides additional payments to make up the difference. Finally, CMS adds 7.1 percent to the OPPS payments for services furnished by rural SCHs beginning in 2006, excluding drugs and biologicals. CMS makes these additional payments to rural SCHs budget neutral by reducing payments to all other hospitals by 0.4 percent.[2]

CMS reviews and revises the APCs and their relative weights annually. The review considers changes in medical practice, changes in technology, addition of new services, new cost data, and other relevant information. The Balanced Budget

Refinement Act of 1999 requires CMS to
consult with a panel of outside experts
as part of this review. CMS also annually
updates the conversion factor by the
hospital market basket index, unless the
Congress stipulates otherwise.

Drugs and biologicals whose costs exceed a
threshold ($65 per administration in 2010)
have separate APCs; these separately paid
drugs and biologicals do not receive outlier
payments. ∎

1   CMS did not impose uniform payment adjustments from
    August 2000 through April 2002, even though pass-
    through payments exceeded the statutory limit.

2   For SCHs, CMS first determines their OPPS payments
    with the 7.1 percent add-on then determines their
    hold-harmless payments based on those augmented
    payments.

Cost of Capital

Learning Objectives

- Describe how organizations determine the need for external financing
- Explain three factors that influence interest rates
- Calculate the present or future value of a lump sum investment
- List the types of external financing available to healthcare organizations
- List and describe the types of investments available to healthcare organizations

Key Terms

Auction rates	Federal funds rate	Point
Bad debt	Funds	Portfolio
Basis	Future value	Present value
Bond	General fund	Prime rate
Book value	Interest	Principal
Call	Interest-bearing	Property
Capital assets	Liquidation value	Refinancing
Capital budget	Lower of cost or	Reinvestment
Certificate of deposit	market	Return on investment
Commercial paper	Market basket	(ROI)
Compounding	Market value	Savings account
Coupon rate	Maturity	Simple interest
Credit line	Money market	Stock
Debt	account	Treasury stock
Depreciation	Net present value	Unrestricted
Discount	Net working capital	donation
Dividends	Par value	Zero coupon bonds
Equipment	Payback period	
Equity	Plant	

Need for Financing

Individuals who want to purchase an automobile or a home cannot usually do so without borrowing money from a financial institution. Similarly, individuals who make large purchases, such as televisions, may prefer to use a credit card rather than pay cash. The ability of an individual to borrow or to obtain a credit card is dependent on the individual's ability to repay the loan. That ability is measured by the individual's credit rating—a score calculated by one of three organizations that track the creditworthiness of individuals: TransUnion, Equifax, or Experian. This credit score was developed by the Fair Isaac Corporation (FICO).

Organizations may also want to purchase automobiles or buildings and may want to make purchases using credit rather than paying cash. There are two fundamental components to an organization's decision to borrow rather than use cash: cash flow from operations as predicted by the operating budget and capital investments as predicted by the capital budget. Planning for these cash needs is rolled up into the cash budget. The ability of organizations to borrow may be determined by the lender itself or by the organization's credit rating.

Cash Budget

As mentioned in chapter 4, the cash budget is the result of planning for the collection of receivables and expenditure of cash to resolve payables. Cash does not always come in at a predictable rate. Organizations provide services that generate revenue; however, the receipt of cash can be delayed for weeks or even months.

The cash budget is derived from the net cash inflows and outflows represented by the operating and capital budgets. The cash and operating budgets were discussed in chapter 4. The operating budget reflects the routine revenue of the organization and the costs associated with generating that revenue: one business cycle. The capital budget involves the acquisition of resources that will serve the organization over a longer term.

Capital Budget

Part of the organization's strategic planning process is the acquisition of fixed assets for the purpose of expansion or replacement of expired resources. Expansion may include addition or modification of existing buildings or the purchase of new **equipment** for new services or enhancement of existing services. Expired resources, such as heating, ventilation, and air-conditioning (HVAC) equipment, vehicles, patient beds, and computers, are replaced routinely. Both expansion and replacement activities are identified and quantified through the capital budget process.

Organizations are generally free to define items of sufficient value to be included in the **capital budget** however they desire. Smaller organizations may define capital items as any purchases of fixed assets in excess of $500 or any projects that involve modification of furniture, fixtures, or buildings. Other organizations may use higher limits. Two factors affect the definition of capital budget items: **depreciation** and **basis.**

If an asset is to be depreciated over a period in excess of one year, it is a long-term asset and should be capitalized. To capitalize an asset means that the asset is recorded at acquisition value on the balance sheet at the time of purchase (see chapter 2) and expensed off over the life of the asset. Under the IRS Alternative Depreciation System, certain assets may be depreciated on a straight-line basis over the recovery period. The General Depreciation System allows faster recovery (IRS 2011). Table 7.1 shows the acquisition and subsequent depreciation of equipment with a useful life of five years.

The analysis of which projects to accept is the subject of chapter 8. Table 7.2 lists some key assets affected by the capital budget process.

A healthcare organization that does not purchase new technology or keep its buildings and services up-to-date risks failure or at least risks losing some of its market share to its competitors. Patients and their families expect healthcare services that are clean, state-of-the-art, and physically attractive.

The capital budget can involve millions of dollars. Therefore, the capital budget process and its accompanying decision making are complex. Consequently,

Table 7.1   Capital asset depreciation

Total Capital Purchase: $150,000 Purchased in January of Year 1			
Year	Depreciation	Accumulated Depreciation	Net Asset Value on Balance Sheet at Y/E
1	$30,000	$30,000	$120,000
2	$30,000	$60,000	$90,000
3	$30,000	$90,000	$60,000
4	$30,000	$120,000	$30,000
5	$30,000	$150,000	$0

Table 7.2 Key components of the capital budget process

Capital budget	Estimates the expenditures to acquire or replace long-term assets
Capital assets, or fixed assets	Otherwise known as **property, plant,** and equipment (PPE); physical assets with an estimated useful life of more than one year and a value that exceeds the organization's stated threshold
Property	Refers to the land the healthcare organization uses for its buildings, parking lots, helipad, and so on
Plant	Buildings and structures that are owned by the organization
Equipment	Automobiles, HVAC units, some furniture, CT scanner (if owned)

healthcare organizations need to be careful and deliberate in how they decide what is needed, what is of greatest priority, and when and how they will make their purchases. The capital budget is a plan that identifies the major asset items that have been assigned a high priority for purchase and the expected source of funds required to make the purchase. Can those asset items be purchased with profits generated in past years, or will the organization have to—or perhaps choose to—borrow the funds to pay for them? Well-planned capital decisions are needed to reach the healthcare organization's long-term goals. Thus, the capital budget reflects planned expenditures usually for at least three years into the future.

Net Working Capital

One of the most important measures of an organization's financial health is **net working capital.** Net working capital is the difference between current assets and current liabilities. For an individual, this could be a comparison between cash in the bank and the outstanding monthly bills.

Current assets are the most liquid assets on the balance sheet. They typically are used within one business cycle (typically a year) and can generally be turned into cash quickly. As defined in chapter 2, current assets include cash, marketable securities, accounts receivable, and inventory.

Current liabilities are the most pressing of the liabilities on the balance sheet. They must be resolved quickly and are generally resolved with cash. They are usually represented on the balance sheet as a payable—for example, accounts payable, salaries payable, or taxes payable.

If an organization has $2 million in current assets and $2 million in current liabilities, then its working capital is zero. The organization is barely able to pay its most pressing obligations. If an unforeseen problem occurred, it would not be able to pay its bills and, without additional funding, could quickly become bankrupt. Even if sales are strong, organizations, such as hospitals, that do not collect cash at the point of sale are at the mercy of purchasers who may not remit funds on a timely basis. Although the buildup of accounts receivable technically increases net working capital, it is the collection of those receivables and thus their timely conversion to cash that actually allows the hospital to meet payroll and pay vendors. Thus, the careful management of the cash budget is a critical factor in maintaining financial stability.

Time Value of Money

All projects and investments are evaluated in terms of their contribution to the organization. Some contributions are measured in terms of increased market share. Others may be measured in the increase of asset value. However measured, the project or investment is expected to result in a positive return on investment. **Return on investment** (ROI) is the benefit derived from the project or investment. For the purpose of this discussion, the general term investment refers to the purchase or project and the return is measured in US dollars.

ROI has two components that are measurable in dollars: cash inflows that derive from the investment and the increase in value of the investment. Cash inflows may be dividends or interest; increase in investment value is determined by the market for the investment.

Some investments generate cash to the investor. A savings account is the simplest example of such an investment. The investor deposits cash with the financial institution, which invests the collective deposits and pays the depositors less than the financial institution earns. If the financial institution makes profitable investments, it can pay a higher rate to the depositors.

Dividends are a portion of the value of an entity that is paid out to shareholders of an organization. Dividends are based purely on the performance of the company, in contrast to interest, which is typically determined at the beginning of an investment.

Interest-Bearing Instruments

A savings account is an example of an **interest-bearing** investment instrument. In other words, **interest** is calculated based on the value of the account (the **principal**). Table 7.3 illustrates the calculation that affects two types of accounts that bear interest: the **certificate of deposit** and the **savings account.** A certificate of deposit is a special type of interest-bearing account in which the deposit amount is fixed at the beginning of the period. The depositor agrees to leave the deposit in the account for a specified amount of time.

Table 7.3 shows the interest paid on a savings account for a year. This is an example of **simple interest,** which is the calculation of interest based solely on the principal. Simple interest is calculated by multiplying the principal by the interest rate.

Generally, simple interest is expressed as the annual interest rate. To determine the periodic (monthly, quarterly) interest rate from the annual interest rate, divide the annual interest rate by the appropriate portion of the year. One month of simple interest is the annual interest rate divided by 12. Five months of simple interest is the annual interest rate divided by 12, times 5. Table 7.4 shows 6 percent simple interest for 1 through 12 months.

The depositor has two options for the disposition of the interest or cash inflow from the deposit: leave the cash and let it continue to earn a return, or withdraw the cash and invest it elsewhere. If the investor leaves the cash in the account, the cash is subject to compounding.

Table 7.3   Calculation of simple interest

Deposit: $100,000 Annual Interest Rate: 6%		
Month	**Principal Balance**	**Interest Payment**
1	$100,000	
2	$100,000	
3	$100,000	
4	$100,000	
5	$100,000	
6	$100,000	
7	$100,000	
8	$100,000	
9	$100,000	
10	$100,000	
11	$100,000	
12	$100,000	$6,000 ($100,000 × 6%)
Ending balance	$106,000	

Table 7.4 Calculation of simple interest over less than a year

Deposit: $1,000 Annual Interest Rate: 6%		
Maturity	**Principal Balance**	**Interest Payment**
1 month	$1,000	$5 = ($1,000 × 0.06)/12
2 months	$1,000	$10 = (($1,000 × 0.06)/12) × 2
3 months	$1,000	$15 = (($1,000 × 0.06)/12) × 3
4 months	$1,000	$20 = (($1,000 × 0.06)/12) × 4
5 months	$1,000	$25 = (($1,000 × 0.06)/12) × 5
6 months	$1,000	$30 = (($1,000 × 0.06)/12) × 6
7 months	$1,000	$35 = (($1,000 × 0.06)/12) × 7
8 months	$1,000	$40 = (($1,000 × 0.06)/12) × 8
9 months	$1,000	$45 = (($1,000 × 0.06)/12) × 9
10 months	$1,000	$50 = (($1,000 × 0.06)/12) × 10
11 months	$1,000	$55 = (($1,000 × 0.06)/12) × 11
12 months	$1,000	$60 = (($1,000 × 0.06)/12) × 12

Compounding

If an account is subject to **compounding,** the interest generated from the investment is added to the value of the account in order to determine the amount of interest in each subsequent period. This **reinvestment** of the interest increases the return on the investment over the simple interest earned on the original investment.

To illustrate this point, table 7.5 calculates one year of interest on an account that begins with a one-time investment of $1,000 and a stated interest rate of 6 percent (section A). In the simple interest column, the investment earns $60, which is calculated and distributed at the end of the year for a five-year total interest earned of $300. This investment would be enhanced by compounding annually, as illustrated in table 7.5, section B. In the compound interest column (section C), the investment earned $348.85. Here, the interest is calculated monthly and the value of the interest is added to the principal, creating a new principal amount at the beginning of each month.

Periodic compounding results in a higher rate of return than simple interest. Even though the stated interest rate in the example is 6 percent, the depositor earned more than 6 percent on the original principal investment because the interest was reinvested each month. In fact, the total return on investment for the compounded account was 6.98 percent. While the extra $48.85 in this

Table 7.5 Simple versus compound interest

A. Simple interest—Distributed at the end of each year

Year	Principal Balance	Interest Payment—Distributed
1	$1,000	$60 = ($1,000 × 6%)
2	$1,000	$60 = ($1,000 × 6%)
3	$1,000	$60 = ($1,000 × 6%)
4	$1,000	$60 = ($1,000 × 6%)
5	$1,000	$60 = ($1,000 × 6%)
Ending balance	$1,000	
Total interest		$300

B. Compound interest—Distributed at the end of each year

Year	Principal Balance	Interest Payment—Distributed
1	$1,000	$60 = ($1,000 × 6%)
2	$1,060	$63.6 = ($1,060 × 6%)
3	$1,124	$67.416 = ($1,124 × 6%)
4	$1,191	$71.46096 = ($1,191 × 6%)
5	$1,262	$75.7486176 = ($1,262 × 6%)
Ending balance	$1,338.23	
Total interest		$338.2255776

C. Compound interest—Reinvested at the end of each month

Month	Principal Balance	Interest Payment—Distributed
1	$1,000	$5 = $1,000 × (6%/12)
2	$1,005.00	$5.03 = $1,005.00 × (6%/12)
3	$1,010.03	$5.05 = $1,010.03 × (6%/12)
4	$1,015.08	$5.08 = $1,015.08 × (6%/12)
5	$1,020.15	$5.10 = $1,020.15 × (6%/12)
6	$1,025.25	$5.13 = $1,025.25 × (6%/12)
7	$1,030.38	$5.15 = $1,030.38 × (6%/12)
8	$1,035.53	$5.18 = $1,035.53 × (6%/12)
9	$1,040.71	$5.20 = $1,040.71 × (6%/12)
10	$1,045.91	$5.23 = $1,045.91 × (6%/12)
11	$1,051.14	$5.26 = $1,051.14 × (6%/12)
12	$1,056.40	$5.28 = $1,056.40 × (6%/12)
13	$1,061.68	$5.31 = $1,061.68 × (6%/12)
14	$1,066.99	$5.33 = $1,066.99 × (6%/12)
15	$1,072.32	$5.36 = $1,072.32 × (6%/12)
16	$1,077.68	$5.39 = $1,077.68 × (6%/12)

Month	Principal Balance	Interest Payment—Distributed
17	$1,083.07	$5.42 = $1,083.07 × (6%/12)
18	$1,088.49	$5.44 = $1,088.49 × (6%/12)
19	$1,093.93	$5.47 = $1,093.93 × (6%/12)
20	$1,099.40	$5.50 = $1,099.40 × (6%/12)
21	$1,104.90	$5.52 = $1,104.90 × (6%/12)
22	$1,110.42	$5.55 = $1,110.42 × (6%/12)
23	$1,115.97	$5.58 = $1,115.97 × (6%/12)
24	$1,121.55	$5.61 = $1,121.55 × (6%/12)
25	$1,127.16	$5.64 = $1,127.16 × (6%/12)
26	$1,132.80	$5.66 = $1,132.80 × (6%/12)
27	$1,138.46	$5.69 = $1,138.46 × (6%/12)
28	$1,144.15	$5.72 = $1,144.15 × (6%/12)
29	$1,149.87	$5.75 = $1,149.87 × (6%/12)
30	$1,155.62	$5.78 = $1,155.62 × (6%/12)
31	$1,161.40	$5.81 = $1,161.40 × (6%/12)
32	$1,167.21	$5.84 = $1,167.21 × (6%/12)
33	$1,173.04	$5.87 = $1,173.04 × (6%/12)
34	$1,178.91	$5.89 = $1,178.91 × (6%/12)
35	$1,184.80	$5.92 = $1,184.80 × (6%/12)
36	$1,190.73	$5.95 = $1,190.73 × (6%/12)
37	$1,196.68	$5.98 = $1,196.68 × (6%/12)
38	$1,202.66	$6.01 = $1,202.66 × (6%/12)
39	$1,208.68	$6.04 = $1,208.68 × (6%/12)
40	$1,214.72	$6.07 = $1,214.72 × (6%/12)
41	$1,220.79	$6.10 = $1,220.79 × (6%/12)
42	$1,226.90	$6.13 = $1,226.90 × (6%/12)
43	$1,233.03	$6.17 = $1,233.03 × (6%/12)
44	$1,239.20	$6.20 = $1,239.20 × (6%/12)
45	$1,245.39	$6.23 = $1,245.39 × (6%/12)
46	$1,251.62	$6.26 = $1,251.62 × (6%/12)
47	$1,257.88	$6.29 = $1,257.88 × (6%/12)
48	$1,264.17	$6.32 = $1,264.17 × (6%/12)
49	$1,270.49	$6.35 = $1,270.49 × (6%/12)
50	$1,276.84	$6.38 = $1,276.84 × (6%/12)
51	$1,283.23	$6.42 = $1,283.23 × (6%/12)
52	$1,289.64	$6.45 = $1,289.64 × (6%/12)
53	$1,296.09	$6.48 = $1,296.09 × (6%/12)

(continued)

Table 7.5   Simple versus compound interest *(continued)*

Month	Principal Balance	Interest Payment—Distributed
54	$1,302.57	$6.51 = $1,302.57 × (6%/12)
55	$1,309.08	$6.55 = $1,309.08 × (6%/12)
56	$1,315.63	$6.58 = $1,315.63 × (6%/12)
57	$1,322.21	$6.61 = $1,322.21 × (6%/12)
58	$1,328.82	$6.64 = $1,328.82 × (6%/12)
59	$1,335.46	$6.68 = $1,335.46 × (6%/12)
60	$1,342.14	$6.71 = $1,342.14 × (6%/12)
Ending balance	$1,348.85	
Total interest		$348.85

example may not seem extraordinary, consider the effect against a larger principal. A $100,000 original investment would generate an additional $4,885 just by compounding.

Discounted Instruments

Some investments do not earn interest by multiplying the rate by the principal, but rather by subtracting the interest from the ending value to arrive at an investment amount. In this scenario, the investment pays $100,000 at the end of the period and the investment is **discounted** from that **par value** or ending amount. Interest is calculated based on the *discount rate,* which is different from the rate of return. For example, a one-year, $10,000 instrument discounted at 5 percent would be sold for $9,500 (10,000 – (10,000 × 5 percent)). However, the return on investment is based on the invested amount of $9,500. So, the $500 interest is a 5.2632 percent return on the $9,500 investment (500/9500). Table 7.6 illustrates the calculation of a three-month and a one-year investment, discounted at 6 percent, with a maturity value of $100,000.

The most notable of the discounted investment instruments are US Treasury Bills. These investments are sold in increments of $10,000 with the purchase price discounted from the ending or par value of the bill. US Treasury Bills are considered the safest type of investment and are therefore offered at very low returns on investment. As will be discussed later, the level of risk inherent in an investment has a direct impact on the rate of return of that investment.

Calculating Total Value

The calculation of return on investment is relatively simple when a short period of time is involved. However, for longer periods of time, there are mathematical formulas that can assist in the process of determining the present or future

Table 7.6   Interest on discounted investments

One-year investment	
Discount rate	6%
Investment × 106% =	$100,000
Investment =	$100,000/(1 + 6%)
Investment =	$94,339.62
Three-month investment	
Discount rate	6%
Investment × (106%/4) =	$100,000
Investment =	$100,000/(1 + (6%/4))
Investment =	$98,522.17

value of an investment loan. Individuals benefit from understanding these calculations because they are used to determine mortgage and automobile loan payments, for example. Similarly, organizations and financial institutions use them for the same purposes and for determining pricing of various investments.

Because the mathematics of value calculations is beyond the scope of this text, the examples below use Microsoft Excel to aid the reader in actually performing the calculations discussed. A list of key terms associated with these calculations is listed in table 7.7.

Money is expected to grow in value over time, assuming that it is invested. The **present value,** or today's cash, if invested at a specified rate, will earn interest and become some higher, **future value.** This was illustrated in table 7.3. A present value of $100,000, invested at 6 percent for one year, became the future value of $106,000. Conversely, in order to have $106,000 at the end of the year, if the interest rate is 6 percent, the investor must deposit $100,000.

Table 7.7   Key terms in calculating interest and value

Compound	Process of reinvesting distributed interest back into the interest-earning balance
Discount	Price of the investment is less than the par value
FV	Value of the investment at maturity
Par value	Face or noninterest portion of the investment at maturity
Periodic payments (periods)	Number of times interest is paid during the life of the investment
PV	Current value of the investment
Rate	Stated interest rate to be paid by the issuer (borrower)

Future Value

The calculation of interest illustrated in table 7.3 can be expressed as a formula. In this formula, PV is the present value; r is the interest rate; n is the number of payments in the period, and F is the future value (the present value, plus all of the interim payments). It is important to note that this calculation applies to both the borrower and the lender. Using the simple interest example in table 7.3,

$$PV = 100{,}000$$
$$FV = 106{,}000$$
$$r = 6 \text{ percent}$$
$$n = 1$$

If the present value (the amount to be invested) is known, the future value can be calculated using this formula:

$$FV = PV \times (1 + r)^n$$

Using a $100,000 investment for one year at 6 percent,

$$FV = 100{,}000 \times (1 + .06)^1$$
$$FV = 100{,}000 \times (1.06)$$
$$FV = 106{,}000$$

Here, the period is "year" and the investment was for one year.

This same formula can be used to calculate the compound interest example in table 7.5, section B. This time the number of periods is five, and the dollars below are larger to illustrate the effect of compounding.

$$FV = 100{,}000 \times (1 + .06)^5$$
$$FV = 100{,}000 \times (1.06)^5$$
$$FV = 100{,}000 \times 1.3382256$$
$$FV = 133{,}822.56$$

Table 7.8 compares each year of the original example (table 7.5, section B) to the formula.

In the preceding examples, the investor deposited an amount into the savings account. The amount deposited is the present value (PV) of the investment.

Table 7.8   Interest compounded annually

Comparing manual calculation of compound interest to formula			
Compound interest—Reinvested at the end of each year			
Year	Principal Balance	Interest Payment	Formula: FV = PV × (1 + r)^n
1	$1,000	$60.00 = ($1,000 × 6%)	$1,000
2	$1,060.00	$63.60 = ($1,060.00 × 6%)	$1,060.00 = $1,000 × 1.06
3	$1,123.60	$67.42 = ($1,123.60 × 6%)	$1,123.60 = $1,000 × 1.06 × 1.06
4	$1,191.02	$71.46 = ($1,191.02 × 6%)	$1,191.02 = $1,000 × 1.06 × 1.06 × 1.06
5	$1,262.48	$75.75 = ($1,262.48 × 6%)	$1,262.48 = $1,000 × 1.06 × 1.06 × 1.06 × 1.06
Ending balance	$1,338.23		$1,338.23 = $1,000 × 1.06 × 1.06 × 1.06 × 1.06 × 1.06

Interest is calculated beginning with the present value. The present value is the investment and the payments the interest earned.

Present Value

The future value formula also works for the determination of the present value when the future value is known. For example, discounted investments state the discount rate and the par or payment at maturity. The investor must calculate the cost of the investment using the same calculations as previously, solving for the present value.

Step 1: Begin with the *FV* formula.

$$FV = PV \times (1 + r)^n$$

Step 2: Divide both sides of the equation by $(1 + r)^n$.

$$\frac{FV}{(1 + r)^n} = PV \times \frac{(1 + r)^n}{(1 + r)^n}$$

Step 3: The $(1 + r)^n$ cancels out on the right side, leaving:

$$\frac{FV}{(1 + r)^n} = PV$$

Since the goal was to solve for *PV,* flip the equation around so that *PV* is on the left. Now, the known values can be plugged in to determine the present value of an investment that is sold at a discount.

$$PV = \frac{FV}{(1+r)^n}$$

Consider the previous example; the future value of the investment is $133,822.56, the interest rate 6 percent, and the number of periods is 5.

$$PV = \frac{133,822.56}{(1+0.06)^5}$$

$$PV = \frac{133,822.56}{1.3382256}$$

$$PV = 100,000$$

Adjusting for Multiple Payments in a Year

The future value calculation is used to determine compound interest on an investment with a single investment at the beginning and a lump sum payment at maturity. Similarly, the present value calculation is used to determine the initial investment amount when the lump sum payment at the end represents the investment plus the total interest to maturity. The preceding examples use whole years for the periods.

If the instrument pays interest at a different rate—semiannually or monthly, for example—the formula must be adjusted to reflect the frequency of compounding. A five-year investment with semiannual payments at 6 percent would look like this:

$r = 3$ percent (the 6 percent interest, divided by 2 because there are two semiannual payments each year)

$n = 10$ (there are two payments each year multiplied by 5 years, for a total of 10 payments)

Assuming an initial investment of $100,000, enter the stated values and rates into the future value formula:

$$FV = PV \times (1+r)^n$$

$$FV = 100,000 \times (1+r)^n$$

$$FV = 100,000 \times (1+.03)^{10}$$

$$FV = 100,000 \times 1.3439164$$

$$FV = 134,391.64$$

Table 7.9 shows the individual calculations, by period, that prove the formula calculation.

Other Useful Formulas

One way of calculating the value of an investment is to compare it to other investments using the concept of **net present value.** The net present value of an investment is the present value of any income stream, less the present value of any outflow of cash. This calculation is important for the comparison of investments or projects that have differing investments and cash flows. Project

Table 7.9   Interest compounded semiannually

Comparing manual calculation of compound interest to formula		
Compound interest—Reinvested at the end of each semiannual period		
Year / Principal Balance	Interest Payment	Formula: $FV = PV \times (1 + r)^n$
1 — $1,000	$30.00 = ($1,000 × 3%)	$1,000
6 mos — $1,030.00	$30.90 = ($1,030.00 × 3%)	$1,030.00 = $1,000 × 1.03
2 — $1,060.90	$31.83 = ($1,060.90 × 3%)	$1,060.90 = $1,000 × 1.03 × 1.03
6 mos — $1,092.73	$32.78 = ($1,092.73× 3%)	$1,092.73 = $1,000 × 1.03 × 1.03 × 1.03
3 — $1,125.51	$33.77 = ($1,125.51 × 3%)	$1,125.51 = $1,000 × 1.03 × 1.03 × 1.03 × 1.03
6 mos — $1,159.27	$34.78 = ($1,159.27 × 3%)	$1,159.27 = $1,000 × 1.03 × 1.03 × 1.03 × 1.03 × 1.03
4 — $1,194.05	$35.82 = ($1,194.05 × 3%)	$1,194.05 = $1,000 × 1.03 × 1.03 × 1.03 × 1.03 × 1.03 × 1.03
6 mos — $1,229.87	$36.90 = ($1,229.87 × 3%)	$1,229.87 = $1,000 × 1.03 × 1.03 × 1.03 × 1.03 × 1.03 × 1.03 × 1.03
5 — $1,266.77	$38.00 = ($1,266.77 × 3%)	$1,266.77 = $1,000 × 1.03 × 1.03 × 1.03 × 1.03 × 1.03 × 1.03 × 1.03 × 1.03
6 mos — $1,304.77	$39.14 = ($1,304.77 × 3%)	$1,304.77 = $1,000 × 1.03 × 1.03 × 1.03 × 1.03 × 1.03 × 1.03 × 1.03 × 1.03 × 1.03
Ending balance — $1,343.92		$1,343.92 = $1,000 × 1.03 × 1.03 × 1.03 × 1.03 × 1.03 × 1.03 × 1.03 × 1.03 × 1.03 × 1.03

Figure 7.1　Net present value of two investments

◇	A	B	C	D	E
1					
2					
3					
4					
5					
6			Investment A		Investment B
7			$50,000 3% bond		$100,000 2.5% bond
8					
9		Annual Cash Inflows	1500		25000
10			1500		25000
11			1500		25000
12			1500		25000
13		Payment at Maturity	51500		125000
14					
15		Expected rate of return = 5%			
16					
17			$45,670.52		$186,589.53
18					
19		Formulas on line 17	=NPV(5%,C9:C13)		=NPV(5%,E9:E13)
20					

Figure 7.2　Calculating loan payments

◇	A	B	C	D	E	F	G
1							
2							
3							
4		Mortgage Amount	$	200,000			
5		Interest Rate		5%			
6		Number of years		30			
7							
8		Payment		($1,073.64)			
9							
10		Formula in cell D8		=PMT(D5/12,30*12,200000)			
11							
12		Note: Excel returns a negative value, because the payment is an outflow of cash					
13							

comparison is discussed in chapter 8. Figure 7.1 shows the net present value of two different investments. The investment with the higher net present value would be more desirable from a purely financial perspective. However, other factors must be considered, such as alternative uses for the cash and the liquidity of the two investments.

The present value may also be the deposit on a purchase and the payments represent both interest and payments toward the full amount. In the case of an automobile loan or a mortgage, the desired calculation is typically to solve for the payment amount. Figure 7.2 shows the calculation of payments on a 30-year $200,000 mortgage at 5 percent.

Inflation and Interest Rates

In a growing economy, the price of goods and services, on average, will rise. The reason for this varies. In general, the economy is growing because the demand for goods and services is increasing. Higher demand pushes prices higher, which in turn increases the costs of producing goods and services, which prompts companies to raise prices further, and so on. From an economic standpoint, a small amount of inflation is not a bad thing because it signals growth and active markets. Extremely high inflation is not good because it signals problems in the economy: a breakdown in the market, such as the dot-com bubble, or failure of the country's monetary system, for example. The opposite of inflation is deflation, in which demand is falling and consequently prices are falling.

The consumer price index (CPI) is one measure of inflation/deflation. There are two indices calculated by the US Bureau of Labor Statistics that fall under this heading. One index is a measure of urban consumers—about 87 percent of the US population; the other measure is a subset of that population. Both of these indices measure prices of a set **market basket** of goods and services at a point in time. The percentage change from one point in time to the next is the consumer price index (Bureau of Labor Statistics 2011). Anticipated inflation affects financial markets. In the United States, the Federal Reserve sets interest rates: specifically, the rates at which financial institutions can borrow directly from the Federal Reserve Bank or loan to each other, through the Federal Reserve Bank. The primary set rate is called the discount rate. Qualified banks may borrow directly from the Federal Reserve Bank at the discount rate. The Federal Open Market Committee of the Federal Reserve Bank meets face-to-face eight times a year (about every six weeks) to discuss whether interest rates are correct. They may also meet more frequently via conference call. The decision whether to raise or lower interest rates is based on many factors, including inflation (Federal Reserve 2011).

Tied closely to the discount rate is the **federal funds rate,** which is the rate at which banks lend their excess reserves to each other for very short periods of time, usually overnight or one day. Banks lend money to their best customers at a slightly different rate, called the **prime rate.** The prime rate is set higher than the federal funds rate. Most interest rates for other borrowers are established as some percentage over prime. Although the prime rate is set by the banks themselves, it does not vary significantly from one bank to another (Federal Reserve 2011).

The rate at which borrowers can obtain loans in any form depends on a variety of factors, including the expected interest rates during the life of the loan and the borrower's ability to pay back the loan.

Credit Ratings

As mentioned at the beginning of this chapter, organizations are subject to the same type of scrutiny as individuals with respect to their creditworthiness. The ability of the borrower to obtain a loan or other financing, as well as the interest rate to be earned or paid, is determined by the organization's credit rating. The credit rating is a reflection of the opinion of reputable experts about the ability of the organization to pay its debts. An organization with a good credit rating is a less risky investment and will enjoy lower borrowing rates than an organization with a lower credit rating. This relationship between risk and return is expressed in the capital market equation, as represented in figure 7.3. The lower the risk, the lower the expected return. The higher the risk, the higher the expected return on investment.

An organization that has the highest rating will be able to borrow money at the lowest possible rates. This is good for the organization, because it is therefore able to finance operations and projects relatively inexpensively. On the other hand, the return on investment for the lender is not very high: low risk, low return. A financial institution that takes depositors' savings and lends the money to a low-risk borrower will earn low interest on the loan and in turn pay even lower interest to the depositors.

Financial institutions have policies regarding the level of risk that they will take with the funds available to them. Savings account depositors do not typically expect a bank, for example, to take high risks with their money in order to obtain higher interest rates. On the contrary, they expect their deposits to be safe. However, a small amount of risk is necessary in order for the financial institution to earn more than their depositors expect to be paid. So, the

Figure 7.3   The relationship between risk and return

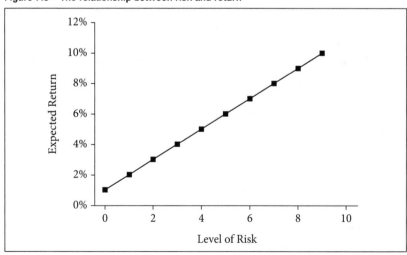

financial institution will maintain a broad range of investments that sustains a reasonable rate of return.

The failure of some banks and other financial institutions in recent years was largely due to the excess amount of risk that the institutions accepted in the investment of their depositors' funds. For example, some banks granted mortgages to individuals with insufficient collateral or for payments in excess of normal limitations.

The best-known experts in the corporate credit rating business are Moody's, Standard & Poor's, and Morningstar. Financial institutions and investment managers also maintain their own analysis departments. The advantage of being rated by one of the organizations described below is that they are independent of the companies they rate. See table 7.10 for examples of ratings by the major independent credit rating organizations that follow.

Moody's

Moody's Investors Service (Moody's) is a subsidiary of Moody's Investment Corporation. Moody's provides customers with credit ratings, research, and risk analysis. According to Moody's, "The firm's ratings and analysis track debt covering more than 110 countries, 12,000 corporate issuers, 25,000 public finance issuers, and 106,000 structured finance obligations" (Moody's 2011).

Standard & Poor's

Standard & Poor's (S&P) publishes credit ratings, indices, investment research, and risk evaluations and solutions. It rates both stocks and mutual funds. "In 2009, we [S&P] published more than 870,000 new and revised credit ratings. Currently, we rate more than US$32 trillion in outstanding debt" (Standard & Poor's 2011).

Morningstar

Morningstar "provides stock market analysis; equity, mutual fund, and ETF research, ratings, and picks; portfolio tools; and option, hedge fund, IRA, 401k, and 529 plan research" (Morningstar 2011).

Types of Financing

Organizations do not always have the cash they need to finance their strategic goals or even to meet payroll on occasion. There are many different ways to

Table 7.10   Examples of ratings by major independent credit rating organizations

Morningstar	
AAA	Extremely Low Default Risk
AA	Very Low Default Risk
A	Low Default Risk
BBB	Moderate Default Risk
BB	Above Average Default Risk
B	High Default Risk
CCC	Currently Very High Default Risk
CC	Currently Extreme Default Risk
C	Imminent Payment Default
D	Payment Default
Moody's	
Aaa	Obligations rated Aaa are judged to be of the highest quality, with minimal credit risk.
Aa	Obligations rated Aa are judged to be of high quality and are subject to very low credit risk.
A	Obligations rated A are considered upper-medium grade and are subject to low credit risk.
Baa	Obligations rated Baa are subject to moderate credit risk. They are considered medium grade and as such may possess certain speculative characteristics.
Ba	Obligations rated Ba are judged to have speculative elements and are subject to substantial credit risk.
B	Obligations rated B are considered speculative and are subject to high credit risk.
Caa	Obligations rated Caa are judged to be of poor standing and are subject to very high credit risk.
Ca	Obligations rated Ca are highly speculative and are likely in, or very near, default, with some prospect of recovery of principal and interest.
C	Obligations rated C are the lowest rated class and are typically in default, with little prospect for recovery of principal or interest.
Standard & Poor's	
AAA	Extremely strong capacity to meet financial commitments. Highest Rating.
AA	Very strong capacity to meet financial commitments.
A	Strong capacity to meet financial commitments but somewhat susceptible to adverse economic conditions and changes in circumstances.
BBB	Adequate capacity to meet financial commitments but more subject to adverse economic conditions.
BBB−	Considered lowest investment grade by market participants.
BB+	Considered highest speculative grade by market participants.

BB	Less vulnerable in the near term but faces major ongoing uncertainties to adverse business, financial, and economic conditions.
B	More vulnerable to adverse business, financial, and economic conditions but currently has the capacity to meet financial commitments.
CCC	Currently vulnerable and dependent on favorable business, financial, and economic conditions to meet financial commitments.
CC	Currently highly vulnerable.
C	Currently highly vulnerable obligations and other defined circumstances.
D	Payment default on financial commitments.

Sources: Morningstar (http://news.morningstar.com/pdfs/corp_credit_rating_factsheet.pdf). Moody's (http://www.moodys.com/ratings-process/Ratings-Definitions/002002). Standard & Poor's (http://www.standardandpoors.co/ratings/definitions-and-faqs/en/us#def_1). All ratings and descriptions are the copyright of the respective organizations.

obtain funding for both operations and projects. In this section, we will discuss some of the key financing alternatives and how they work.

Debt

Debt is a broad term that means something is owed to another party. On the balance sheet, debts are liabilities. Current liabilities include accounts payable, salaries payable, and taxes payable. In the noncurrent liabilities, organizations may have mortgages and other long-term loans. One way organizations can raise funds for capital projects is through debt financing. Typically, the financing strategy will mirror the underlying reason for the financing: either short term or long term. The strategic goals of the organization drive whether the organization will seek equity or debt financing.

Short Term

Short-term debt consists of instruments that must be repaid within a year. They are listed in the current liabilities section of the balance sheet. This section may also include the portion of long-term debt that is due in the current fiscal year.

As discussed earlier in this chapter, the organization must develop a cash budget in order to determine its needs for the fiscal year. Occasionally, the amounts due on salaries, for example, may exceed the cash in the bank. Perhaps there has been a slowdown in collections or a major payer is late with a remittance. Either way, the organization must fulfill its obligations to employees. To accomplish that, the organization may decide to negotiate a **credit line,** usually with a financial institution. A credit line is a fixed amount of cash that is available to the borrower for short-term needs. It is a loan that is not used until it is needed and it is repaid when funds are available. To use the funds, the borrower *draws* on the loan. A credit line typically has no fixed **maturity** date. Maturity is the date on which the loan must be repaid. Instead, a credit line contract will have language that requires the borrower to evidence its continuing creditworthiness. Failure to do so could mean the end of the credit or possibly an increase in the interest rate, for example.

A credit line is a loan and may be secured or unsecured. Secured loans are guaranteed against an asset. A credit line could be secured against accounts receivable, for example. Unsecured loans have no underlying guarantee. The benefits of a secured loan are primarily to the lender. Secured loans obtain preferential treatment in bankruptcy proceedings: their funds are considered before any payments to unsecured creditors.

Another type of instrument with which organizations can raise funds is **commercial paper.** Commercial paper is an unsecured debt instrument with a maturity of less than nine months (270 days). Companies may use commercial paper as an alternative to a credit line. Commercial paper may be issued by companies to fund inventory purchases or general operations, for example. It can be issued with a longer maturity or for the purchase of fixed assets; however, such commercial paper would require Securities and Exchange Commission (SEC) involvement. Typically, organizations issue short-term commercial paper. Commercial paper may be traded in the secondary markets at prevailing interest rates.

Example: Ninety-day commercial paper is issued by the organization at a discount from par value for a discount rate of 4 percent. A par value of $1 million would be purchased for $990,099 by the lender (1,000,000/(1 + (4%/4)). On the balance sheet, the borrower now has cash of $990,099 and a current liability of $1,000,000. At maturity, the borrower would pay $1 million to the lender— the purchase price plus the interest of $9,901. If the discount rate in the marketplace goes down, the lender may choose to sell the commercial paper to another party (the secondary market). Say the interest rate goes down to 3% two months later. There are now 30 days left to maturity. The investor (lender) can hold the paper to maturity or sell it to another (secondary) investor. If sold, the secondary investor would pay the original lender $997,506 (1,000,000/(1+(3%/12)). The secondary investor would then obtain the $1 million from the original borrower.

Interest calculations on short-term debt depend on the instrument. A credit line may charge interest on the average drawn over the period of time while commercial paper is issued at a discount.

Long Term

Organizations that want to obtain financing for purchases or projects with repayment over a long period of time (in excess of one year) may choose to issue **bonds.** Bonds are long-term debt instruments and appear on the balance sheet as long-term liabilities. Most bonds are interest bearing, so periodic interest payments are made by the borrower over the life of the bond. Funding through bond issuance requires the participation of several parties: the investment banker, the SEC, and the marketplace.

An investment banker helps the organization obtain approval from regulatory agencies for the bond issuance. The investment banker also helps to determine the correct interest rate for the bond and to find the appropriate market for the bond. The SEC must approve a bond issuance that is offered to the general public.

The market determines the price of the bond. Although the interest rate paid by the issuer (the borrower) will typically remain constant throughout the life of the bond, the price paid by investors will vary depending on the market rates at the time of purchase. So, even at issuance a bond may sell for more or less than the principal if the market rate is different from the face value. Some bonds are actually issued at **auction rates.** In other words, the market defines the interest rate at the time of issuance. While this avoids the problem inherent in setting a rate in advance, the interest rate may be more than the organization is prepared to pay. Again, the investment banker will play an important role in assisting the organization to navigate this market.

Originally, bonds were issued in paper form. There were "coupons" attached to the bond, which investors submitted to the issuer for payment periodically—usually twice a year. In today's market, a clearinghouse keeps track of the owners of the bonds as ownership may change many times over the life of the bond. The world's largest such clearinghouse is Depository Trust & Clearing Corporation, located in New York City (Depository Trust & Clearing Corporation 2011). The periodic interest rate paid by the issuer to bondholders is still called the **coupon rate.** Bonds that are issued without an interest rate are called **zero coupon bonds.**

Although technically bonds may be sold by any organization, the regulatory restrictions and marketability make this a strategy that is appealing to larger corporations and municipalities.

The issuance of a bond raises cash for the organization. Here is the organization's balance sheet before the bond issuance:

Assets		Equity	
Cash	$10,000,000	Fund balance	$10,000,000
Liabilities			
	$0		

Here is the balance sheet after the issuance of $10 million in bonds with a 4 percent coupon rate:

Assets		Equity	
Cash	$19,500,000	Fund balance	$9,500,000
Liabilities			
Bond	$10,000,000		

In this example, the organization received $9,500,000 in cash, net of $500,000 in costs associated with the issuance. Note that the bond itself has no impact on the fund balance (other than the expenditure for issuance). This is an important consideration for some organizations as will be discussed in the equity section that follows. Bonds are contractual obligations to repay and may carry a variety of restrictions and covenants. For example, cash received from bonds that are issued for a specific purpose may be used only to fulfill that purpose. So, a bond issued for the purpose of funding construction of a facility expansion cannot be used for general operating expenses.

Another strategy for long-term financing is to borrow against collateral, such as a building. A long-term loan against such a structural asset is a mortgage. Again, there is no impact on the fund balance of an initial mortgage loan, but the interest paid on the balance of the loan is tax deductible.

Equity

As discussed in chapter 2, the balance sheet contains three sections: assets, liabilities, and equity. **Equity** is the net value of the organization: assets minus liabilities. The equity section of the balance sheet identifies both the owner-ship structure of the organization and also the cumulative earnings of the organization.

Retained Earnings/Fund Balance

Part of the equity section of the balance sheet is the cumulative earnings of the organization. In a for-profit organization, this is represented by the retained earnings account. In a not-for-profit organization, it is called the fund balance.

At the end of each fiscal period, the organization's income statement (state-ment of revenue and expenses) represents the net income or net loss due to its activities in the period. Organizations may use this cumulative income to fund continuing operations and any expansion. Organizations with sufficient retained earnings or fund balance may not need to seek external funding for operations or projects. The cost of financing in this manner is the opportunity cost of leaving the funds invested rather than spending them on the project.

Impact of Charitable Donations

Donations may be received by any healthcare organization. However, those donations are tax-deductible by the donor only if the recipient enjoys tax-exempt status (see chapter 1). Tax issues are discussed later in this chapter.

Donations to a tax-exempt organization increase the organization's cash and its fund balance. **Unrestricted donations** will increase the **general fund.** Other donations may be restricted. Restrictions on the use of donations create an obligation on the part of the organization to comply with the restriction. Typical restrictions include specified projects and additions to already existing restricted funds. Restricted donations are discussed in chapter 1.

Partnership

Not-for-profit organizations are not owned by individuals. They are run in trust for the benefit of the community that they serve. Consequently, not-for-profit organizations cannot raise funds by selling ownership shares of the orga-nization to other parties. For-profit organizations, however, are characterized by the depth and breadth of their ownership.

At the inception of a for-profit organization, an investment is made to fund the business. This investment is the ownership interest in the organization. At its simplest, the owner puts $10,000 into the business, which results in a balance sheet that looks like this:

Assets		Equity	
Cash	$10,000	Owner's equity	$10,000
Liabilities			
	$0		

In this example, there is only one owner, who has 100 percent interest in the equity of the firm. If the owner wants to expand the business and does not have any additional cash to invest, the owner can take a loan. Loans are short-term or long-term liabilities and appear on the corresponding section of the balance sheet along with notes and bonds. If this owner takes a $5,000 loan at start-up, it has this effect on the balance sheet:

Assets		Equity	
Cash	$15,000	Owner's equity	$10,000
Liabilities			
Loan	$5,000		

Another way that the owner can raise funds is by sharing ownership in the firm with others. The owner can take on a partner and share ownership that way. The ownership is divided according to a written agreement between the partners. For the purpose of this example, a 50 percent ownership is granted to the new partner. Ownership could be merely an investment for the new partner, or the original owner could be obligated to share management responsibilities with the new partner, depending on their contractual agreement.

Assets		Equity	
Cash	$25,000	Partners' equity	$20,000
		(Owners' interest at 50%/50%)	
Liabilities			
Loan	$5,000		

Common Stock

If sharing management responsibilities with another owner is not an acceptable alternative, the owner could take on multiple investors and thereby limit the interest each investor might have in the day-to-day operations of the firm. In other words, the owner could sell equity shares in the firm. The owner could sell 10,000 shares at $1 each to 10,000 different individuals in order to raise $10,000, which would have the following effect on the balance sheet:

Assets		Equity	
Cash	$25,000	Owner's equity $20,000	
		(Common stock shares: 20,000 @ $1)	
Liabilities			
Loan	$5,000		

In this example, the original owner has a 50 percent ownership interest in the company. Other investors all together have the other 50 percent; however, the ownership is spread among 10,000 different individuals, each of whom has less than 1 percent equity investment in the company. A person with such a small investment in this company would be unlikely to want to be involved in the day-to-day management of the company.

The owner has now raised the funds to begin operations. At the end of the year, the owner has generated $1,000 in net income and the balance sheet looks like this:

Assets		Equity	
Cash	$10,000	Owner's equity $20,000	
Inventory	$1,000	(Common stock shares: 20,000 @ $1)	
Accounts rec.	$5,000	Retained earnings $1,000	
Equipment	$12,000		
Liabilities			
Accounts payable	$3,000		
Loan	$4,000		

The owner can do one of two things for the common stockholders: declare a dividend or retain the earnings in the business. Many businesses never declare a dividend and the only reward to common stockholders is the increase in the **market value** of the stock. Think about the **liquidation value** of this company. The liquidation value is the amount that the owners would receive if they sold the company in its entirety: all assets and all liabilities. Assume the assets could be liquidated at **book value** or the amount recorded in the balance sheet and the liabilities settled as stated above. Instead of a net value of $20,000, the net value is now $21,000. That means each common stock share is worth $1.05: an increase of 5 percent. Theoretically, an owner could sell his or her share to another investor for $1.05. The original investor's return is 5 percent and the new investor's cost basis is $1.05. Note that this secondary market transaction has no impact on the balance sheet of the company.

The price of a **stock** at any given time is a combination of factors that net to whatever someone is willing to pay for it. In the secondary market, the price of the stock is not relevant to the organization except as an indicator of investor perception. Many millions of dollars have changed hands on the expectation of a company's future performance—regardless of the historical results of operations. For example, A1 Braces earned a 5 percent return in its first year of operation. If the market expects that the demand for braces will increase 10 percent and that A1 Braces will keep pace with that demand, then the share price could rise accordingly. When the expectations of the market exceed the ability of the underlying companies to meet those expectations, the stock is overpriced. Once the market realizes its mistake, the price will fall to more realistic levels. This phenomenon occurred in the late 1990s when the market overpriced Internet companies, resulting in what is commonly called the dot-com bubble. The bubble burst in 2000 when investors realized their error and prices plummeted.

While market perception is a factor in the price of a stock, the technical calculation is the present value of the future earnings. Although stock pricing is beyond the scope of this text, it is important to note that there are mathematical formulas for the valuation of stocks that inherently include variables such as desired rate of return and expected growth. But even the mathematical calculation of what one should pay for a stock today is not an accurate predictor of what that stock will be worth tomorrow, as expectations change.

For the issuer of the stock, the value of the stock in the market is not reflected on the balance sheet of the company but will be mentioned in the footnotes to the financial statements. The only time the market price of the shares will appear on the balance sheet is when the company buys or sells its own stock. These purchased shares are called **treasury stock** and have a separate place on the balance sheet. Then, if these shares are sold again, the amount received will also be recorded in this same place. An excellent resource for understanding the equity section of the balance sheet is AccountingCoach.com (Averkamp 2011).

To the investor, all marketable securities held as investments appear on the balance sheet as current assets. At the end of any fiscal reporting period, the market value of the investments is determined and the balance sheet may be adjusted to reflect the current market value rather than the cost of the securities, if the value of the securities has declined. This **lower of cost or market** process provides the users of the financial statements with a more conservative estimate of the value of the assets of the organization in a declining market.

Preferred Stock

As noted previously, common stock shares may or may not pay dividends. Some organizations may find it beneficial to sell stock shares that not only always pay dividends, but they pay a guaranteed dividend as well. These shares are called preferred stock and take precedence over common stock shares in terms of the payment of dividends.

Dividends on preferred stock may be cumulative or noncumulative. This is specified at the time of issuance. Cumulative dividends mean that all preferred stock dividends must be paid to preferred shareholders before any dividends may be paid to common shareholders. For example: A company doesn't pay any preferred dividends in 2009. At the end of 2009, it owes preferred shareholders $150,000. In 2010, the company declares a dividend and has $400,000 to distribute. It must pay all of the dividends in arrears to the preferred shareholders first. That leaves $250,000. Then, it must pay the preferred dividend—say, another $150,000. That leaves $100,000 it can pay to common shareholders.

Noncumulative dividends must still be paid prior to dividends on common shares. However, if the company does not declare a dividend in a particular year, it just skips that dividend on preferred shares. In the preceding example, there would be no dividend declared for preferred shareholders in 2009. In 2010, there would be $250,000 available for common shareholders after the preferred dividend payment.

Refinancing

Over the course of a loan agreement, the prevailing interest rates may change. If the change is favorable, the organization may seek to pay off the loan. If there is insufficient cash available to do so, the organization may choose to refinance.

Refinancing is the replacement of an existing loan or debt instrument with a different one. Desirably, the new arrangement is on better terms than the old one. Individuals do this frequently with mortgage loans when interest rates are lower than the original mortgage loan rate. The **payback period** for the processing cost of refinancing must be taken into consideration. For an individual refinancing a mortgage, the cost of refinancing consists of the title search, filing fees, bank processing fees, and often a small percentage of the loan amount—from a fraction of a **point** (percentage of the total loan) to several points, depending on the terms of the agreement. Table 7.11 shows the calculation of the payback period for a 30-year $200,000 loan at 6 percent that is refinanced to 5 percent. For an organization refinancing a long-term bond, the calculation is similar but the dollars are larger. Issuance of a new bond costs the same as the issuance of the old one, so that process and cost must be considered. Further, if the old bond does not have a **call** feature—the ability of the issuer to pay off the principal to investors prior to the maturity date—then the issuer will have to purchase back its own bonds in the secondary market. Either way, the transaction costs must be considered.

Sale of Accounts Receivable

Another aspect of debt is related to accounts receivable. In every organization, some percent of receivables will never be collected. Receivables that are uncollectible are called **bad debt.** As part of their overall financial strategy, organizations routinely account for their historical experience with bad debt by reducing their reported receivables by their experiential percentage. Bad debt is problematic only when it threatens to exceed historical experience. Therefore,

Table 7.11   Refinancing a mortgage—payback period

At inception	
Principal	$200,000
Term	30 years
Rate	6%
Current payment	($1,199.10) = PMT(6%/12, 30 × 12, $200,000)

Several years later	
Current principal	$195,000
Refinancing cost	$2,500 (interest, title, filing, attorney fee)
New rate	5%
New payment	($1,046.80) = PMT(5%/12, 30 × 12, $195,000)

Current payment minus new payment	$152.30 cash flow savings
Refinancing cost divided by cash flow savings	16.42 months before new payment begins to have positive cash flow

monitoring of collections as well as the unbilled amounts is extremely important. Healthcare facilities have to contend not only with the prospect of not being able to collect legitimate receivables (in the case, for example, of indigent care), but also for being unable to collect receivables due to tardy claims. Thus, particular attention must be paid to timely action on claims denials.

Collection of receivables is a problematic issue for companies that do not collect payment at the point of sale. Healthcare organizations are particularly susceptible to problematic collections, partly because the source of payment is not always known or even accurate at the point of care. For example, a patient may present in the emergency room unconscious and is registered self-pay. Upon investigation, it is determined the patient is covered by commercial insurance. After discharge, it is further determined that the patient's insurance lapsed but the patient is eligible for Medicaid and is in the process of applying. In this example, the hospital's expectation of reimbursement changed at every step.

Another reason that collection is difficult is that the patient's responsibility for payment is not always known at the point of care. The patient may have a script for a test that is not covered by Medicare, based on the diagnosis listed on the script. Even if the patient signs an advance beneficiary notice, the patient will not be billed until after the test is done and it is determined whether the diagnosis provided is correct.

Finally, the healthcare organization may not have the right staffing to follow up on collections. Building a strong financial counseling and collections staff is complex and may not be efficient for the organization.

When collections become a problem, the organization can outsource the collection activity. Another alternative is to sell the accounts receivable. If the organization sells the accounts receivable, it becomes the responsibility of the purchaser to collect from the debtor. Because of the cost and difficulty of collections, the receivables are not worth the full value stated on the balance sheet. They will be sold at a discount from book value.

Tax Implications

There are a number of tax considerations for both the issuer and the investor. To the bond issuer, the interest paid to the bondholders is tax-deductible. However, the dividends paid to stockholders are not. The latter is one source of the term "double taxation" in reference to corporations. The corporation's income is taxed; then, the already net-of-taxes dividend is also taxed on the stockholder's side as income.

Similarly, the interest paid on loans is also tax-deductible. So, a mortgage rate of 5 percent is overall slightly lower because the deduction reduces the organization's tax liability. The deductibility of interest, however, is not a primary reason for obtaining debt financing as opposed to withdrawing from general funds to complete a project. The opportunity cost of lost income from investments must be weighed against the cost of bond issuance.

Another tax consideration for the investor is the status of the issuer. Some bonds, such as those issued by municipalities, are tax-exempt at the state level. Their coupon rates often reflect this and are slightly lower than those of corporate bonds.

Cash Management and Investment Strategies

The scenarios described in this chapter have focused on the raising of cash and funding of shortfalls. Organizations also have the need to invest available cash. Just as organizations may issue the instruments discussed earlier in this chapter, organizations may also purchase them, within the limits of their investment policy. Just as individuals do, the organization would open an account with a financial institution, deposit funds, and instruct the institution as to how to invest those funds. In addition to stocks, bonds, and possibly commercial paper, organizations have other options and variations on those options. Some reasons a healthcare organization may have the need to invest include:

- Charitable foundation donations
- Very short-term cash surplus
- Project funding received before the expenditures are due

Every organization that has the need to invest, whether short-term or long-term, should have an investment policy that guides the responsible individuals in their daily decision making. For example, a simple policy listing the types of approved investments may be sufficient. In organizations that have long-term investment needs, a broader policy may be needed that outlines the specific strategies and investment tools that may be utilized. A charitable foundation, for example, may receive millions of dollars that are not going to be expended immediately. Such a foundation would need a policy that states exactly how those dollars may be invested, including such details as the minimum ratings of debt instruments and a prohibition on certain aggressive strategies, such as short sales (selling a security one doesn't own in anticipation of purchasing it back at a lower price), as well as specific benchmarks against which the returns on investment are measured. An investment policy may even include a prohibition on the investment in securities from certain countries whose human rights record is not consistent with the organization's values.

Interest-Bearing Accounts

Financial institutions offer many different variations of depositor accounts. The simplest of these is the *interest-bearing account.* An interest-bearing account works like the savings account described earlier in this chapter. Funds are deposited and earn interest at a posted rate, usually on the average balance during the period. The underlying source of the interest is the general investment activity of the financial institution. There are usually no restrictions on the deposit and withdrawal of funds from this type of account. Checking accounts can be interest bearing. Savings accounts are inherently interest bearing.

Another type of interest-bearing account is the **money market account.** The underlying source of the interest in a money market account is short-term securities such as commercial paper or shares in funds that trade in these short-term securities (see "Money Market and Other Funds," following). These accounts typically do not have a stated interest rate. They earn whatever is the prevailing interest rate associated with those securities, minus the financial institution's fee for managing the portfolio. Although these accounts typically have no restrictions on the deposit of funds, there may be restrictions on the timing and amount of withdrawals. Financial institutions may exact penalties against an account with excessive withdrawals in a particular time period.

Certificates of Deposit

A certificate of deposit (CD) is a security issued by a bank or other financial institution. CDs are interest bearing and have specific maturities, which range from months to years. Because the financial institution is guaranteed access to those funds for the period, the interest rate on these deposits may be slightly higher than on an unrestricted savings account.

Banks and other financial institutions use the funds raised from certificates of deposit to finance their day-to-day activities. Their purpose is similar to commercial paper and these securities are also available in the secondary market.

Organizations can purchase CDs either directly from the financial institution or secondarily through a broker. A less risky way to purchase CDs is by purchasing shares in a money market fund, as described next.

Money Market and Other Funds

Money market **funds** are pooled investments in short-term securities, such as commercial paper and CDs. Financial institutions determine the investment strategy of the fund and open the fund to investors. As cash is received from various investors, the fund managers purchase securities that are consistent with the investment strategy of the fund. Funds may have limitations on the number of investors, the minimum purchase, and the total number of available shares. Investors may purchase shares in the fund directly or through a broker.

There are funds that invest in virtually any available type of security. A particular stock fund may target only stocks of companies that routinely pay dividends; another stock fund may target only stocks issued by non-US companies. There are stock funds that purchase the exact stocks that compose the Dow Jones Industrial Average and others that mirror other indices. Important considerations in purchasing shares in a fund include the risk of the underlying investments and the management fee charged by the fund manager. In addition to the management fee, there may be a purchase fee or a sales fee. The sales fee may be waived if the investor stays in the fund for a specified period of time.

Investment in managed funds is one way to reduce the risk of a particular investment. The purchase of shares in a particular company carries the inherent risk of loss if the company does not do well. That risk is lowered if the particular company is only one of many that are owned by the fund.

Managed Portfolios

Organizations that have large-dollar, long-term investment needs may want to consider customized, managed **portfolios.** Such a portfolio differs from a fund because the organization actually owns the securities, not just a share in the pool of securities. Portfolios may be managed in a variety of ways. Two common strategies are the individual portfolio and the shared portfolio.

An individual portfolio is managed specifically for the organization. It is entirely customizable for the organization. The organization has a direct relationship with the portfolio manager, who could theoretically be an employee of the organization.

A shared portfolio is different in that the portfolio strategy is directed by a portfolio manager who executes the strategy across the accounts of many investors. So, Company A invests $500,000 and Company B invests $1,000,000. They have both chosen Strategy X. The portfolio manager then purchases exactly the same securities for both Company A and Company B. The only difference is that Company B owns twice as many.

Summary

Organizations often need to obtain funding from external sources to meet their cash needs for routine operations and to finance capital investments. For debt financing, the cost of financing is a factor of the interest rate and the duration of the investment. Equity financing does not have the same repayment obligations that debt financing has; however, sale of equity shares affects the ownership and sometimes the management of the organization. An organization's ability to obtain financing is affected by its credit rating and by its tax status. Not-for-profit organizations cannot issue stock but may obtain debt financing and may accept tax-deductible donations. For-profit organizations may obtain equity or debt financing, but donations are not tax-deductible to the donor. There are two sides to financing: the seller and the purchaser. Organizations may be on either side of the transaction: borrowing to fund cash shortfalls and investing surplus cash, for example.

CHECK YOUR UNDERSTANDING

1. Items to be included in the capital budget are best defined as:
   a. Fixed assets costing more than $500
   b. Items that are depreciated
   c. Items that are depreciated under the IRS Alternative Depreciation System
   d. Items included in the organization's criteria for capital budget
2. A certificate of deposit with a principal of $3,000 that earns 6 percent annual interest has a maturity of three months. What is the interest at maturity on this account?
   a. $18
   b. $45
   c. $60
   d. $180

3. A savings account at Big Bank earns 2 percent interest, compounded monthly. If the initial deposit is $5,000, what is the value of the account at the end of two months?
   a. $5,008.34
   b. $5,016.68
   c. $5,100.17
   d. $5,202.00

4. A one-year Treasury bill with a value at maturity of $10,000 on September 30 is selling at a discount rate of 1.5 percent. What is the purchase price of the bill if it is purchased on June 30?
   a. $7,200.00
   b. $7,462.50
   c. $9,850.00
   d. $9,852.22

5. What is the interest earned on a five-year, $50,000 investment at 4 percent interest, compounded annually?
   a. $52,000.00
   b. $60,000.00
   c. $60,832.65
   d. $61,049.83

6. Which of the following is a reason that a healthcare organization might have the need to invest?
   a. Short-term cash shortfall
   b. Charitable foundation donations
   c. Acquisition of a new building
   d. Bond coupon payment due

7. What federal body sets the discount rate, at which banks may borrow directly from the central bank?
   a. Federal Open Market Committee of the Federal Reserve Bank
   b. DHHS
   c. The US Congress
   d. Bureau of Labor Statistics

8. The most important factor in determining whether to lend money to an organization is its:
   a. Balance sheet
   b. Net patient service revenue
   c. Credit rating
   d. FICO score

9. Of the following instruments, which is a not-for-profit hospital most likely to choose in order to finance a three-year facility expansion project?
   a. Revolving credit line
   b. Commercial paper
   c. Common stock
   d. Bond
10. A hospital had $5,000,000 in donations, which it invested in a 5 percent coupon bond with a maturity of five years from the date of purchase. The market interest rate at the time of the purchase was 4 percent. What is the semiannual interest payment that the hospital will receive?
   a. $20,000
   b. $25,000
   c. $40,000
   d. $50,000

References

Averkamp, Harold. 2011. Stockholder's equity. AccountingCoach.com. http://www.accountingcoach.com/online-accounting-course/17Xpg01.html.

Bureau of Labor Statistics. 2011. Consumer Price Index, frequently asked questions. http://www.bls.gov/cpi/cpifaq.htm.

Depository Trust & Clearing Corporation. 2011. About DTCC, our business: An overview. http://www.dtcc.com/about/business/index.php.

Federal Reserve Board of Governors. 2011. Federal Open Market Committee, about the FOMC. http://www.federalreserve.gov/monetarypolicy/fomc.htm.

FICO. 2011. http://www.fico.com/en/Pages/default.aspx.

IRS. 2011. Publication 946. Figuring depreciation under MACRS. http://www.irs.gov/publications/p946/ch04.html.

Moody's Corporation. 2011. http://www.moodys.com/Pages/atc.aspx.

Morningstar. 2011. http://www.morningstar.com.

Standard & Poor's. 2011. http://www.standardandpoors.com/about-sp/main/en/us.

Capital Investment Decisions

Learning Objectives

➤ Define capital investment
➤ Discuss how the cash flows of an investment project differ from its accounting profits
➤ Identify and discuss the four main cost analysis methods used in practice to compare capital investments
➤ Discuss various techniques for assessing risk in capital projects

Key Terms

Accounting rate of return	Internal rate of return (IRR)
Average rate of return (ARR)	Lease
Break-even analysis	Net present value (NPV)
Cannibalistic side effect	Net working capital
Capital	Operating cash flow (OCF)
Cash flow	Opportunity cost
Cash flow from assets (CFFA)	Payback period
Discounted cash flow	Stand-alone principle
Discounting factor	Sunk costs
Incremental cost	Synergistic side effect

Capital Purchases

The concept of a **capital** budget was introduced in chapter 7. The first step in capital budgeting is to determine the projects that must be funded in the next three to five years. Healthcare providers are faced with a large number of capital needs such as medical equipment, facility expansion, satellite clinic construction, computer hardware, and so forth. Each capital expenditure should be analyzed to determine if the purchase or construction is an efficient use of the provider's resources.

The access to capital funding is dependent on the financial position of a provider. A strong financial position allows a provider to access capital funding through loans or bonds at a competitive rate. Even providers with strong balance sheets must ration capital expenditures to some extent. The costs and benefits of each capital project should be compared to alternative projects and also to the cost of capital to determine the best use of the limited resources.

Project Cash Flow Analysis

Cash flow analysis is commonly used to compare capital projects and assess their potential influence on the financial position of the provider. The statement of cash flow is one of the four standard components of the financial statement. The statement of cash flow takes information from the income statement and balance sheet and translates it into a report of movement of cash in and out of the entity's funds during the reporting period. A cash flow analysis for a capital project essentially creates a report of the flow of cash into and out of the entity for the project under consideration.

The **stand-alone principle** is used when performing a cash flow analysis for a project. The stand-alone principle states that each project should be analyzed in isolation, considering only the cash flow that is impacted by the project. Applying the stand-alone principle allows an unbiased view of the impact of the project in isolation from other factors that might be impacting the provider and comparison of that figure to the cost of capital. For instance, if a provider is performing a cash flow analysis for the purchase of a new MRI machine that will be installed into a space that is currently occupied by the provider, the cost of leasing that space should not be considered. If a new space must be leased to house the new equipment, then that is an incremental cost due to the project and that cost should be considered. An **incremental cost** is a cost that is incurred by a change in business. The cost of leasing the space to house the new MRI machine is incremental because it is incurred only due to the acquisition of the new equipment.

An accurate cash flow analysis requires a methodical review of all of the incremental costs and revenue directly associated with the project. Any cash flow that occurs whether or not the project is completed should be excluded from the analysis. **Sunk costs** should be excluded from the analysis. Sunk costs are those costs that would have been expended even if the project is not pursued. One example of sunk costs is feasibility studies. If a provider hired a consultant to perform a market analysis to determine if there was a need for additional capacity in various services, and that study determined that more MRI capacity was needed in the community, the cost of the market analysis would be considered a sunk cost and should be excluded in the analysis of the MRI machine purchase.

Financing costs should also be excluded from a cash flow analysis. The cash flow produced by the project is compared to the acquisition cost based on the **net present value.** The cost of capital or financing costs will be used to assess the affordability of the project, but it is not included in the cash flow analysis.

Opportunity costs should be included in a cash flow analysis. Opportunity costs are those benefits that are given up or extra costs incurred by pursuing one project over another. For instance, if the new MRI machine will be placed in an area that now houses vending machines, then the revenue lost for removing the vending machines should be considered an opportunity cost. In general, any revenue that would be lost due to the project's completion should be considered an opportunity cost.

The cost of side effects should also be considered in a cash flow analysis. In our MRI machine purchase example, one side effect of the purchase may be a decrease in volume at one of the provider's other MRI sites. If the new machine is placed in a more convenient location than where current services are offered, then the provider may experience a shift in services to the new site and not an incremental increase in volume. The shift in volume away from the current site would be a **cannibalistic side effect.** Side effects may also have a positive impact on the project. The new patients coming to the facility to use the MRI machine will likely need to park. If the provider owns its own parking facility, then the incremental revenue due to the new patients may be considered a source of cash. This is sometimes called a **synergistic side effect.**

The impact on **net working capital** should also be included in a cash flow analysis. Net working capital is defined as current assets minus current liabilities. Most projects require some sort of start-up costs. They may include a down payment for financing or the purchase of initial inventory of supplies. These costs will be replaced as the project is implemented and becomes operational, but the initial costs should be included in the analysis because they will influence the ability of the provider to pursue other opportunities during the start-up period. The impact on net working capital may be thought of as an internal loan to the project.

The impact on the tax liability due to a project should also be incorporated into the cash flow analysis. Since most physician practices and some other provider types are for-profit entities, it is important to understand the tax implications of a capital project. Capital purchases are reflected on an entity's financial statement as a depreciation expense. That expense will offset some of the revenue produced by the project and will lower the net revenue. Since tax liability is based on net revenue, decreasing net revenue will decrease tax liability and improve the cash flow for a project.

Table 8.1 lists common cost categories and guidance on their inclusion in a cash flow analysis.

Pro Forma Financial Statements

The first step in evaluating capital projects is compiling the information to build pro forma financial statements. In the investing world, pro forma describes a method of calculating financial results to emphasize either current or projected figures. Table 8.2 displays a pro forma income statement and figure 8.1 shows a simple balance sheet for the purchase of new MRI equipment.

In the scenario presented in table 8.2 and figure 8.1, a provider is considering the purchase of an MRI machine. The projected annual volume of procedures is 1,000. The projected gross revenue is $250,000 based on the current average

Table 8.1   Types of cost

Type of Cost	Include in Cash Flow Analysis?
Sunk costs	No
Opportunity costs	Yes
Side effects (positive and negative)	Yes
Impact on net working capital	Yes
Tax effect	Yes

Table 8.2   Pro forma income statement—MRI machine purchase

Revenue (1,000 tests @ $250 each)	$250,000
Variable costs (supplies @ $50/unit)	$50,000
Gross profit	= $200,000
Fixed cost (staff)	$50,000
Depreciation ($300,000/5 years)	$60,000
EBIT (earnings before interest & taxes)	= $90,000
Taxes (not-for-profit entity = 0% tax rate)	$0
Net income	= $90,000

Figure 8.1   Pro forma balance sheet

	Year 0	Year 1	Year 2	Year 3	Year 4	Year 5
Net working capital	$10,000	$0	$0	$0	$0	$0
Net fixed assets	$300,000	$240,000	$180,000	$120,000	$60,000	$0

reimbursement per test of $250 and the projected 1,000 procedures. The variable cost per procedure is $50. The cost of an additional technologist to staff the machine is $50,000. The cost of the machine is $300,000. The useful life of the machine is five years and there is no salvage value at the end of the useful life. If straight-line depreciation is used, the depreciation expense is $300,000/5 or $60,000 per year. This shows up as an expense in the income statement and also as the amount of the decrease in net fixed asset value in the balance sheet. The provider is a not-for-profit entity with no tax liability. These figures taken together leave the provider with $90,000 in estimated net income, according to this pro forma. Operating the MRI machine will also require an initial investment of $10,000 from net working capital to purchase supplies. This figure is presented in the pro forma balance sheet.

Notice that the pro forma statements include only the balance sheet and income statement: items that are influenced by the project under consideration. The pro forma figures must be converted into cash flow to perform the cash flow analysis for this project.

Cash Flow Calculations

The project cash flow is called the **cash flow from assets** (CFFA). The formula has two components: **operating cash flow** (OCF) and the change in assets during the life of the project.

$$\text{Operating Cash Flow} = \text{EBIT} + \text{Depreciation} - \text{Taxes}$$
$$\text{CFFA} = \text{Operating Cash Flow} - \text{Capital Spending} - \text{Net Working Capital}$$

From the MRI example, the OCF = $90,000 + $60,000 - $0 = $150,000. Recall from chapter 3 that EBIT is the earnings before interest and taxes. Since depreciation is not a cash event, that figure is added to the net income to determine the OCF. The impact on net fixed assets must also be taken into consideration in the cash flow calculation. The largest change in fixed assets is due to the

Figure 8.2   Cash flow analysis

Cash Flow Source	Year 0	Year 1	Year 2	Year 3	Year 4	Year 5
Operating		$150,000	$150,000	$150,000	$150,000	$150,000
From assets	($310,000)					$10,000
Total	($310,000)	$150,000	$150,000	$150,000	$150,000	$160,000

actual expense for the MRI machine. This occurs at the beginning of the project. The net working capital is a cash outflow at the beginning of the project but will be cash inflow at the end of the project. The projected overall cash flow for the MRI machine project is presented in figure 8.2.

The cash flow analysis in figure 8.2 may now be used to determine if the project is a favorable investment.

Cost Benefit Analysis

A structured cost-benefit analysis is an excellent tool for deciding which capital projects are the best investment for a provider. Cash flow analysis quantifies one aspect of the benefits of a project. There are a number of strategies for analyzing the costs and benefits of capital projects. Four alternatives are presented here:

1. **Payback period**
2. **Average rate of return**
3. Net present value
4. **Internal rate of return**

There may be intangible, nonmonetary benefits that should be factored into capital planning decisions. The purchase of new technology and equipment may improve a provider's reputation in the community. This may provide a marketing edge and allow the provider to attract more patients or even doctors who wish to use the new technology or a particular brand of implants. These factors should be weighed along with the quantitative methods presented in this text prior to making a final decision.

Payback Period

The payback period for an investment is the amount of time it takes for the accumulated cash flow to exceed the initial investment—in other words, how long until investors make their money back. As a simple example, suppose a physician decides to invest $5,000 in a new electronic health record (EHR) system. The vendor supplying the system assures the physician that the system will run on his current computer network and increase his cash flow by $2,500 per year. The payback period on the EHR investment is $5,000/$2,500 = 2 years.

The payback period must be compared to some standard value that is acceptable to an entity or may be compared between two competing capital projects. If the payback period is below the standard value or the competing project, then the investment is acceptable. If the net annual cash flow is constant over the useful life of the investment, the general formula for the payback period is as follows:

$$\text{Payback Period} = \frac{\text{Investment Amount}}{\text{Net Annual Cash Flow before Taxes}}$$

In many cases the net annual cash flow may vary by year. In our MRI machine example, the net annual cash flow for the useful life of the machine is found in figure 8.2. The accumulated cash after year 1 is $150,000; after year 2 it is $300,000 and after year 3 it is $450,000. The initial investment is $310,000. The payback of the initial investment occurs between years 1 and 2. Since the net cash flow for the years surrounding the payback period is a constant $150,000, we can use the formula above:

$$\text{Payback Period} = \frac{310,000}{150,000} = 2.07 \text{ years}$$

The calculation of the payback period in situations where the net cash flow is not consistent over the analysis period is slightly more complex. Suppose we change the MRI machine example to reflect a 10 percent increase in the cash flow each year. The net cash flow for year 1 is $150,000, for year 2 is $165,000, and for year 3 is $181,500. The payback is best calculated using a table as found in figure 8.3. Note that after year 1 the investment balance is $160,000. This figure is less than the year 2 net cash flow. The payback is 1 plus 160,000/165,000 of a year or 1.97 years.

The methodology of using a table to calculate the payback period is applicable in both the special case of equal net annual cash flow and the unequal case. If the required payback period for this provider was two years, then the criteria would be met in both of these scenarios and the investment is considered to be favorable.

Figure 8.3   Net cash flow payback calculation

Year	Net Cash Flow	Investment Balance
0	$0	$310,000
1	$150,000	$160,000
2	$165,000	($5,000)
3	$181,500	($186,500)

The payback period is a measure of investment performance that is easy to understand. Since it is based on cash flows, it favors investments with a high level of liquidity (those that produce immediate cash). The disadvantages of the payback period are that it ignores the time value of money and it requires an arbitrary cutoff point to be determined by executive leadership or the board of directors. The payback period does not consider any cash flows after the payback is complete and is therefore biased against projects that may take longer to mature and begin to produce cash.

Average Rate of Return

The average rate of return (ARR) is another method for making capital project decisions. The average rate of return is also referred to as the **accounting rate of return.** The ARR is defined as the average accounting profit divided by the average accounting value of the investment. The formula typically used to calculate ARR is as follows:

$$\text{Average Rate of Return} = \frac{\text{Average Net Income}}{\text{Average Investment Amount}}$$

Note that the numerator in the ARR formula is the average net income, not the average cash flow. Recall that net income includes depreciation expense, so the ARR will be dependent on the depreciation method used by the entity.

For the MRI machine example, the average net income per year is $90,000 based on the pro forma income statement found in table 8.2. The initial investment is $300,000 and final investment amount is –$10,000 after five years. The average investment amount is ($310,000 + –$10,000)/2 = $150,000. The ARR for this investment is then as follows:

$$ARR = \frac{90,000}{150,000} = 0.6 \text{ or } 60 \text{ percent}$$

The ARR for this investment may be compared against competing capital projects to see if it is more or less favorable. The ARR may also be compared to the provider-wide ARR to determine if the investment has a return comparable to the norm at the facility.

The ARR has some significant limitations (Ross et al. 2011, 240):

1. It is not a true rate of return because the time value of money is ignored.
2. Comparisons use an arbitrary benchmark or cutoff.
3. It is based on accounting net income and book values instead of cash flow and market value of the investment.

The ARR does have some advantages in that it is fairly easy to calculate and the needed information for the provider-wide ARR is available in the financial statements of the entity. The ARR is very similar to the calculation of the return on assets ratio presented in chapter 3.

Net Present Value

The difference between a capital investment's market value and its cost is called the net present value (NPV). The NPV is another method of comparing the value of competing investments or capital projects. To calculate the NPV we must first explore the concept of **discounted cash flow** (DCF).

Discounted cash flow is related to the time value of money. The present value (PV) of $100 is $100, but the future value (FV) of $100 is more than $100 due to inflation. Suppose a hospital chief financial officer (CFO) knows that he will need $100,000 to buy new laboratory equipment in one year. How much money should the CFO put aside now if he knows he can earn 5 percent by investing the funds for 12 months? In this case, the CFO needs to know the PV of the investment to ensure that the FV is $100,000. According to the formulas presented in chapter 7, the PV may be calculated by the following:

$$PV = \frac{FV}{(1+r)^n} = \frac{100,000}{(1+0.05)^3} = \frac{100,000}{1.05} = \$95,238$$

Present value is essentially the inverse of future value. To calculate the present value of a cash amount, the future value is discounted by the interest rate. Similarly, to calculate the present value of cash flow that occurs in the future we must discount the value by the present value factor. The calculation that estimates the present value of future cash flow is called DCF valuation.

The example of the CFO saving for laboratory equipment may be expanded to a multiyear calculation. Suppose instead of one year, the CFO finds out that the purchase of the new equipment is in three years. The equipment cost is still $100,000 and the annual rate of return for his investment is 5 percent. The present value to be invested is as follows:

$$PV = \frac{FV}{(1+r)^n} = \frac{100,000}{(1+0.05)^3} = \frac{100,000}{1.158} = \$86,384$$

The figure $1/(1+r)^n$ is referred to as the **discounting factor** or present value factor. The discounting factor in the three-year example is $1/1.158 = 0.8638$. The discounting factor in the one-year example is $1/1.05 = 0.9524$. The discounting factor decreases as the number of periods increases or the interest rate increases. Table 8.3 displays present value factors for calculating the discounted value of $1 in future cash flow. Notice that the first and third rows in the 5 percent column match the PV factors calculated in the previous examples.

The calculation of the NPV of a capital investment involves calculating the DCF valuation of the cash flow projected from the pro forma financial statements. Returning to the MRI machine example, the cash flow analysis displayed in figure 8.4 can be expanded to include a calculation of the DCF valuation. The first step is to determine the discounting factor to be used. The discounting rate should be based on the provider's cost of capital. If the provider in our example is able to borrow money for the purchase of the MRI machine at an interest rate of 5 percent, then 5 percent should be used as the discounting rate. The discounting factor for each year at 5 percent is selected. Figure 8.4 shows the calculation of the DCF valuation and NPV for the purchase of the MRI machine.

Table 8.3   PV factors for various years and interest rates

Life of Investment in Years	Interest Rate					
	1%	3%	5%	7%	9%	10%
1	0.9901	0.9709	0.9524	0.9346	0.9174	0.9091
2	0.9803	0.9426	0.9070	0.8734	0.8417	0.8264
3	0.9706	0.9151	0.8638	0.8163	0.7722	0.7513
4	0.9610	0.8885	0.8227	0.7629	0.7084	0.6830
5	0.9515	0.8626	0.7835	0.7130	0.6499	0.6209
6	0.9420	0.8375	0.7462	0.6663	0.5963	0.5645
7	0.9327	0.8131	0.7107	0.6227	0.5470	0.5132
8	0.9235	0.7894	0.6768	0.5820	0.5019	0.4665
9	0.9143	0.7664	0.6446	0.5439	0.4604	0.4241
10	0.9053	0.7441	0.6139	0.5083	0.4224	0.3855

Figure 8.4   Discounted cash flow analysis—scenario 1

Cash Flow Source	Year 0	Year 1	Year 2	Year 3	Year 4	Year 5
Operating		$150,000	$150,000	$150,000	$150,000	$150,000
From assets	($310,000)					$10,000
Total	($310,000)	$150,000	$150,000	$150,000	$150,000	$160,000
PV factor	0	0.9524	0.9070	0.8638	0.8227	0.7835
DCF valuation	($310,000)	$142,860	$136,050	$129,570	$123,405	$125,360

The NPV for this example is the sum of the DCF valuation row or $347,245. Since this is a positive number, the investment in the MRI machine is favorable and should be pursued. Figure 8.5 demonstrates the impact of the cost of capital on the NPV of an investment. In this second scenario the discounting factor is increased to 10 percent. This could occur if a provider did not have a strong enough balance sheet to merit the lowest interest rates for a loan or did not earn a favorable bond rating. The NPV for the equivalent cash flow assumptions and a 10 percent cost of capital is $264,827 versus the NPV of $347,245 when the cost of capital is 5 percent. This is a significant difference in investment value over a relatively short period of time.

The strengths of NPV are that it takes the time value of money into consideration and uses a realistic cost of capital as the test to determine if an investment is favorable. It also considers the cash flow during the entire investment period. One disadvantage of NPV is that it is not easy to explain to an audience that does not have a financial background.

Internal Rate of Return

The internal rate of return (IRR) is closely related to NPV. The IRR is the discounting rate that results in a NPV of zero. In other words, the IRR is the cost of

Figure 8.5   Discounted cash flow analysis—scenario 2

Cash Flow Source	Year 0	Year 1	Year 2	Year 3	Year 4	Year 5
Operating		$150,000	$150,000	$150,000	$150,000	$150,000
From assets	($310,000)					$10,000
Total	($310,000)	$150,000	$150,000	$150,000	$150,000	$160,000
PV factor	0	0.9091	0.8264	0.7513	0.6830	0.6209
DCF valuation	($310,000)	$136,364	$123,967	$112,697	$102,452	$99,347

Table 8.4   NPV for various discounting rates for MRI example

Discounting Rate	NPV
5%	$347,245
10%	$264,827
20%	$142,611
30%	$58,029
40%	($2,866)

capital that results in a **break-even analysis** return on the investment. In calculating the NPV, an assumption must be made about the cost of capital. If the IRR is used as a criterion for choosing an investment, the investment is favorable if the IRR is less than the cost of capital or higher than an investment return threshold for the provider.

The calculation of IRR is difficult to perform without the assistance of spreadsheet software. The value can be calculated by trial and error by using a calculator. In the case of our MRI machine example, we know that the IRR must be higher than 10 percent because the NPV for a discounting rate of 10 percent is positive. Table 8.4 displays data that may be used to find the IRR for this example. Since the NPV changes from positive to negative between 30 percent and 40 percent, the IRR must be in that range. The NPV for a discounting rate of 39 percent is $2,420 and for 39.5 percent is ($243). The IRR for this example is approximately 39.5 percent.

Figure 8.6 shows the relationship between NPV and discounting rate for the MRI machine example. The point where the line crosses the NPV = 0 axis represents the IRR value, or 39.5 percent in this case.

One advantage of the IRR is that it essentially calculates a break-even point for the investment—that is, if funds may be acquired for less than the IRR, then the investment will have a positive return. The IRR also shows the return on the original investment, which is a more intuitive concept for those less experienced in finance to grasp. A disadvantage of the IRR is the difficulty in performing the calculation.

Figure 8.6　Relationship between discounting rate and NPV

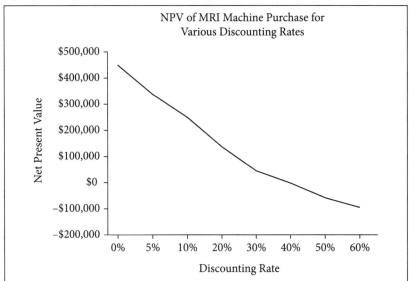

Lease versus Purchase

A **lease** option may be available to providers that are interested in acquiring new equipment. The lease versus purchase decision is not only a financial decision. Some leases leave the maintenance and management of the equipment as the responsibility of the lessee. Some leases include a guaranteed proportion of uptime. or time that the equipment will be in working condition. All of the terms of the lease should be considered prior to deciding which method of equipment acquisition is right in a particular situation. The cash flow approach used to quantify the return on investment for capital projects may be used to determine if leasing or buying is a better choice from a financial point of view.

From a financial statement perspective, a lease is very different from a purchase. Purchased equipment is recorded as a fixed asset and appears on the balance sheet in the asset portion. The depreciation of the purchased equipment for the reporting period is recorded as an expense on the income statement. Leases may be treated as operating or capital leases depending on the rights transferred to the lessee. In an operating lease, the lessor transfers the right to use the item to the lessee, but the item must be returned at the end of the lease period. Since the lessee does not own that item, it appears as an operating expense on the income statement and has no impact on the balance sheet. In a capital lease, the lessee takes on more ownership rights and responsibilities for the item. Items that are acquired via a capital lease are recorded as assets and liabilities on the balance sheet. There are accounting guidelines that determine how a lease should be classified. This discussion will be limited to operating leases. The different accounting treatment of purchased and leased equipment will influence the NPV calculation for an investment. Recall from earlier in this chapter:

$$\text{Project Cash Flow} = \text{Operating Cash Flow} - \text{Capital Spending} - \text{Net Working Capital}$$

Not-for-Profit Organizations

In a not-for-profit entity, the operating cash flow is reduced by the lease payments in the lease versus buy decision. The capital spending becomes zero under a lease. The net working capital is likely unchanged.

Consider the MRI machine purchase from earlier in this chapter. If we assume the cost of capital for the provider is 5 percent, then the NPV of the project is $347,245 if the machine is purchased (see table 8.4). What if the machine could be leased for $60,000 per year for five years? How would the NPV change? The pro forma income statement would change because leased equipment is not depreciated. The revised pro forma income statement is presented in figure 8.7. The project cash flow under the lease scenario is $100,000 − $0 − $10,000 = $90,000.

The discounted cash flow analysis and NPV calculation change to the values displayed in figure 8.8. The NPV for the lease situation is $387,481 versus $347,245 for the previous buy alternative with a 5 percent discount rate. Note

Figure 8.7   Pro forma income statement—MRI machine lease versus buy

	Buy	Lease
Revenue (1,000 tests @ $250 each)	$250,000	$250,000
Variable costs (supplies @ $50/unit)	$50,000	$50,000
Gross profit	= $200,000	= $200,000
Fixed cost (staff + lease payment)	$50,000	$100,000
Depreciation ($0 under lease)	$60,000	$0
EBIT (earnings before interest & taxes)	= $90,000	= $100,000
Taxes (not-for-profit entity = 0% tax rate)	$0	$0
Net income	= $90,000	= $100,000

Figure 8.8 Discounted cash flow analysis—MRI machine lease

Cash Flow Source	Year 0	Year 1	Year 2	Year 3	Year 4	Year 5
Operating		$90,000	$90,000	$90,000	$90,000	$90,000
From assets	($10,000)					$10,000
Total	($10,000)	$90,000	$90,000	$90,000	$90,000	$100,000
PV factor		0.9524	0.9070	0.8638	0.8227	0.7835
DCF valuation	($10,000)	$85,716	$81,630	$77,742	$74,043	$78,350

that there is a significant difference in the year-to-year cash flow for the lease situation because the lease payments reduce the cash flow in the pro forma.

The lease versus buy decision may come to different conclusions in for-profit versus not-for-profit providers. Often it is the treatment of depreciation expense and the tax rate that make the difference in the two scenarios. As an example, consider two physician practices that are considering the acquisition of a new computer system to support their new electronic medical record system. Both are considering the same computer system that costs $50,000. They can each lease the system for $10,000 per year over five years. Suppose the useful life of the computer system is five years and that both practices use straight-line depreciation. Both practices can obtain a 7 percent loan to fund the purchase of the computer systems. One practice, Docs, Inc., is a for-profit entity and the second practice, Treat-em, is a not-for-profit entity. The following tables outline the NPV analysis of lease versus buy for these two practices.

> **Step 1:** Create pro forma financial statements for each entity in the buy scenario—income statement in figure 8.9. The capital expenditure of $50,000 is added to both balance sheets.
> **Step 2:** Convert the pro forma income statements to cash flow analysis—figure 8.10.
> **Step 3:** Perform a DCF valuation to calculate NPV—figure 8.11.
> **Step 4:** Create pro forma financial statements for each entity in the lease scenario—income statement in figure 8.12. The capital expenditure of $50,000 is added to both balance sheets.
> **Step 5:** Convert the pro forma income statements in figure 8.12 to cash flow analysis—figure 8.13.
> **Step 6:** Perform a DCF valuation to calculate NPV—figure 8.14.

The leasing option has a better NPV for both practices. Notice that the tax impact of the depreciation in the purchase option and the lease expense in the

Figure 8.9 Docs, Inc. and Treat-em profit and loss figures—buy scenario

	Docs, Inc. (For-Profit)	Treat-em (Not-for-Profit)
Revenue (no additional revenue)	$0	$0
Variable costs (none)	$0	$0
Gross profit	= $0	= $0
Fixed cost (IT support)	$5,000	$5,000
Depreciation ($50,000/5)	$10,000	$10,000
EBIT (earnings before interest & taxes)	= ($15,000)	= ($15,000)
Taxes (34% tax rate)—offset taxes on other revenue	($5,100)	$0
Net income	= ($9,900)	= ($15,000)

Figure 8.10 Docs, Inc. and Treat-em operating expenses—buy scenario

	Docs, Inc.			Treat-em		
Year	Operating	From Assets	Total	Operating	From Assets	Total
0		($50,000)	($50,000)		($50,000)	($50,000)
1	$100		$100	($5,000)		($5,000)
2	$100		$100	($5,000)		($5,000)
3	$100		$100	($5,000)		($5,000)
4	$100		$100	($5,000)		($5,000)
5	$100		$100	($5,000)		($5,000)

Figure 8.11 Docs, Inc. and Treat-em total cash flow—buy scenario

	Docs, Inc.			Treat-em		
Year	Total Cash Flow	PV Factor @ 7%	Discounted Cash Flow	Total Cash Flow	PV Factor @ 7%	Discounted Cash Flow
0	($50,000)	N/A	($50,000)	($50,000)	N/A	($50,000)
1	$100	0.9346	$93	($5,000)	0.9346	($4,673)
2	$100	0.8734	$87	($5,000)	0.8734	($4,367)
3	$100	0.8163	$82	($5,000)	0.8163	($4,081)
4	$100	0.7629	$76	($5,000)	0.7629	($3,814)
5	$100	0.7130	$71	($5,000)	0.7130	($3,565)
NPV			($49,490)			($70,501)

Figure 8.12   Docs, Inc. and Treat-em profit and loss figures—lease scenario

	Docs, Inc. (For-Profit)	Treat-em (Not-for-Profit)
Revenue (no additional revenue)	$0	$0
Variable costs (none)	$0	$0
Gross profit	= $0	= $0
Fixed cost (IT support + lease payment)	$15,000	$15,000
Depreciation (N/A for lease scenario)	$0	$0
EBIT (earnings before interest & taxes)	= ($15,000)	= ($15,000)
Taxes (34% tax rate)—offset taxes on other revenue	($5,100)	$0
Net income	= ($9,900)	= ($15,000)

Figure 8.13   Docs, Inc. and Treat-em operating expenses—lease scenario

Year	Docs, Inc.			Treat-em		
	Operating	From Assets	Total	Operating	From Assets	Total
0						
1	($9,900)		($9,900)	($15,000)		($15,000)
2	($9,900)		($9,900)	($15,000)		($15,000)
3	($9,900)		($9,900)	($15,000)		($15,000)
4	($9,900)		($9,900)	($15,000)		($15,000)
5	($9,900)		($9,900)	($15,000)		($15,000)

Figure 8.14   Docs, Inc. and Treat-em total cash flow—lease scenario

Year	Docs, Inc.			Treat-em		
	Total Cash Flow	PV Factor @ 7%	Discounted Cash Flow	Total Cash Flow	PV Factor @ 7%	Discounted Cash Flow
0		N/A			N/A	
1	($9,900)	0.9346	($9,253)	($15,000)	0.9346	($14,019)
2	($9,900)	0.8734	($8,647)	($15,000)	0.8734	($13,101)
3	($9,900)	0.8163	($8,081)	($15,000)	0.8163	($12,245)
4	($9,900)	0.7629	($7,553)	($15,000)	0.7629	($11,444)
5	($9,900)	0.7130	($7,059)	($15,000)	0.7130	($10,695)
NPV			($40,592)			($61,503)

lease option causes the for-profit entity to have a more favorable NPV for both scenarios. Since no additional revenue is projected for the implementation of the EHR system, it is not surprising that the NPV is negative for all four calculations.

The decision to lease or buy equipment is dependent on the tax status of an organization, the useful life of the item purchased and the cost of capital for the provider considering the acquisition. The more favorable option is not obvious without a careful analysis. The framework presented here allows the provider to compare the NPV of the various alternatives.

Summary

The financial position of healthcare providers makes the acquisition of capital a critical business decision. Providers operate on very small margins and must have objective quantitative criteria for deciding which projects will help improve their financial position. Formulating pro forma financial statements and projecting the impact on cash flow of various capital projects provide a framework for evaluating alternatives. The four methods of measuring the return on investment—payback period, average rate of return, net present value, and internal rate of return—all provide a standardized method to assess the potential value of capital projects.

CHECK YOUR UNDERSTANDING

1. Depreciation should be added to net income in converting the income statement to a cash flow analysis. (True/False)
2. Financing costs should be included in a cash flow analysis. (True/False)
3. A pro forma income statement estimates the impact of a change in the current financial situation. (True/False)
4. A discounted cash flow analysis considers the time value of money. (True/False)
5. One of the strengths of a payback period analysis is that it considers the net income for the life of the item purchased. (True/False)
6. Which of the following variables is not included in the calculation of net present value of an investment?
   a. Cash flow
   b. Present value
   c. Useful life of item
   d. Payback period

7. If a new X-ray machine costs $10,000 and the estimated increase in cash flow is $5,000 per year, what is the payback period?
   a. 6 months
   b. 1 year
   c. 2 years
   d. 3 months

8. If the discounting rate for an investment increases, then the net present value of that investment:
   a. Does not change
   b. Increases
   c. Decreases
   d. Not enough information

9. Which of the following attributes of an organization is most important to consider when making a lease versus buy decision?
   a. Net income
   b. Depreciation method
   c. Tax status
   d. Value of the item to be leased or purchased

10. A change in net working capital directly impacts which portion of the financial statement?
   a. Balance sheet
   b. Income statement
   c. Statement of cash flow
   d. None of the above

Reference

Ross, Stephen, Randolph Westfield, and Bradford Jordan. 2011. *Essentials of Corporate Finance,* 7th ed. New York: McGraw-Hill/Irwin.

Answer Key

Check Your Understanding 1

1. False	6. c
2. False	7. a
3. True	8. a
4. False	9. a
5. False	10. a

Check Your Understanding 2

1. True	6. a
2. False	7. b
3. False	8. a
4. False	9. c
5. False	10. a

Check Your Understanding 3

1. False	6. b
2. True	7. d
3. True	8. c
4. False	9. b
5. False	10. b

Check Your Understanding 4

1. c	6. d
2. a	7. d
3. a	8. d
4. c	9. b
5. a	10. d

Check Your Understanding 5

1. False
2. False
3. False
4. True
5. True

6. c
7. c
8. d
9. c
10. a

Check Your Understanding 6

1. False
2. True
3. True
4. False
5. True

6. a
7. b
8. c
9. d
10. a

Check Your Understanding 7

1. d
2. b
3. b
4. d
5. c

6. b
7. a
8. c
9. d
10. b

Check Your Understanding 8

1. True
2. False
3. True
4. True
5. False

6. d
7. c
8. c
9. c
10. a

Glossary

A

Accountable care organization (ACO):   An organization of healthcare providers accountable for the quality, cost, and overall care of Medicare beneficiaries who are assigned and enrolled in the traditional fee-for-service program

Accounting rate of return: The projected annual cash inflows, minus any applicable depreciation, divided by the initial investment

Accounts payable (A/P):   Records of the payments owed by an organization to other entities

Accounts receivable (A/R):   1. Records of the payments owed to the organization by outside entities such as third-party payers and patients 2. Department in a healthcare facility that manages the accounts owed to the facility by customers who have received services but whose payment is made at a later date

Accrual-based accounting: A method of accounting that requires business organizations to report income in the period earned and to deduct expenses in the period incurred

Accrued expenses: Expenses recognized on the books before they are paid; they are the opposite of a prepaid expense and are typically periodic in nature—examples include utilities, rent, and payroll taxes

Advance beneficiary notice (ABN):   A statement signed by the patient when he or she is notified by the provider, prior to a service or procedure being done, that Medicare may not reimburse the provider for the service, wherein the patient indicates that he will be responsible for any charges

Affordable Care Act (ACA):   Legislation that included a number of initiatives intended to extend coverage and eliminate many of the practices of health insurers that compromised the level of coverage offered to individuals

Allocation: Assigning or spreading a common cost among several cost centers, such as when a hospital spreads the cost of housekeeping among patient rooms, nursing stations, labs, and administrative offices

Ambulatory payment classification (APC):   A categorization of CPT/HCPCS codes that is used for payment under the hospital outpatient prospective payment system (OPPS)

Asset management: Ratios that measure how effective a facility is in utilizing its assets to improve the facility's financial health

Assets: The human, financial, and physical resources of an organization

Auction rates: Market-defined interest rates at the time of issuance; typically used in the context of bonds

Average: The value obtained by dividing the sum of a set of numbers by the number of values

Average age of plant: The ratio that measures the age of the facility's fixed assets to assess the need for replacement

Average rate of return: The average accounting profit divided by the average accounting value of the investment

B

Bad debt: The portion of the receivables of an organization that is uncollectible

Balance billing: A reimbursement method that allows providers to bill patients for charges in excess of the amount paid by the patients' health plan or other third-party payer (not allowed under Medicare or Medicaid)

Balance sheet: A report that presents the assets, liabilities, and net assets of an organization at a specific point in time

Balanced Budget Act (BBA) of 1997:   Public Law 105-33 enacted by Congress on August 5, 1997, that mandated a number of additions, deletions, and revisions to the original Medicare and Medicaid legislation; the legislation that added penalties for healthcare fraud and abuse to the Medicare and Medicaid programs and also affected the hospital outpatient prospective payment system (HOPPS) and programs of all-inclusive care for the elderly (PACE)

Basis: The original cost of a fixed asset

Bell-shaped curve: *See* normal distribution

Benchmarking: The systematic comparison of the products, services, and outcomes of one organization with those of a similar organization; or the systematic comparison of one organization's outcomes with regional or national standards

Bill hold: The number of days, determined by the hospital, that a claim will remain on the list of discharged and not final billed (DNFB) accounts waiting for late charges, coding, error correction, and final documentation

Board of directors: The elected or appointed group of officials who bear ultimate responsibility for the successful operation of a healthcare organization

Bond: Contractual obligation to repay; may carry a variety of restrictions and covenants

Book value: The full value of an asset according to its balance sheet account balance; this amount represents the original cost minus any accumulated depreciation

Bottom-up: A variation on the traditional budget model in which a department would develop its budget based on its own, known contractual obligations and expectations; the departmental budgets are then combined to form the full organizational budget

Break-even analysis: A financial analysis technique for determining the level of sales at which total revenues equal total costs, beyond which revenues become profits

Budget cycle: The complete process of financial planning, operations, and control for a fiscal year; may overlap multiple fiscal years

Budget variance: When the actual performance is different from the budget

C

Call: The ability of the issuer to pay off the principal to investors prior to the maturity date

Cannibalistic side effect: A negative side effect of a capital project. For instance, a shift in volume away from the current site due to the creation of another site

Capital: Cash or goods used to generate income

Capital assets: Physical assets with an estimated useful life of more than one year

Capital budget: The allocation of resources for long-term investments and projects that involve the purchase of capital assets

Capitalization ratio: A measure of the proportion of the assets that were funded by debt

Capitated rate: A managed care term that refers to the fixed amount a physician or other healthcare provider is paid to provide services to a patient or a group of patients over a pre-specified period of time; often expressed as a per-member-per-month (PMPM) amount

Carve-outs: Applicable services that are cut out of the contract and paid at a different rate or via a different methodology

Case-mix index: The average relative weight of all cases treated at a given facility or by a given physician, which reflects the resource intensity or clinical severity of a specific group in relation to the other groups in the classification system; calculated by dividing the sum of the weights of MS-DRGs for patients discharged during a given period by the total number of patients discharged

Cash-based accounting: A method of accounting that is used most frequently in a sole proprietorship or a small business environment that recognizes income and expense transactions when cash is received or cash is paid out

Cash budget: A forecast of needs for available funds throughout the year

Cash flow: The availability of money to pay the organization's bills (receipts minus disbursements)

Cash flow from assets: A transfer of funds coming into a company's possession that are generated by the company's assets

Catholic Health Association (CHA):   An association whose purpose is to assist its members through education, facilitation, and advocacy and to advance the mission of the Catholic church through the ministry of providing optimal health services and programs to the people and communities they serve

Centers for Medicare and Medicaid Services (CMS):   The division of the Department of Health and Human Services that is responsible for developing healthcare policy in the United States, administering the Medicare program and the federal portion of the Medicaid program, and maintaining the procedure portion of the International Classification of Diseases, ninth revision, Clinical Modification (ICD-9-CM); called the Health Care Financing Administration (HCFA) prior to 2001

Certificate of deposit: A security issued by a bank or other financial institution typically paying a fixed interest rate and requiring the investor to leave the funds deposited for a set term

Charges: In healthcare, a price assigned to a unit of medical or health service, such as a visit to a physician or a day in a hospital; may be unrelated to the actual cost of providing the service

Charity care: Services for which healthcare organizations do not expect payment because they previously determined the patients' or clients' inability to pay

Claims corrections: Technical coding or charging errors or missing charges on claims that can delay billing for days or weeks

Commercial paper: An unsecured debt instrument with a maturity of less than nine months (270 days)

Commercial payer: A private health insurance payer (not a government payer)

Common size: Standardized values in financial statements that enable comparisons from year to year or facility to facility

Community benefit: The positive impact that a not-for-profit hospital has on the community it serves

Compounding: Interest generated from an investment is added to the value of the account in order to determine the amount of interest in each subsequent period

Consumer: A person who purchases and/or uses goods or services; in healthcare, a patient, client, resident, or other recipient of healthcare services

Contractual allowance: The difference between what is charged by the healthcare provider and what is paid by the managed care company or other payer

Controllability: A characteristic of cost that is generally within the control of the department manager

Controllable costs: Costs that can be influenced by a department director or manager

Cost: 1. The amount of financial resources consumed in the provision of healthcare services 2. The dollar amount of a service provided by a facility

Cost centers: Groups of activities for which costs are specified together for management purposes

Cost shifting: The cost of caring for government insurance beneficiaries is shifted to the private insurance market

Coupon rate: The periodic interest rate paid by the issuer to bondholders

Coverage ratio: A measure of the ability of the facility to pay debt based on its current level of income

Credit line: A fixed amount of cash that is available to the borrower for short-term needs

Critical access hospitals (CAHs):   1. Hospitals that are excluded from the outpatient prospective payment system because they are paid under a reasonable cost-based system as required under section 1834(g) of the Social Security Act 2. Small facilities that give limited outpatient and inpatient hospital services to people in rural areas

Current assets: Cash and other assets that typically will be converted to cash within one year

Current ratio: The total current assets divided by total current liabilities

D

Days cash on hand: Combines figures from the balance sheet and income statement; it represents the number of days of operating expenses that the organization holds in cash or cash equivalents

Days in patient accounts receivable: A measure of the average number of days that a facility takes to collect for services provided to patients

Debt: Incurred when money is borrowed and must eventually be paid

Debt performance: Ratios used to judge the creditworthiness of a firm

Debt ratio: The total liabilities divided by the total assets

Debt to equity ratio: In for-profit firms, a measure of the investment in the firm by lenders and suppliers versus the investment by shareholders; in not-for-profit facilities, a measure of the amount of debt compared to the amount collected via charitable contributions and grants

Decision theory: The expected cost of investigating and not investigating a budget variance are calculated and compared to determine the most cost-effective alternative

Decision tree: A structured data-mining technique based on a set of rules useful for predicting and classifying information and making decisions

Depreciation: The allocation of the dollar cost of a capital asset over its expected life; it represents the decrease in value of a capital asset over its life

Desired earnings: The percentage resulting from dividing the net income before taxes by net service revenue

Desired rate of growth: The increase in equity or fund balance

Direct method allocation: In this allocation method, all overhead (non–patient service) costs are distributed across all revenue-producing cost centers, according to a predetermined percentage

Discharged and not final billed (DNFB): A report that includes all patients who have been discharged from the facility but for whom, for one reason or another, the billing process is not complete

Discount: 1. The application of lower rates of payment to multiple surgical procedures performed during the same operative session under the outpatient prospective payment system; the application of adjusted rates of payment by preferred provider organizations 2. Reducing the payment in the hospital outpatient prospective payment system (HOPPS) (payment status indicator = T). In the CMS discounting schedule, Medicare will pay 100 percent of the Medicare allowance for the principal procedure (exclusive of deductible and copayment) and 50 percent (50 percent discount) of the Medicare allowance for each additional procedure. For example, if two CT scans (APC group 0349) are performed in the same visit, the first is reimbursed at the full APC group rate, the second at 50 percent of the APC group rate.

Discounted cash flow: The calculation that estimates the present value of future cash flow

Discounting factor: The factor by which a future cash flow must be multiplied to obtain the present value

Disproportionate share payment: A statutory adjustment to the Medicare inpatient payment rate based on the proportion of inpatient days paid via Medicaid

Dividends: The portion of an organization's profit that is distributed to its investors

Double-entry bookkeeping system: Used to record financial transactions in accounting systems; each asset or input of value must have a corresponding liability or output of value for the equation to remain in balance

Double step-down allocation: A method of cost allocation that allows the allocation of overhead departments to any department in the first step; the second step is identical to step-down allocation

E

Earnings before interest and taxes (EBIT): The net income plus interest or taxes paid during the year

Equipment: A long-term (fixed) asset account representing depreciable items owned by the organization that have value over multiple fiscal years (for example, the historical cost of a CT scanner is recorded in an equipment account)

Equity: Securities that are shared in the ownership of the organization

Equity statement: Details the changes in the equity found on the balance sheet either year-to-date or from one year to the next

Exempt: Specific groups of employees who are identified as not being covered by some or all of the provisions of the Fair Labor Standards Act

Expenses: Amounts that are charged as costs by an organization to the current year's activities of operation

F

Favorable variance: The positive difference between the budgeted amount and the actual amount of a line item, that is, when actual revenue exceeds budget or actual expenses are less than budget

Federal funds rate: The rate at which banks lend their excess reserves to each other for very short periods of time, usually overnight or one day

Federal Poverty Guidelines (FPG):   A set of income criteria used to determine whether a patient is eligible for discounted services or may be eligible for federal assistance; the FPG are updated annually by HHS

Fee-for-service: A payment system in which the payer pays a set fee for a particular item or service when it is dispensed to a patient

Financial accounting: The mechanism that organizations use to fully comprehend and communicate their financial activities

Financial ratios: Used to analyze the relationships between data elements found on the financial statements

Financial statement: A statement comprised of balance sheets, income statements, statements of cash flow, and statements of shareholder equity or equity statements, typically using footnotes to explain circumstances and clarify the methods used to account for those circumstances

Fiscal year: Any consecutive 12-month period an organization uses as its accounting period

Fixed asset turnover: A measure of the amount of revenue produced by each dollar of fixed assets or property and equipment

Flexible budget: A type of budget that is based on volumes of services and that may "flex" up or down as volumes fluctuate during the budget year

Formulary: A listing of drugs, classified by therapeutic category or disease class; in some health plans, providers are limited to prescribing only drugs listed on the plan's formulary. The selection of items to be included in the formulary is based on objective evaluations of their relative therapeutic merits, safety, and cost.

For-profit: A category of organization in which owners or shareholders profit from the operation of the firm

Funds: Money or assets that can be converted to money

Future value: The total dollar amount of an investment at a later point in time, including any earned or implied interest

G

General fund: The primary or catchall fund of a nonprofit organization or governmental agency

Generally accepted accounting principles (GAAP): An accepted set of accounting principles or standards and recognized procedures central to financial accounting and reporting

Geometric mean length of stay: A measure of the typical length of stay that is not as impacted by outliers as the arithmetic mean or average; see statistical texts for the formula

Government payer: Healthcare programs administrated by federal, state, or local government agencies, including Medicare, Medicaid, TRICARE, State Children's Health Insurance Program (SCHIP), and others

Gross domestic product (GDP): A statistic that economists use to measure the value of all products a country produces

Gross revenue: The total amount of money an organization takes in

Grouper: A computer software program that assigns prospective payment groups on the basis of clinical codes

H

Health maintenance organization (HMO): An entity that combines the provision of healthcare insurance and the delivery of healthcare services, characterized by: (1) an organized healthcare delivery system to a geographic area, (2) a set of basic and supplemental health maintenance and treatment services,

(3) voluntarily enrolled members, and (4) predetermined fixed, periodic pre-payments for members' coverage

High-deductible health plan: A health plan where the subscriber must pay a significant amount of money prior to receiving any coverage from the insurance company

Horizontal analysis: A method of analysis that transforms the figures on the financial statements into statistics that may be used to measure performance for the same facility over the course of time; also known as trend analysis

Hospital Cost Reporting Information System (HCRIS): The CMS database that is used to compile Medicare cost reports for public release and analysis

---

I

Income: Inflow of cash or cash equivalents resulting from work (provision of services), capital (interest or profit), or land (rent or profit)

Income statement: A statement that summarizes an organization's revenue and expense accounts using totals accumulated during the fiscal year

Incremental cost: A cost that is incurred by a change in business

Indemnity plans: Health insurance coverage provided in the form of cash payments to patients or providers in return for the payment of a premium; these plans typically require a higher premium than other plan designs, but they allow the most flexibility in patient choice of provider

Indirect medical education payment: A statutory adjustment to the Medicare inpatient payment system that provides teaching hospitals with additional payments to offset the cost of maintaining medical educational programs

Intensity of service: A statistic that measures the level of diagnostic and therapeutic services required to treat a set of patients

Interest: 1. The cost of borrowing money; payment to creditors for using money during the term of a loan 2. The income from an investment

Interest-bearing: An investment instrument, such as a savings account, in which interest is calculated based on the value of the account (principal); simple interest is calculated by multiplying the interest rate by the principal amount

Internal rate of return (IRR): The rate that makes the net present value calculation equal zero; it represents the break-even point for the time value of money for an investment

Inventory: Goods on hand and available to sell, presumably within a year (a business cycle)

IPPS PC Pricer: Medicare software that calculates the prospective payment a hospital is paid to cover the cost of treating the typical patient for a particular disease related group

L

Labor pool: The available group of trained workers in the economy

Lease: A contract in which the owner of a property agrees for another person to use the property for a fee

Liability: 1. A legal obligation or responsibility that may have financial repercussions if not fulfilled 2. An amount owed by an individual or organization to another individual or organization

Liquidation value: The amount that the owners would receive if they sold the company or an asset in its entirety: all assets and all liabilities

Liquidity: The degree to which assets can be quickly and efficiently turned into cash; for example, marketable securities are generally liquid, the assumption being that they can be sold for their full value in a matter of days, whereas buildings are not liquid because they cannot usually be sold quickly

Long-term assets: Assets whose value to the organization extends beyond one fiscal year; for example, buildings, land, and equipment are long-term assets

Long-term liabilities: Liabilities that have a due date past one year after the ending date of the report

Lower of cost or market: A process that provides the users of financial statements with a conservative estimate of the value of the assets of the organization in a declining market

M

Managed care: 1. Payment method in which the third-party payer has implemented some provisions to control the costs of healthcare while maintaining quality care 2. Systematic merger of clinical, financial, and administrative processes to manage access, cost, and quality of healthcare

Managerial accounting: The development, implementation, and analysis of systems that track financial transactions for management control purposes, including both budget systems and cost analysis systems

Margin: The profit or net income a firm earns divided by the revenue

Market basket: Mix of goods and services in a particular market sector or category

Market share: The percentage of available business that is captured by the organization in the area primarily served by the organization

Market value: The price at which something can be bought or sold on the open market

Matching: A concept that enables decision makers to look at expenses and revenues in the same period to measure the organization's income performance

Maturity: The date on which an obligation must be repaid

Medicaid: An entitlement program that oversees medical assistance for individuals and families with low incomes and limited resources; jointly funded between state and federal governments and legislated by the Social Security Act

Medicare: A federally funded health program established in 1965 to assist with the medical care costs of Americans 65 years of age and older as well as other individuals entitled to Social Security benefits owing to their disabilities

Medicare Cost Report: Each hospital participating in Medicare must submit a cost report on an annual basis

Medicare severity diagnosis-related groups (MS-DRGs):   The US government's 2007 revision of the DRG system, the MS-DRG system, better accounts for severity of illness and resource consumption

MedPAC: An agency that advises Congress on Medicare payment issues, tracks a number of statistics regarding hospital financial performance, and releases the results in their annual data book

Money market account: An interest-bearing account with an underlying source in short-term securities such as commercial paper or shares in funds that trade in short-term securities

N

Net assets: The organization's resources remaining after subtracting its liabilities

Net patient service revenue: The gross patient revenue or total amount charged to patients minus any discounts that the facility may negotiate with third-party payers

Net present value: A formula used to assess the current value of a project when the monies used were invested in the organization's investment vehicles rather than expended for the project; this value is then compared to the allocation of the monies and the cash inflows of the project, both of which are adjusted to current time

Net working capital: The difference between current assets and current liabilities

Nonexempt: All groups of employees covered by the provisions of the Fair Labor Standards Act

Nonoperating activities: Cash flow from noncapital financing activities, capital and related financing activities, and investing activities

Nonoperating gains and losses: *See* nonoperating revenue and expenses

Nonoperating revenue and expenses: Revenue received for activities that are not related to healthcare

Normal distribution: A theoretical family of continuous frequency distributions characterized by a symmetric bell-shaped curve, with an equal mean, median, and mode; any standard deviation; and with half of the observations above the mean and half below it

Not-for-profit: An organization whose proceeds or net income is not paid to any individual or group of individuals

O

Operating activities: Patient care and healthcare operations, which include certain administrative, financial, legal, and quality improvement activities necessary to run a business and support the core functions of treatment and payment

Operating budget: The budget that summarizes the anticipated expenses for a department's routine, day-to-day operations

Operating cash flow: Earnings before interest and taxes, plus depreciation, minus taxes

Operating expenses: Expenses that are required to deliver care to patients or operate the facility

Operating income: Incoming cash representing receipts from and on behalf of patients, payments received during the reporting period for care provided in previous periods, and prepayments for services that may be provided in later periods

Operating margin: A measure of the level of profitability experienced in a firm's operations

Opportunity cost: The benefits that are given up or extra cost incurred by pursuing one project over another

Outlier: 1. A case in a prospective payment system with unusually long lengths of stay or exceptionally high costs (day outlier or cost outlier, respectively) 2. An extreme statistical value that falls outside the normal range

Overhead: The expenses associated with supporting but not directly providing patient care services

P

Par value: The value for which a security can be issued or redeemed

Payback period: A financial method used to evaluate the value of a capital expenditure by calculating the time frame that must pass before inflow of cash from a project equals or exceeds outflow of cash

Payer: The entity that is reimbursing the provider for care

Payer mix: The collection of payers that remit payments to a provider

Per-diem rate: A payment methodology that pays a provider a fixed amount for each day of an inpatient stay

Permanently restricted net assets: Funds permanently restricted by donor or grantor stipulations

Permanent variance: A financial term that refers to the difference between the budgeted amount and the actual amount of a line item that is not expected to reverse itself during a subsequent period

Per member per month (PMPM): The amount of money paid monthly for each individual enrolled in a capitation-based health insurance plan

Physician–hospital organization (PHO):   An integrated delivery system formed by hospitals and physicians (usually through managed care contracts) that allows for cooperative activity but permits participants to retain some level of independence

Plant: Buildings and structures that are owned by an organization

Point: A percentage of a total loan

Portfolio: A set of investments owned by an organization and generally managed by a financial institution

Preferred provider organization (PPO):   A managed care arrangement based on a contractual agreement between healthcare providers (professional and/or institutional) and employers, insurance carriers, or third-party administrators to provide healthcare services to a defined population of enrollees at established fees that may or may not be a discount from usual and customary or reasonable charges

Premium: The amount of money that a policyholder or certificate holder must periodically pay an insurer in return for healthcare coverage

Prepaid expenses: Expenses paid prior to an organization receiving the benefit of the item or service. Amount appears on balance sheet as an asset.

Present value: 1. The current value of an investment required to meet a set target at a future time 2. A value that targets the current dollar investment and interest-rate needs to achieve a particular investment goal

Prime rate: Banks lend money to their best customers at a slightly different rate that is set higher than the federal funds rate

Principal: The amount originally invested

Private fee-for-service: A prepaid health insurance plan that allows beneficiaries to select private healthcare providers; also called an indemnity plan

Private payer: Employer-sponsored plans where the employer may be self-insured or may contract with a health insurance company to provide coverage for their employees

Product: An item or a service (such as healthcare) that can be available for sale in the economy

Profit: The difference between revenues and expenses used to build reserves for contingencies and long-term capital improvements

Profitability: A standard measure of the overall performance of any type of firm

Profit and loss statement: *See* statement of revenue and expenses

Property: The land a healthcare organization uses for its buildings, parking lots, helipad, and so on

Prospective payment system (PPS): A type of reimbursement system that is based on preset payment levels before the service has been provided; specifically, one of several Medicare reimbursement systems based on predetermined payment rates or periods and linked to the anticipated intensity of services delivered as well as the beneficiary's condition

Q

Quick ratio: A measure of a firm's liquidity

R

Refinancing: The replacement of an existing loan or debt instrument with a different one

Reinvestment: Investing the returns on an investment instead of taking a payout of the return after each period; if an account is subject to compounding, the interest generated from the investment is added to the value of the account to determine the amount of interest in each subsequent period

Restricted net assets: Funds permanently restricted by donor or grantor stipulations

Retained earnings: Undistributed profits from a for-profit organization that stay in the business

Retrospective payment system: A type of fee-for-service reimbursement in which providers receive recompense after health services have been rendered

Return on assets (ROA): The return on a company's investment, or earnings, after taxes divided by total assets

Return on equity (ROE): A measure of profitability that takes into consideration the organization's net value

Return on investment (ROI): The return on an investment divided by the cost of the investment

Revenue: The funds generated from providing healthcare services; earned and measurable income

Revenue code: A three- or four-digit number in the chargemaster that represents a department or functional area

Revenue cycle: 1. The process of how patient financial and health information moves into, through, and out of the healthcare facility, culminating with the facility receiving reimbursement for services provided 2. The regularly repeating set of events that produces revenue

Risk: 1. The probability of incurring injury or loss 2. The probable amount of loss foreseen by an insurer in issuing a contract 3. A formal insurance term denoting liability to compensate individuals for injuries sustained in a healthcare facility

Root cause: The underlying event(s) that led to a problem, determined through methodical investigation

S

Savings account: An account that sets aside the cash assets of an organization and pays a set interest rate or return; the amount invested is not at risk

Self-pay: A type of fee-for-service reimbursement in which the patients or their guarantors pay a specific amount for each service received

Sensitivity: The ability of a decision rule to detect a true difference

Short-term investments: Investments likely to be held for less than 12 months; typically short-term bonds or stocks that can be converted to cash quickly

Simple interest: The calculation of interest based solely on the principal

Social Security Act of 1935: The federal legislation that originally established the Social Security program as well as unemployment compensation and support for mothers and children; amended in 1965 to create the Medicare and Medicaid programs

Specificity: The ability of the decision rule not to falsely identify a variance as significant or a false positive

Stand-alone principle: Used when performing a cash flow analysis for a project; measures only the impact of the project and no other attributes of the organization

Standard deviation: A measure of variability that describes the deviation from the mean of a frequency distribution in the original units of measurement; the square root of the variance

State Children's Health Insurance Program (SCHIP): The children's healthcare program implemented as part of the Balanced Budget Act of 1997; sometimes referred to as the Children's Health Insurance Program, or CHIP

Statement of activities: A statement that summarizes an organization's revenue and expense accounts using totals accumulated during the fiscal year; also known as the income statement

Statement of cash flow: A statement detailing the reasons why cash amounts changed from one balance sheet period to another

Statement of net assets: *Also called* balance sheet

Statement of revenue and expenses: A financial statement showing how much the organization makes or loses during a given reporting period; also known as the income statement

Statement of shareholder equity: Details the changes in the equity found on the balance sheet either year-to-date or from one year to the next

Statistical budget: The collective strategic assumptions used by department managers as their framework for developing their operating budgets

Statistical process control: A tool that may be used to identify budget variances that go beyond random occurrences

Step-down allocation: A budgeting concept in which overhead costs are distributed based on a measurement of the proportion of the service used by each patient care department

Stock: A share of the ownership of a corporation

Stop-loss: Shifts the prospective payment into a percentage of charge payment after the charge reaches a fixed threshold

Sunk costs: Those costs that would be expended even if the project is not pursued

Synergistic side effect: A positive side effect of a capital investment

T

Temporarily restricted net assets: Funds temporarily restricted by donor or grantor stipulations

Temporary variance: The difference between the budgeted and actual amounts of a line item that is expected to reverse itself in a subsequent period; the timing difference between the budget and the actual event

Third-party contract: A contractual arrangement between a provider and a payer that outlines the services to be provided to the payer's subscribers and the methodology to determine the payment for services

Third-party payer: An insurance company (for example, Blue Cross/Blue Shield) or healthcare program (for example, Medicare) that pays or reimburses healthcare providers (second party) and/or patients (first party) for the delivery of medical services

Third-party payer settlements: Amounts that payers may have prepaid or owe for services provided to their subscribers

Threshold: A boundary, beginning point, or target amount

Times interest earned (TIE) ratio: Measures the amount of income that is available to pay interest on debt

Top-down: A process flowing from the executive level down to the department or function level that forces departments to conform their budgets to the executive team's expectations

Total asset turnover ratio: Used to measure the turnover or utilization of a facility's assets

Total margin: A measurement of the overall profitability of a firm

Traceability: Refers to whether the cost is directly or indirectly traceable to the service

Traditional budget: A model in which the department is given a projected increase or decrease in expected revenue or expenses for the coming year, usually expressed as a percentage

Transactions: The individual events or activities that provide the basic input to the accounting process

Treasury stock: When a company buys or sells its own stock

Trend analysis: A tool that transforms the figures on the financial statements into statistics that may be used to measure performance for the same facility over the course of time; also known as horizontal analysis

TRICARE: The federal healthcare program that provides coverage for the dependents of armed forces personnel and for retirees receiving care outside military treatment facilities in which the federal government pays a percentage of the cost; formerly known as Civilian Health and Medical Program of the Uniformed Services

U

Underinsured: A set of patients who do not have health insurance coverage and must pay out of pocket for services

Unfavorable variance: The negative difference between the budgeted amount and the actual amount of a line item, where actual revenue is less than budget or where actual expenses exceed budget

Unit price: The cost to produce the unit of volume or the revenue per unit volume

Unrestricted donation: Funds donated to a not-for-profit organization to use in any way the not-for-profit sees fit

Unrestricted net assets: All net assets that are not temporarily or permanently restricted by donor or grantor

US Census Bureau: The federal government agency responsible for the US census

V

Value-based purchasing (VBP): A CMS incentive plan that links payments more directly to the quality of care provided and rewards providers for delivering high-quality and efficient clinical care; incorporates clinical process-of-care measures as well as measures from the Hospital Consumer Assessment of Healthcare Providers and Systems (HCAHPS) survey on how patients view their care experiences

Variability: The dispersion of a set of measures around the population mean

Variance: 1. A disagreement between two figures 2. The square of the standard deviation; a measure of variability that gives the average of the squared deviations from the mean 3. In financial management, the difference between the budgeted amount and the actual amount of a line item; in project management, the difference between the original project plan and current estimates

Variance analysis: An assessment of a department's financial transactions to identify the root cause of the differences between the budget amount and the actual amount of a line item

Vertical analysis: A methodology used to compare financial statements from year-to-year or between facilities. The values in the balance sheet are standardized by the total assets. The values in the income statement are standardized by the operating revenue.

W

Wage index: A ratio that represents the relationship between the average wages in a healthcare setting's geographic area and the national average for that healthcare setting. Wage indexes are adjusted annually and published in the *Federal Register*.

Working capital: The ability to satisfy obligations measured as the net of short-term assets and short-term liabilities

Z

Zero-based budgets: Types of budgets in which each budget cycle poses the opportunity to continue or discontinue services based on available resources so that every department or activity must be justified and prioritized annually to effectively allocate resources

Zero coupon bonds: Bonds issued without an interest rate

Index

Note: Page numbers with *f* indicate figures; those with *t* indicate tables.

I N D E X